Meaning in Suffering

Interpretive Studies in Healthcare and the Human Sciences

Volume VI

Meaning in Suffering

Caring Practices in the Health Professions

Nancy E. Johnston

and

Alwilda Scholler-Jaquish

Volume editors

THE UNIVERSITY OF WISCONSIN PRESS

The University of Wisconsin Press
1930 Monroe Street, 3rd Floor
Madison, Wisconsin 53711-2059

www.wisc.edu/wisconsinpress/

3 Henrietta Street
London WC2E 8LU, England

1   3   5   4   2

Printed in the United States of America

Library of Congress Cataloging-in-Publication Data
Meaning in suffering : caring practices
in the health professions / edited by
Nancy E. Johnston and Alwilda Scholler-Jaquish.
p.   cm.—(Interpretive studies in healthcare and
the human sciences; v. 6)
Includes bibliographical references and index.
ISBN 0-299-22250-0 (cloth: alk. paper)
ISBN 0-299-22254-3 (pbk.: alk. paper)
1. Suffering   2. Medical care   3. Terminal care
I. Johnston, Nancy E.   II. Scholler-Jaquish, Alwilda.   III. Series.
[DNLM: 1. Pain—nursing.   2. Stress, Psychological—nursing.
3. Empathy.   4. Palliative Care—methods.
5. Terminal Care—methods. WY 160.5 M483 2007]
BF789.S8M43   2007
616´.029—dc22   2006031772

Dedicated to our fathers

JAMES ROBERT PORTER
(1919–2006)
and
DONALD LEE SCHOLLER
(1913–2005)

who taught us how to find
meaning in suffering

Contents

Acknowledgments

No volume comes to fruition without the contributions of many people. Although we cannot name all of the generous people who offered their time, wisdom, and talent, we would like to particularly acknowledge the following people:

Nancy Diekelemann and Pamela Ironside for their wise guidance and encouragement.

Kathryn H. Kavanagh for her contribution to this volume, astute counsel, and unfailing friendship.

Nadine Cross for her skillful accompaniment through challenging times.

Christine Sorrell Dinkins for her ability to make excellent ideas sparkle.

The authors for the knowledge and skill that went into producing outstanding manuscripts.

The reviewers who responded generously to our call and offered their insightful comments under tight time constraints.

Our families who assumed extra burdens and gave us gifts of time so that we could work on this volume.

And each other for the journey we have shared. It has taken us to places we never imagined, deepening our mutual trust, respect, and friendship.

Meaning in Suffering

Introduction

NANCY E. JOHNSTON and
ALWILDA SCHOLLER-JAQUISH

Suffering does not happen to us; we happen to suffer. Suffering is what we
choose to do with pain.

Younger, 1995, 55

When we suffer personally, and when we encounter the suffering of
another person, we are confronted with many questions. A taken-for-
granted and apparently robust future now jeopardized leaves in its place
a hollow of uncertainty and fragility. Painfully unsettling, suffering seems
to call forth a natural human proclivity to distance oneself from the specter of vulnerability. Understandably there is a tendency for healthcare
professionals to protect ourselves from the ravages of suffering encountered in the lives of the persons we care for. We do this by relating from a
distance even though this is incongruent with our commitment to remain
engaged and to care compassionately. This volume calls us to strengthen
our capacity to remain fully present to individuals and their families during times of profound loss and also reveals ways in which new possibilities
both arrive and are closed down during suffering.

In the opening chapter Kathryn H. Kavanagh uses narrative ethnography to offer an intimate portrait of one woman's journey with a chronic
illness. She deepens our understanding of the essential facts of suffering,
illuminates how meaning and purpose come to be challenged in a time of
suffering, and reveals how the self comes to be redefined. Laying the
foundation for her interpretive inquiry by developing the metaphor of
quilt, Kavanagh asks how we explore and understand such interrupted

lives. She explores this question by writing that we understand by listening, and further suggests that listening involves "attending to both the dominant and the muted meanings . . . [and] searching for the pain and stories that lie outside expectable discussion."

Ingrid Harris then offers a compelling philosophical approach to suffering. Suggesting that suffering can be a gift, Harris creates awareness of the opportunities that come to sufferer and healer alike. Drawing on the thought of Calvin Schrag, she writes that the way the gift becomes present is through the interaction of the sufferer and the healer. Harris reminds us that meaning is double edged since it is all too often that negative rather than positive meanings are taken up. These negative, destructive meanings close down our ways of being in the world, prevent healing, and distort attempts to regain wholeness. Expanding further on how health professionals can respond "fittingly" in ways that help with the reconstruction of positive meanings, Harris encourages us to consider the infinite number of possible ways our imagination allows us to interpret any event.

Nancy Johnston takes the position that enabling healthcare professionals to come to grips with suffering in a way that helps them to overcome the tendency to care "at a distance" requires a new discourse. This discourse must not only enable us to understand the threats to meaning and purpose that people experience during a time of adversity but it must also generate knowledge about how meaning comes to be restored in the face of great trial and hardship. She also shows how her interpretive phenomenological study contributes such knowledge by illuminating how people reconstruct meaning in situations of adversity and by shedding light on human and healthcare practices that both help and hinder the restoration of positive meanings.

Craig Klugman uses a narrative phenomenological study to reveal how the practice of inviting bereaved people to tell stories of loved ones who are deceased assists individuals to accomplish important grief work. Noting that tellers are often searching for new hope, new interpretations, and new outcomes, Klugman affirms that it is during a "breakdown" that people have the opportunity to grasp new meaning about their lives. Revealing the power of storytelling as a caring health practice, Klugman shows how it enables catharsis, heals wounds, constructs new meanings, restores connections to community, and fosters openness to new experiences.

Bonnie Ewing explores the meaning to dying children of a well-intended social practice—the granting of special wishes to children with a life-threatening illness by the Make-A-Wish Foundation. Addressing the special challenges of gaining access to children's perspectives uncontaminated by adult preconceptions and expectations, Ewing describes a hermeneutical phenomenological study in which children were invited to express their experiences through artwork. Explicating the embedded meanings that were manifested in symbols and images in the children's drawings, she uncovers the shared meanings of children with life-threatening illnesses who have had their special wish fulfilled. In this way she brings to expression experiences that could not otherwise be articulated. Reflecting on the implications of the study, Ewing suggests that conventional treatments intended to perpetuate life should be evaluated carefully against the benefits that can be secured by focusing more intentionally upon the preservation of quality of life for dying children

In the final chapter Shelley Raffin Bouchal offers an ethnography of the human practices of nurses who care for dying individuals. Illuminating the sense of vocation that nurses often bring to their work, she describes the "calling" they experience in helping their patients to live fully while dying. Raffin Bouchal connects us to the realities of pain, loss, and suffering that are inevitably part of the journey by describing the challenges encountered by nurses as they experience intense interpersonal involvement within the context of their patients' limited time horizons. By depicting the human connections, transformations, and social realities that arise on a palliative care unit, Raffin Bouchal reveals how nurses endure suffering, confront death, and reflect on the meaning of life.

This volume, the sixth in the series *Interpretive Studies in Healthcare and the Human Sciences,* presents many voices of suffering and challenges healthcare professionals to respond fittingly to the call to care. As we offer new ways of thinking about suffering, we invite everyone to remain open to the possibilities that arrive with suffering and to become attentive and skillful cocreators of meaning.

References

Cassell, E. J. (1991a). *The nature of suffering and the goals of medicine.* New York: Oxford University Press.

Cassell, E. J. (1991b, May–June). Recognizing suffering. *Hastings Center Report,* 24–31.

Diekelmann, J. (2005). The retrieval of method: The method of retrieval. In P. M. Ironside

(Ed.), *Beyond method: Philosophical conversations in healthcare research and scholarship* (pp. 3–57). Madison: University of Wisconsin Press.

Diekelmann, N. (1991). The emancipatory power of the narrative. In *Curriculum revolution: Community building and activism* (pp. 41–62). New York: National League for Nursing.

Frank, A. W. (2004). Dignity, dialogue, and care. *Journal of Palliative Care, 20,* 207–211.

Frankl, V. E. (1984). *Man's search for meaning.* New York: Washington Square Press. (Original work published 1946)

Fredriksson, L., & Eriksson, K. (2001). The patient's narrative of suffering—a path to health: An interpretive research synthesis on narrative understanding. *Scandinavian Journal of Caring Science, 15,* 3–11.

Gadamer, H.-G. (2003). *Truth and method* (2nd ed.; J. Weinsheimer & D. G. Marshall, Trans.). New York: Continuum. (Original work published 1960)

Heidegger, M. (1977). The question concerning technology. In *The question concerning technology, and other essays* (W. Lovitt, Trans., pp. 3–35). New York: Harper & Row.

Heidegger, M. (1993b). The origin of the work of art. In D. F. Krell (Ed.), *Basic writings* (A. Hofstadter, Trans., pp. 143–203). San Francisco: HarperSanFrancisco. (Original work published 1960)

Madison, G. B. (1990). The philosophical centrality of the imagination: A postmodern approach. In G. B. Madison, *The hermeneutics of postmodernity: Figures and themes* (pp. 178–195). Bloomington: Indiana University Press.

Madison, G. B. (2005). *On suffering.* Unpublished manuscript.

Polkinghorne, D. (1988). *Narrative knowing and the human sciences.* Albany: State University of New York Press.

Picard, C. (1991). Caring and the story: The compelling nature of what must be told and understood in the human dimension of suffering. In D. A. Gaut & M. M. Leininger (Eds.), *Caring: The compassionate healer* (pp. 89–98). New York: National League for Nursing.

Rogers, B. L., & Cowles, K. V. (1997). A conceptual foundation of human suffering in nursing care and research. *Journal of Advanced Nursing, 25,* 1048–1053.

Sahler, O. J. Z., Frager, G., Levetown, M., Cohn, F. G., & Lipson, M. A. (2000). Medical education about end-of-life care in the pediatric setting: Principles, challenges, and opportunities. *Pediatrics, 105,* 575–584.

Schrag, C. O. (2002). *God as otherwise than being: Toward a semantics of the gift.* Evanston, IL: Northwestern University Press.

Schrag, C. O. (2004). Ethics of the gift: Acknowledgement and response. *Symposium, 8,* 195–212.

Schafer, R. (2004). Narrating, attending, and empathizing. *Literature and Medicine, 23,* 241–251.

Steeves, R. H., & Kahn, D. L. (1987). Finding meaning in suffering. *Image: Journal of Nursing Scholarship, 19,* 114–116.

Wuthnow, R. (1991). *Acts of compassion: Caring for others and helping ourselves.* Princeton, NJ: Princeton University Press.

Younger, J. B. (1995). The alienation of the sufferer. *Advances in Nursing Science, 17*(4), 53–72.

1

Meaning in Suffering

A Patchwork Remembering

KATHRYN H. KAVANAGH

Dr. Rain appeared, the bulging pockets on her white jacket straining its center button. She absentmindedly squelched buzzing apparatuses while looking around the room at the four of us and ascertaining our relationships with her patient. She then addressed herself to Joanne: "Well, the chances are about 10% of surviving a year without treatment." She paused. "And about 10% with treatment." She filled the room with jargon and checked to see if we followed; we did, except for Walt, Joanne's husband of 41 years—but he did not interrupt, and we three nurses did not slow down the talk on his behalf. Dr. Rain asked what questions we had. She was careful not to seem pushy about the experimental drug. It was all palliative now.

Joanne had had polymyositis for 20 years, but it was leukemia sounding the death knell. Both the stroke a few weeks earlier and the newly diagnosed leukemia were attributed by the clinicians to past treatments, and here they were pushing another drug. I learned later that Joanne had figured it out. She had written in her diary two years earlier: "I'm convinced it's due to 17 years chemo meds for poly and now the side effects are showing their ugly face" [Diary 2].[1]

Dr. Rain covered everything she could imagine being of use and got from us every question we could produce. Joanne's decision to participate in the drug trial was not a difficult one when there wasn't going to be much time no matter what she did. The talk was of possibilities, not probabilities; the prize was quality of life, not quantity. More "older people" were needed to participate; participation was a contribution. Dr. Rain

chuckled when we bristled at the "older people" language and acknowledged that we four sixtyish folks were on the young side of old.

Joanne communicated a need to commit herself to action, which was
typical Joanne. Walt interjected something about Joanne's ashes going to
a reef in the ocean if and when it came to that. It seemed both a surprising note and an indication that he too was processing all this at deeper
levels. Joanne would go along with the new drug—"What else can I do?"
Only later did I realize that she had broken the poststroke pattern of
stopping after the second word. As soon as it was known that the drug
trial would have another participant, the project director arrived with a
flurry of forms for which she efficiently extracted shaky signatures. Then,
as she attempted a hasty exit, Joanne stopped her. Dr. Rain had returned
with more printouts. I was awed when Joanne, with no reference to
her own plight but ensuring the attention of the supervising physician,
stammered out a compliment about young Dr. Rain's caring presence.

Quilt—A Bedcover Made by Stitching through the Whole: Coming to the Inquiry

> All interpretation is grounded in understanding.
> Heidegger, 1927/1962a, p. 195

Joanne was a quilter, and quilts are storied. Quilting, like hermeneutics, invites ongoing dialogue and makes possible the making, preserving,
and sharing of meaning. Symbolism and openness abound in the gathering of hundreds of individual pieces in their path toward being "singular
plural" (Nancy, 2000). Joanne's quilting lends a metaphor for her story
through its creative organization, its enduring commitment, its colorful
sense of play, and, in more philosophical terms, the situatedness of everyday activities with their embedded knowing, which involves the person-
world that both shapes us and is shaped by us (Heidegger, 1927/1962a).

Challenges were nothing new to Joanne. I had been aware of her
physical limitations for at least a decade. I even brought them up, only to
have Joanne sidestep that conversation with "Oh, it's just a muscular
thing" and a joke about aging. The boundary "draws us by its very withdrawing" (Diekelmann, 2005, p. 3). While a student in a nursing master's
program, Joanne took my healthcare and culture courses and involved

herself in diversity workshops I led. We also shared an interest in sewing and quilting; I teased her about being the only person I knew who owned two Berninas. The Bernina is a Swiss-made sewing machine, and I have owned two in the past 40 years (the first one still works); Berninas are made for serious sewers. Joanne and I occasionally went to quilt shows, but more often we met to discuss culture and nursing, particularly when she encountered people with backgrounds unfamiliar to her. Over the years I watched Joanne go from being ambulatory, albeit unable to "do steps," to needing arms on chairs to push herself up, and finally to an electric cart to get around. One night, outside a diner with a good ramp and wheelchair seating, she demonstrated with pride the lift in her van. Her friend Millie helped her figure out how to pull down the van door after getting the cart inside. I admired Joanne's independence, but I still knew nothing about polymyositis.

After Joanne's son Chris called to tell me she'd had a stroke I visited her whenever I could, following her from her local hospital to a rehabilitation center and then to the cancer unit of a major medical center when leukemia was diagnosed. Watching this highly verbal woman struggle for words, I saw suffering in her living with a chronic debilitating disease now compounded by a stroke and then superimposed with acutely devastating leukemia.[2] What is more, Joanne was not the only one suffering; there was Walt too. Joanne said she would think about writing her story with me. A few weeks later, hospitalized yet again, she said, "Okay, do it." Language serves to substitute no-thing for a thing no longer there (Mairs, 1996), while in the coalescence of thrownness, understanding, and language lies the possibility of being fully human (Diekelmann, 2005, citing Heidegger). Joanne's words came in fragments, patched together like a few more pieces of a quilt. Aware of the impact of the stroke on her linguistic compensations for her physical problems, I thought aphasia had left the "let's" out when she said "do it." Now I am not so sure. How do we explore and understand such interrupted lives? Listening involved attending to both the dominant and the muted meanings. Heilbrun (1988) urges searching for the pain and stories that lie outside expectable discussion. Personal oral narratives in conversational contexts can be emancipating (Borland, 1991; Diekelmann, 1991), as were, according to her daughter-in-law Kristen, the stories that Joanne so loved hearing about her grandchildren.

The oldest of the arts (Cruikshank, 1992), storytelling is at the core of the search for meaning. Stories are never simple and always have multiple perspectives. Nor do they involve only individuals. For example, Joanne was to be in the hospital only four days for the experimental treatment. The first dose of the drug was inserted into Joanne's intravenous line. The combination of the extra fluids and who knows what else—the clear liquid looked so innocent up there in its little plastic bag—set Joanne's heart racing and her chest heaving. Walt ran for a nurse: "She's in trouble!" It was a small blip in medical history, but it was terrifying. Joanne thought her chest was going to explode, and Walt thought she was going to die. Later, when Walt spoke of going home exhausted after Joanne's first treatment, I asked whether he had finally got some rest and whether he had called their sons Skip and Chris—both adults, married, and fathers. The answer to both questions was no. Instead, he said, he "cried half the night." This was suffering cosuffered.

When Joanne agreed to our study, I, a medical anthropologist, started keeping field notes. Inquiry requires thick description, careful listening, and reading between the lines. Notes of my visits, for instance, went like this:

The medical center wanted Joanne treated like an out-patient and Joanne wanted to go home. I was to visit her today, but I got a message from Walt that her schedule had again been changed. Last week they ended up at the cancer unit four days, sometimes for hours at end, and sometimes with nothing getting done to or for Joanne when they were there. There seems to be little consideration of the effort involved in Walt's getting Joanne up and fed, bathed, clothed, and out to the van for the forty-minute trips into the city. Where would Joanne be without Walt? He says she is tired, she gets tired of sitting and waiting: "Everything hurts." Who gives the health system the authority to put a person on hold like that?

Their lives revolved around good days, bad days, but few predictable days—or even hours. Joanne and Walt lived in response to her physical condition, no longer merely around it. That meant Joanne could not attend the speech therapy and physical therapy sessions that symbolized for her the climb back to normalcy after the stroke. Joanne had little residual paralysis, but she was frustrated with her speech and cognitive impairment. Walt took her to work with a woman who had worked with other quilters who had had strokes—Joanne was excited. Her daughter-in-law Kathleen described it: "She was getting her energy back. It was as if she said, 'Okay, now I've had my cry and I'm moving on.'" But she had the chance to visit the sewing coach only once. Her condition and the "new drug" overwhelmed any quality of life.

Finding the Materials, Revealing the Pattern: The Inquiry

As if unfolding toward an ethos of the unknown, flexibility characterizes the crazy quilts of lives today. The paths of our existence are no longer limited by old rhythms of production and procreation but are instead indeterminate and full of myriad commitments and new beginnings. Continuity is the exception; adapting to discontinuity is an emerging problem of the era (Bateson, 1990). Composing a life involves continual reimagining of the future and reinterpretation of the past. While our lives are generally longer and more filled with possibilities than ever before, we are also more likely to engage in a day-to-day process of self-invention than in one of discovery. Then along comes a catastrophic diagnosis and prognosis. I wanted to know how one bears pain and uncertainty or the immediate reality of nausea and vomiting so violent that it seems it will not stop. Where is the meaning in such compromised existence? Hampl (1999) says pain has strong arms. As individuals and as a couple, Joanne and Walt were clearly in its grip.

How easy it is to wish for a trajectory of healing and improving health; how powerless one feels knowing that whatever will happen will happen. For most of us living everyday lives, the notion of being at the mercy of what our bodies can or cannot do is merely a mental exercise. As parts of a modern society we spend little time contemplating bodily functioning, let alone mortality. How often do we think about what tattered remnants of life constitute humanity when the whole is damaged? These questions are harder to know, perhaps, when our culture splatters mortality across the media with such indifference as to render it meaningless. Isak Dinesen wrote: "All suffering is bearable if it is seen as part of a story" (cited in Metzger, 1992, p. 47). I wrote in my notes: "What is the story here? Will it all be over before it begins?"

When Joanne agreed to work with me on her story, I told her we would make it her memoir, since that genre depicts the author's life vividly, affectively, and uniquely (Tedlock, 2000). Memoir creates a window into a life, acknowledging the importance of a historical perspective and highlighting a point of view (Frank, 2000). I pondered the task of cowriting a memoir with someone severely compromised in communication. Can a woman who can get out only every third word "write" a memoir? Not that Joanne ever particularly liked writing. Now she was very ill and could barely sign her name, and construction of the quilt squares she was working on when she had the stroke eluded her. But the stroke was only a new wrinkle in the old problem. Years earlier Joanne wrote: "Also went to speech evaluation. Didn't do well—there is a lot of facial and throat and tongue involvement" [Diary 1]. Now the brain conspired with the muscles against speech. During her hospitalizations she learned the risks and frustrations of the staff's not knowing what she meant or wanted. Joanne clung tightly to Walt's presence; his interpretation of her speech and needs proved more valid and reliable than anyone else's. Did her discomfort distract her from concern about the future or exacerbate it? Cure was beyond our purview; how might we help her heal? Could I hear these things if Joanne communicated them to me? Joanne's memoir evolved into narrative ethnography, which combines life history and memoir.

Final Stitches

In the midst of life we are in death.
  Book of Common Prayer, 1928, p. 332

The dwindling sands in Joanne's hourglass evoked for me the hungry ghosts of Buddhist iconography. Portrayed as beings with huge bellies that serve as storehouses for all they can possibly consume, their throats are as narrow as needles. Whatever they put in their mouths leaves them unsatisfied, so they perpetually devour anything they can (Levitt, 2003). I likened the task of representing Joanne in her story to the ritual feeding of the hungry ghosts; I wanted to understand everything I could of her experience. Despite their dissatisfied natures, hungry ghosts are fed the food of awakening directly from the Buddha's bowl, making new realizations possible. The narrow place, having an opportunity to be expressed, becomes a path of freedom. I wanted Joanne to share with me her stories about suffering. Joanne's work and her play were purposeful, and she kept at them, staving off suffering's victory when it would make accomplishment impossible (Cassell, 1991b). How was that? The storyteller picks the material and knows where she is and where she intends to go. It would be *her* voice, *her* characters, *her* worldview (See, 2002) while I wrote—but that was not to be. Yet suffering and transcendence are among the things most at stake in daily experience; they deserve to be the focus of study (Kleinman, 1995).

Walt called. "Joanne was pronounced at 8:15 this morning." After a harrowing month Joanne's friend Ski wrote in the notebook the family kept at Joanne's bedside: "She had Walt, Skip, and Chris at her side. It was [a] peaceful and beautiful death—just as she would have wanted it." Later a friend said, "She got tired. She just got too tired and could not do any more."

Notes from the funeral:

The church is a work in progress, the ceiling a patchwork of squares in transition or missing. Joanne would have appreciated that. She is there, her cremains under one of her most colorful quilts. A couple hundred people gathered to celebrate her existence and to grieve her departure. They look a homogeneous lot; Joanne would have voted for more diversity in the congregation. There are beautiful stories shared by those closest to Joanne. Stories about her more recent years— storms of ill health and her insistent striving for that rainbow, her spirit of joy and bursts of creativity, the flaming red hair proclaiming her philosophy of life, her stubbornness and culinary disasters. But most of the stories were about her caring, her being the consummate people person, her many years in nursing, and her desire for a legacy. This went beyond not speaking ill of the dead; people respected Joanne.

Ski, Joanne's longtime friend, coworker, and cosurvivor of various nursing education programs, told a story about Joanne tipping over an equipment tray to prevent some eager doctor from doing something completely misguided to his patient. Ski wound around her own neck a fuchsia feather boa she'd bought for Joanne; we all knew she would have loved its flagrant flamboyance. Joanne was known for her thoughtful gifts, carefully selected and often self-crafted to reflect highly individual interests and tastes. I thought about Joanne and Walt planning to buy their grandsons tickets for *The Lion King* at the Hippodrome in the spring, which Joanne would not see. There were stories of the polymyositis and of loving her through the hard times. One of her sons made reference to her love of human diversity and how she encouraged them to go and meet people unlike themselves—to meet them where they were and to "always remember to *bring back a piece of fabric.*"

Probability suggests that women are more likely than men to endure the loss of that "tangible 'we'" of a life partner (Mairs, 1994, p. 134).

Because his own father and several uncles died young, Walt "set Joanne up," paying off the mortgage and anticipating that she would outlive him by years. Instead, Joanne was 62 when she died. Falling off the actuarial charts invites both wry outrage and a loneliness felt by one whose life unfolds out of sync (Mairs, 1993). Joanne worked part-time until the stroke, but her coworkers knew nothing of the polymyositis. How was it that Joanne chose to live 20 years of suffering as she did? That others close to Joanne knew so little about her health status was one of those absences that begs retrieval (Diekelmann, 2005). Walt gave me two diaries that Joanne began in 1985 when a physician suggested she journal her increasingly unsettling health experiences. The earlier small book is inscribed: "Given to me by Charlotte from a yard sale for $.25," and the later one: "Diary of a/my disease." Joanne used them primarily as medical journals. She typically added entries when she experienced health problems; when in remission, she seldom wrote in them. I transcribed both handwritten diaries, translating the medical jargon for Walt.

I then interviewed Joanne's closest friends and her family: her husband, sons, daughters-in-law, and grandsons. I initiated an ongoing conversation with Karen, Joanne's friend, who is a psychologist. Each of these individuals spent an average of three or more hours with me in personal or phone interviews or, in the therapist's case, ongoing e-mails.[3] I encouraged each participant to use his or her own words and format. Each understood the nature of the inquiry and my intent to write and submit this manuscript, and each was invited to communicate additional stories—most did. All of the interviews were transcribed with wide margins for notes. Strong patterns quickly emerged.

Through Joanne's story I sought to examine the phenomenological nature of sickness with the goal of deepening our grasp of human suffering. "[T]he quotidian truths of a body in trouble" (Mairs, 1996, p. 10) are not generalizable but rather interpretations of particular participants in particular situations. Stories are like babies: holding someone else's baby does not make it yours, but holding it does instill responsibility—in this case, for understanding and representing (Kavanagh, 2005). Written texts are never without ambiguity (Cruikshank, 1992), so it was a leap of faith on the part of those people closest to Joanne to share their stories with me. Additionally, given my own relationship with Joanne, I was challenged to attend to others' perspectives and not confuse them with my own. No one's self-reflection is only a private, subjective act; it too comes with interpretation and theories. So I initiated the interviews and shaped the story, asking participants what meanings they made of their experiences and observations, while I sought the metathemes and used them to stitch the story together much as Joanne did quilt blocks.

The open-ended questions around which the interviews unfolded focused on description of Joanne's experience with suffering and polymyositis and how that diagnosis led her to reinterpret her self and her life, the participants' interpretations of the meaning of what happened, and how Joanne dealt with support. I noted in the interviews that Joanne's diary entries indicated that she did not expect to be cured, and I asked about healing and how being a nurse might have influenced Joanne's response to chronicity. Everyone viewed Joanne as a doer; she was constantly busy with work, family, crafts—something. I asked the study participants about Joanne's need to be productive and to leave a legacy. I also asked about humor (another trait everyone who knew her associated with Joanne), depression, and what Joanne expected would happen to her over time. Finally, I asked what, if anything, Joanne's experience taught us about being human and how her needs might have been better met. As I amassed the three narrative sets (the diaries, the interviews, and the field notes) I compiled a fourth text of notes from related readings. Writing and interpreting meant moving back and forth among and across the texts, pulling threads and themes together—an experience much like creating a quilt design.

Gathering and Assembling Pieces

Colors—more colors than the sun has . . .

Silko, 1981, p. 65

The course of events in Joanne's life proved to me that interpretive inquirers need "sterner stuff" than fiction writers (Zinsser, 2004). Interpretive inquiry is about interpreting, communicating, visualizing, representing, and translating harsh realities of living (James, Hockey, & Dawson, 1997), such as Walt's having been charged for nine days' worth of medications *after* Joanne died and, as if to deepen the wound, the bill working its way to a collection agency. As the arbitrator of Joanne's story I was concerned with the practices of representing, which always simplify unnaturally, with fusing the ethnographic with the biographical to find voices for a "multiplicity of meanings" (Heidegger, 1968, p. 71); and with how even the organization of text affects meaning (Wallman, 1997). I strove to hear how others made sense of Joanne's reality. However, this could no longer be the process of my assisting her creation of her own memoir. Nor is it a life story or life history, focused as this "patchwork remembering" is on only the final third of Joanne's life and on interpretations of her suffering that were stitched together after her death. The sheer complexity of the whole convinced me that her quilting indeed supplied a telling metaphor for the whole. While suffering destroys communication (Younger, 1995), Joanne created a voice in her quilts.

Quilters often refer to their work as therapy and their immediate sisterhoods of coquilters as support groups. Joanne belonged to two quilting clubs, combining relaxing social interaction with artful productivity. The timelessness of quilts and quilting gave Joanne a refuge from disease-related phenomena. Like most quilters, she always had numerous projects under way; it was the sewing and quilting that mattered. There is an old story about completing projects presaging the end of life; quilters joke that they will live forever if they never finish anything (Detrixhe, 2004). After the stroke I got Detrixhe's *Zen and the Art of Quilting* (2004) so Joanne and I could read parts of it together. On page 5 it says: "Life is suffering." In this version of Buddhist philosophy various "keys to happiness" lead one to overcoming suffering. Names of chapters and quilt patterns affirm this: "Let Not Your Heart Be Troubled"; "All Things Must Pass."

Making quilts is often an act of defiance. Hung over clotheslines, quilts have sent many a message about safety and risk during times of social stress or war. They become voices, historical and personal records, and the preservers and prompts of memories. Quilting is highly ritualized, precise, and repetitious. Ritual has the ability to evoke emotion, bind individuals to past experiences, and bring people together in shared experience (Mead, 1972). Everything from exploring to completing quilt stitching is about possibilities. Making a quilt is very much in the here and now: selecting the colors and patterns; handling the cloth moment to moment; threading needles; pulling the needle and thread through layers of fabric and batting, rocking it in and out of the cloth. Joanne did much of her quilting by hand, which is an activity both absorbing and mind freeing, essentially meditation in a quest for self-understanding: being in quiet surroundings, sitting still, and repeating mental patterns. "Zen quilts" are created out of a desire to make them rather than to have them; they invite sewing with more spirit than rules (Detrixhe, 2004). Joanne often e-mailed me about quilts she was working on, her descriptions sharing a way of living the coming of memories (Heidegger, 1977).

Quilting is not an exact science. It is about letting possibilities unfold and is best approached with a sense of adventure and imagination. It takes basic supplies, faith, and commitment. Perfection is not the goal; people claim that a structurally perfect quilt brings bad luck to the quilter, so one piece is often intentionally mismatched or misplaced (Detrixhe, 2004). Nonetheless, standards among ardent quilters are high. Joanne had at least one quilt with some piece so out of place (for that particular pattern) that she clearly considered it a mistake. Walt showed me the quilt; we searched, but we couldn't find the piece. But Joanne knew it was there.

Unworkable Pieces and Patches, a Body in Trouble: Polymyositis

The body is a dwelling place; it is the "non-I that protects the I" (Bachelard, 1969).[4] But the body with polymyositis has been colonized, often irrevocably. People want to believe that the world is inherently balanced, orderly, and just, that things will work out the way they should. But a "just" world goes beyond predictability to one in which people get what they deserve (Lerner, 1980). Real life has no such obligations. Joanne wrote: "I have no warnings, never know an hour from now how I'll feel" [Diary 2]. Her friends said in varied versions, "She was morbidly afraid of losing control." Polymyositis is about losing control.

Polymyositis is a systemic connective-tissue disease characterized by inflammation and degeneration of the muscles. It is basically a malfunction of the immune system; the cells that normally fight infection mistakenly attack the muscle fibers of the body. The muscles of the limbs close to the torso are most affected, so the shoulders and hips are usually impacted first. The disease progresses symmetrically along both sides of the body, with increasing weakness, pain, and stiffness. The muscles of the head, hands, and feet are typically unaffected.

The condition is rare; incidence estimates range from 0.5 to 10 per million people. Most often it appears among women between the ages of 40 and 60. The cause of polymyositis is unknown, but it is thought to be triggered by a virus. The primary symptoms, which accrue over months and often begin with sensations of coldness in the hands and feet, are fatigue, muscle weakness and wasting, pain and a general feeling of discomfort, stiffness, and difficulty raising the arms over the head, rising from a sitting position, or climbing stairs. Joanne wrote:

Since it is difficult to explain this verbally, I am writing out what I know. At the onset of my physical problems, my hand/fingers turned a funny purple color. 10/85 Shortly after came tendonitis, left wrist in early Nov. . . . Saw doctor at rheumatology, who saw no association between Reynaulds [Raynaud's disease] and tendonitis. "Maybe in twenty years from now we'll look back and say yes." Severe left lateral knee discomfort. . . . Changed jobs, expected complete return to normal in several weeks, but upper body muscle weakness began as well as tendonitis both ankles, especially left. After push from Walt, Millie, Ski—made appointment with Dr. C. . . . I'm slower to move and don't feel well. [Diary 1]

Nearly 50% of the muscle fibers are destroyed before the symptomatic weakness is pronounced. The symptoms tend to wax and wane, but people with the disease are frequently sick. Among those in whom the disease persists, clumsiness and a wide, flat-footed gait become characteristic. Due to the vagueness of symptoms and rarity of the condition, diagnosing polymyositis is difficult and trying. Immersed in weeks of diagnostic workup, Joanne wrote:

I felt nauseated and had tingling, started to wretch and feel AWFUL. . . . The WORST I've ever felt. . . . I even said "shit" a few times. . . . Fingers purple. . . . Skip's especially upset. He knew "something went wrong." God love him. I'm scared too. . . . [Diary 1]

It was the mid-1980s, and Joanne feared she might be HIV-positive. What nurse has not experienced a finger-stick or some other high-risk event that, prior to the days of understanding HIV/AIDS well, might even have been forgotten? She wasn't HIV-positive, but the "worst" got worse.

Blood tests measure cell counts and antibody titers, since polymyositis is characterized by the overproduction of particular autoantibodies and muscle enzymes in the bloodstream. Electromyography involves thin needle electrodes inserted through the skin to measure the electrical activity of the muscles and nerves, and magnetic resonance imaging (MRI) scans reveal inflammations and help guide muscle biopsies, which reveal destruction of muscle fibers and inflammatory cellular responses, while chest X-rays detect lung involvement. Joanne wrote: "I signed permit for bronch[oscopy]—now that freaks me out," and

[W]e went down hill from there. . . . The prep for bronch was awful.—Gag and gag. They passed scope with some difficulty, then didn't monitor my respirations well during procedure—I couldn't convince them I wasn't getting enough air. . . . Was finally placed in face mask. . . . Cough cough cough and gasp gasp gasp . . . Friday 10/10 All appointments cancelled due to my state of fatigue. [But then] I hacked and coughed from 5 AM to 10 PM—exhausted, crying, the **worst** experience of my life . . . pain pain pain and all docs tell me is cough is important. Bullshit. I need some rest and freedom from pain. [Diary 1]

Despite the vagueness of etiology and diagnosis, there is consistency in the treatment of polymyositis. High dosages of corticosteroid medications are given to dampen the activity of the immune system and reduce inflammation. These are followed by maintenance regimens of prednisone, often indefinitely. It is not uncommon for corticosteroids to contribute to muscle weakness or to be ineffectual, so other immunosuppressant medications are used. Joanne wrote: "I'm in 25 percentile that doesn't respond. Still no exercise; how frustrating . . ." [Diary 1]. During those periods when the muscles are not actively inflamed physical therapy is advised to help strengthen them, although their scarred condition makes this painful.

Polymyositis is typically slow in its progression, during which muscle tissue is replaced by functionless scar tissue. Five-year survival rates are estimated to be as high as 80%, and nearly 50% of people with polymyositis recover fully. Those in whom the disease persists eventually become wheelchair-bound or bedridden. Patients are advised to minimize the risk of infections and, because of the extra strain on muscles, against weight gain, something that is particularly difficult when on prednisone and not exercising. Joanne, a nurse in clinical practice and an enthusiastic eater, did not manage to comply with either of those recommendations. The flexors of the neck may be severely affected in polymyositis, causing an inability to raise the head, which was pronounced in Joanne's case. Eventually, the muscles of the internal organs (involving cardiac and pulmonary function) and of the throat (leading to trouble with swallowing) are affected.

A Counterpane Sewn without Needle and Thread: Suffering

My challenge was not to do the impossible—but to learn to live with the possible.

Bender, 1996, p. 85

We don't understand the mystery of life very well. In Western philosophy sufferers are usually portrayed as subjects of tragedy and objects of compassion (Spelman, 1997). Aristotle differentiated himself from Plato by finding a place for grief, even cultivating it. Secular society approaches suffering as something to be eliminated. Medical efforts are dedicated to relieving suffering (or at least pain), and governments profess to intervene in conditions that result in human suffering. Yet despite our best efforts, millions of people suffer from myriad causes. The Navajo tell stories about suffering in the form of monsters. Earth mother Changing Woman's son, Monster Slayer, dealt with most of them, but the elders point out wisely that they are never completely gone (Schwarz, 1997). There are still sickness and aging and sometimes lice; these are facts of living and dying and being. We see only problems to be solved, and the typical solution is to find palliative retreats so that our stressful way of life is not compromised. Modern medicine extends life and reduces physical pain, but suffering is not reducible to physical and material terms (Moore, 2002, p. 94). We scapegoat objects of blame—smoke, fat, microorganisms, stress.

Suffering is a human condition that resists, through the bearing of pain or distress, the flow of living (Kleinman, 1995). Although we often choose to think of such turmoil as aberrant, life is inevitably patched and quilted with losses and falls along with exhilarating achievements and loving pride (Moore, 2002). Suffering dominates the here and now, wielding (like disease) both a heavy presence and vulnerability—for instance, when a physician's offhand question exacerbated Joanne's fears: "'You mean you really took 70 mgm [of] Prednisone since April? **Why?**' This set up more doubt for me—did I do the right thing?" [Diary 1].

The experience of suffering is the product of both the phenomenology of the individual self/body experience and the shared social body of symbolic representation. Viewed close up, this understanding of human suffering is difficult to express (Kleinman, 1995). Suffering can also be exaggerated by anticipation or nonrecognition; it is often overlooked among people who are not taken seriously. Joanne was acutely aware that middle-aged women are often viewed as malingerers, "cspccially if fat." Add "disabled" to that, and the stereotype takes on grave connotations of "damaged goods" (Phillips, 1990). Phenomena such as weakness, fatigue, and nausea show only in one's responses to them. Joanne's relationship with sickness reveals her intent to limit its impact on her life and the risk that it be misinterpreted as "all in my head."

Ragged "Squares," Failing Seams: Pain and Other Responses to Suffering

Sickness requires consideration of both disease and illness. In the intersubjectivity of body/self and health/ill health, *disease* is distinguished by physiological dysfunction or deviation from a biological or medical norm, while *illness* is the meaning and experience of sickness. One may be ill without disease and have disease without being ill. The phenomenology of illness refers to experiential meanings (Kaufmann, 1988), that is, signification and interpretation. Suffering both tests and prompts learning who we are and of what we are capable (Hall, 2004).

There is no doubt that we can (or can fail to) recognize suffering in others (Cassell, 1991b). While technical and theological explanations cannot make up for ignoring suffering (Kushner, 1989), the phenomenon often arouses pity, which uses the suffering of someone else to produce a feeling in oneself (Arendt, 1977). Compassion, in contrast, involves empathy—being so stricken with the suffering of another that one suffers as the other does. Unlike pity (merely an exchange about suffering), compassion is about cosuffering—knowing and entering pain (Davis, 1981). Not all suffering involves physical pain, but Arendt (1959) describes it as the "most private" and "least communicable" (p. 46) of human experiences. In the talk that connects people and creates a common world, compassion is often marked by muteness around pain and suffering (Arendt, 1977). With the experience of intense physical pain inseparable from the sufferer's lived reality, the significance of pain changes with social context, and its unfairness dwells in the eye of the beholder. Attempts to explain experience with pain come up short. Some see it as part of a larger plan, others as statistical probability or random patterning, but lives get twisted and end. There are innumerable stories of pain and people who suffer. Joanne wrote:

It took 1 ½ hours to start [an intravenous in] my left arm—seventh stick done by Dr. C. **I hurt like hell. I wonder when I'll cry.** Oh, it's so hot during the procedure. I listened to classical music; it helped but I had to <u>be still</u> for four hours. The muscles want to move when they know they cannot. Damn. [Diary 1]

All experiences of pain, grief, and loss are ontically the same, while type, intensity, cause, duration, and other characteristics vary. One might search for justice and fairness, but "pain is the price we pay for being alive" (Kushner, 1989, p. 64); there are no exceptions for "deserving" people. The question "Why did it happen?" is often better replaced with "What do I do now that it's happened?" As participants at home in the world, pain— intersubjective and constitutive of the lived flow of experience—takes over. Configured as suffering, it evokes intractable existential questions essential to understanding human conditions and needs. Such questions are positioned and interpretive. They are also, Kleinman (1995) cautions, vulnerable to reductionist analyses. When pain is only a problem, response is only heroic (Moore, 2002). That may cure, but it does not heal; that is, it may resolve disease without instilling a sense of well-being and meaning, while suffering threatens the *whole person* (Cassell, 1991a). Joanne wrote:

10/31 The end of an era—I shall move on to other unknowns but I'm resolved not to be disappointed that I'm not cured. I shall cope. I pledge not to be always cranky. I pray for gracefulness. I am supported by the love and encouragement of loved ones, co-workers and F——— the rest!! Come on world, here we go again. [Diary 1]

The Crooked "Square": Disablement

A good friend, like an old quilt, is both a treasure and a comfort.

Motto on a note tablet

A master status like suffering, disability is strongly linked to social inclusion and exclusion and to personal identity shaping social worlds (Albrecht & Verbrugge, 2000). There is an etiquette to taking care from others that demands a great deal of sociability. With changes in technology and attitude today's social models are constructed on the principle that disability is socially mediated and not a trait of the individual. Still, people assume that all the disabled have to deal with in their lives is their disability—that they are defined by it. In a society that equates physical soundness with beauty and vitality disablement spells serious shortcomings. One is not allowed to lament one's state (Mairs, 1996); instead, one searches for an other who treats the disability as a safe topic of conversation. We can only imagine what it was like for Joanne, a nurse who took care of others, to find herself forced to be dependent. We are all set against ideals flashed on glossy covers and screens. Working bodies can compensate for perceived deficiencies, but when the body does not work, the self wants not to own the parts, while the brain of the troubled body dreams that body into working life, reinforcing disappointment (Mairs, 1996). Yet there remains a societal insistence that disabled individuals "emerge from the shadows" to be visible and present (Mairs, 1996, p. 127).

There is greater recognition today of diversity among people labeled "disabled" and fewer limits in terms of access and opportunity. Persons with degenerative conditions, however, face recurrent demands for revision of self-definition. This is where suffering and disability intercept; not only must one mourn the loss of the "old me" while confronting someone who seems a stranger in one's being, but the disease and suffering "progress" while the self suffers. Those transformations of identity may leave one craving social contact, even at the risk of awkward encounters. Joanne's friends shared stories of having to feed Joanne at tailgate parties (Joanne loved football games) because she could not lift her arms and liberating her from public restroom cubicles when she discovered she could not get up from the toilet: "I'm measurably weaker; can't get up off toilet seats, steps are almost impossible. Arms feel like they're glued to my body" [Diary 1]. But she was determined to be there, although from a wheelchair or electric cart one's perspective of the world is from waist level—other people's eyes pass over your head; you are literally beneath their notice (Mairs, 1996). But Joanne would be there if she could possibly make it happen. She took her grandsons to so many events that, after her death, they worried that they would not know what to do when they no longer automatically headed for the handicap seating sections. Joanne, says Kristen, became a very involved grandparent immediately upon the birth of the oldest grandchild, Brendon. "I think she knew it wasn't going to be forever."

There is no guidebook; one draws one's own map as one proceeds along the journey. No disabled person gets immediately to where she is today; it takes "time and grieving" (Mairs, 1996, p. 134)—and verve. When Joanne was diagnosed with polymyositis, she dyed her hair a wild red and kept it that way. She and Walt nurtured an enduring and spirited myth about the "vat of red dye buried in the backyard" and "Pierre," the stylist Walt filled in for. The red had to be neither convincing nor fashionable; its flamboyance pleased Joanne as a declaration that "I am here." Eventually, her long hair, worn piled on her head, had to be cut when her weak arms could no longer manage it, but it stayed stoplight red. When Joanne was diagnosed with leukemia, her friend Janet sent her a big box full of small gifts, one to open each day. Among them were "gaudy flash-trash earrings. I knew she'd love them." Everybody considered Joanne to be both vibrant and good at expressing herself. She kidded that she did not have ulcers, she gave them. Joanne's daughter-in-law Kathleen, a dance teacher who had a mother of her own, considered "Joanne a mom because she was open-minded, raw, blunt, and outspoken—and so current. She used her energy for living. Rather than channeling it into anger or frustration or sadness, she channeled it into presence and productivity."

Disability is part of a binary with its privileged opposite, ability, which makes life messy. Kathleen lost her father after a long battle with cancer a year prior to Joanne's death. Thinking of her father's gradual decline, Kathleen said, "It was like there was nothing wrong with Joanne; she was such a whole person. I thought she would be here forever. . . . I never thought of her as sick. . . . It was the dominance of her personality. She couldn't pick up [her granddaughter] Addy and felt bad, but she was somehow fragile without being frail." The other daughter-in-law, Kristen, adds, "Joanne did more with 24 hours than anyone else could. If I had her body, I think I would have allowed it to do me in much sooner than she did." How does one make sense of a life so provisional that abilities and disabilities come and go? Years earlier, Joanne wrote: "Able to do steps up and down without help but S-L-O-W; am reaching more but can't do underarms. Sometimes family feels I don't need them anymore" [Diary 1]. Only the self knows its own pain and its reasons to grieve. The miracle is not that the incurable disease disappears or that the terminally ill person lives but that the family survives around the disease, that handicaps do not doom relationships.

In the social eye some disabilities are more acceptable than others. Those that are vague, chronic, and distorting are least acceptable. Culturally, such notions are perpetuated through traditions linking fate with virtue and grace. Bent and misshapen, ugly bodies are wicked witches—and there is no way to atone. Some 80% of Americans claim that individuals can do anything if they want to and try hard enough (Wuthnow, 1991); it takes *visible* evidence—a missing limb, perhaps—to release them from that expectation. Most also think that people usually bring suffering on themselves, and they equate disability with helplessness. Whatever the scenario, the ending is assured: good triumphs over evil, and the wicked witch is made to suffer (Lerner, 1980). Our cognitions create balance where there is none. Misfortune and sickness are interpreted as signs of badness. The message is mute but clear: the disabled person is an accident that ought not to have happened (Mairs, 1996). We protect ourselves from the realities of suffering.

Most people with disabilities don't feel especially sorry for themselves, but neither are they particularly brave. On the other hand, suffering affects a person's sense of connectedness and has at its root a feeling of being forced into submission (Hauerwas, 1979; Younger, 1995). In our busy lives Joanne occasionally felt abandoned:

[E]xcept for Walt, Skip and Chris, all handle their guilt about me when **all** their other tasks are done. It's "oh, by the way, there's poor Joanne. I don't have anything else to do so I'll call her, or god forbid, go see her." . . . I am weaker; I'm almost ready to give in. 7/2 Work is more difficult—I'm pushing especially to get in and out of car. . . . 7/10 It's taking two people to get me up the steps now. Turning point—didn't trip, didn't faint, but while standing in bathroom, I simply collapsed—hit my head on tile floor. [Diary 1]

Living with a disability means that everything takes inordinate planning and work. Feeding and clothing oneself can exhaust body and spirit. Incapacities become the source of "grief inconsolable" and are probably incomprehensible to "anyone still rushing from one good deed to the next and wishing for a chance to put up her weary feet" (Mairs, 1996, p. 80). At times one has to take satisfaction in stasis or in sedentary activities such as sewing.

With a progressively debilitating condition each change requires readjustment to body image and altered needs: "The trouble with degenerative disease is that no accommodation is ever final" (Mairs, 1996, p. 88). This is exacerbated when people feel isolated; being in contact with other sufferers can be positive. At NIH (National Institutes of Health) Joanne wrote: "I met Shirley tonight; another poly patient from Alabama. She's much worse than I, has had poly far longer, but looks a lot like me! A lot of same feelings it's great to share" [Diary 1]. And later: "We're all scared" [Diary 1]. Joanne was not alone with her demons. Grieving, depression, and anger exaggerated by endless waiting, bad news, and ambiguity about courses of action might be shared—cosuffered. Several of her roommates died while Joanne was at NIH for six weeks of diagnostic workup, but she felt she had benefited from being with them. Joanne was determined "not to go down like that." This is where the most intuitive communication—that ideal of understanding spouse, close friends, and family that evolves in affection and intimacy over long periods of time—offers inexpressible comfort (Mairs, 1996). Chris says, "After the diagnosis the four of us became very close." Nevertheless, one feels empty when disability precludes performing even trivial things for others. Often disability means that one must live more publicly than the able-bodied do. Joanne had to discipline herself to turn herself over to others, even strangers. How insufferable is that for a nurse who takes pride in the care she gives others?

Joanne did not contain her disease as one would a tumor that could be removed. She was neither the disease nor Joanne-plus-polymyositis; it was something integrated with her body. Would it be different if the condition were the only way she'd ever known? Or if she did not know it was degenerative and that, no matter how bad her symptoms were at any given time, there was a good chance they would be worse the next day? Polymyositis was shoving Joanne toward muscular catastrophe while forcing the realities of decrepitude and decay into a social world that works hard to avoid them. Only a new paradigm that defines people with disabilities in terms of what they *can* do will impede the imposition of expectations of dependency. Joanne helped construct that way for us by living her abilities and not being defined by polymyositis.

The Dominant Color and Pattern: Agency

Planning for death is difficult; we adore a sense of control.
                                        Mairs, 1993, p. 211

Western culture, in its positivistic and reductionistic preoccupation with science, does not facilitate the integration of mind, body, and spirit. Individuals committed to holism must seek out and develop for themselves what it takes to pursue that quest. In addition to privileging biological and rational approaches in living and in the conventional biomedical paradigm, much is taken for granted. The physical processes of healthy people typically impinge little on their sense of well-being, so they come to believe they are in control of them (Mairs, 1996). Yet, in reality, being one's own agent is challenging. Joanne wrote:

I got up to bathroom—it feels good to have ability to make decisions again. Put underwear on for first time in two days. Am sitting in chair writing this at 3 AM. . . . I'm starting to see the real purpose of this experience, whereas I was smug and sassy in the beginning—I have been stripped of all control, have truly suffered pain, and think I will have to adjust to chronic state of illness but I am developing my esteem in that regard. It's OK—I must ask for strength to ENDURE. [Diary 1]

The mind, active and in control, is supposed to be able to direct what the body does. Invoking the aid of others invites new ideas about suffering and the forfeiting of preconceptions, such as how one is not a victim but a moral agent (Spelman, 1997). Presenting oneself as in need of help but also as someone who makes decisions and judgments implies being capable of making judgments about those who help, even as they do so. Joanne wrote: "No attempt to pamper me—just 'You're going to CAT [scan] for kidney films.' . . . To CAT. The tech was awful, put me flat when I said I couldn't tolerate [it]. Not **one** time did he explain what he was going to do. Ironically, I was asked to fill out an evaluation and I **did**" [Diary 1]. Over time "I can do it myself" becomes less a statement of fact and possibility and more an elusive desire. Mairs (1996) writes that when your body does not move "without batteries beneath your butt" there is a good chance you will "cherish what little [you] have on any given day, in the full knowledge that on some tomorrow it will inevitably be less" (p. 38).

While members of many cultures emphasize *being* (e.g., focusing on who their ancestors were or family is or being oriented toward the present and experiencing the moment), Americans more often focus on *doing*, to the extent that performing tasks overshadows meaning and experience. We tend to be oriented to action, to see ourselves as our own best source of information and opinions, and to believe that we should solve our own problems. Hence, not only is the individual the locus of decision making, but we generally hold ourselves responsible for decisions made: "Individualism is the perception of the self as the cultural quantum in society" (Steward & Bennett, 1991, p. 13).

I'm beginning to get cranky and concerned that staff doesn't tune into pathophysio[logical] and emotional needs. People aren't computing and I need to do more analyzing of me and tell them what to do. Wake up, Joanne, that's a fact. . . . My ability to think clearly and make good decisions has been hampered by this disease process. I have been so overwhelmed with/by what's happening to me that I'm not thinking straight. Today I was **emphatic about no major procedures** until after the weekend pass, also who's looking after the central line? . . . If he couldn't convince me [about safety of procedures], then I shouldn't have consented. It's as simple as that, but boy, was I stupid. . . . It is possible that I will abort [the workup program] by next week. . . . But you know how I feel about quitting anything. [Diary 1]

What got her through this bad stretch? "Then Skip and I went to White Flint Plaza to the fabric store. It's the first time I've been out in **11** days. It felt wonderful but exhausting. I think I'll stay with the program" [Diary 1]. Chris attributes his brother (who says, "I'm so like my mother I almost *am* my mother!") with having had an almost psychic connection with Joanne: "He felt her NIH 'death'" when she had the "terrible reaction to the bronchoscopy." Skip told Chris they had to "get over there right away," and they did.

Modern minds are in continuous transformation, always moving toward completion (Finkler, 1994). This may be a mythic individualism, but great credence is given to being one's own person, even "inventing" the self. Some see this as a break from family and community (e.g., Bellah, Madsen, Sullivan, Swindler, & Tipton, 1985), but we also talk about community while cherishing individual freedom (Wuthnow, 1991). The American quest for autonomy and self-actualization thrives. Self-reliance is the cultural ideal, although the old "fierce, utilitarian self-reliance" has, to an extent, given way to more expressive forms (Steward & Bennett, 1991, p. 137). Individualism is associated with comfort and freedom from outside constraints on personal expression. Aesthetic judgments are frequently equated with personal preferences—the colors in a quilt, the length of the stitches, the harmony experienced when doing something valued (Cassell, 1991b). Aesthetic experience has strong links with acting against suffering (Richard, 1957). Joanne wrote:

Oh how I HATE hospitals. I am totally dependent there and HATE to ask for help for such simple things as in and out of bed. [Diary 1]

Who knows anymore? I'm still an experiment and nothing really works. I am depressed—fed up is a better word. . . . Should I keep pushing? I'm running out of energy and don't know what to do about it. I work hard. My work is purposeful. I'm more of a load for Walt, I can't seem to keep up. We're up to three grans [grandsons Brendon, Connor, and Devon] now and they are a delight but sometimes exhausting. Sewing is my outlet but I miss having friends around—Millie in Kentucky, Jan in West Virginia. [Diary 1]

How are the seemingly paradoxical elements of personal freedom, individual success, and the pursuit of self-interest reconciled with the need
to care and for care in the culture? Some question whether compassion—
to suffer with or, at the very least, to feel with—is really possible in American society, but caring for others is not opposed to individualism. Rather,
caring is a metaphor for self-identity; fulfillment provides the strength,
identity, and self-esteem needed for an individual to care (Wuthnow,
1991). Humans have a desire to give and receive love; caring is the essence of humanity and the basic constitutive phenomenon of human
existence (Watson, 1988). An ontological model of health implies a way
toward something closer to wholeness, even as we live out our incom-
pleteness (Diekelmann, 2005). As suffering and health are natural parts
of life, suffering is a part of health. Health, then, can be understood only
in relation to suffering (Eriksson, 1994). While communion with others is
the basis for human society (Buber, 1958), courage, wisdom, uncondi-
tional caritas, and responsibility for mindfulness and personal integrity in
action are idealized (Eriksson, 1994).

About a year before Joanne had the stroke Chris and Kathleen had a
baby girl, Addison. Joanne was crushed that she could no longer safely
care for children alone as she once had. At times like that Joanne admitted "hating the polymyositis." Still, she found tremendous satisfaction in
her sewing. She wrote: "I love [working] part time—have had plenty of
time to catch up on unfinished projects, love quilts x 3, outfits for Addy—
smocked one; it's beautiful!" When Joanne and Walt, believing in "being
present for hard times and good," went to help out when Kathleen's
father died, "[t]he outfits I made [Addy] fit fine and the smocked romper
looks adorable—truly a work of love. . . . Stopped at a fabric shop only for
a quarter hour" [Diary 2].

Joanne was driven to make things and to make things happen. One of
those things was living *around* polymyositis. She was not about to be defined by this uninvited phenomenon, but neither could she get rid of it.
There were times when Joanne was "this close to being on a ventilator,"
Carol says as she holds her fingers an inch apart. "She was terrified of
being on a ventilator, terrified." Joanne knew all about the eventual internal involvement of polymyositis, but she was determined to maximize the
time she had. "Selflivingworkingsewing" was her mantra, her interpretation of and adaptation to the world in which she found herself, her way of
being human. I had no idea when I began this inquiry how artfully she

had fashioned the quilt that was her life. If living life is an improvisatory art (Bateson, 1990), Joanne's jazzy quilts have much to teach us.

Female children search for role models but often have difficulty imagining female characters that matter. Joanne grew up with a mother who provided a great deal of confusion and little positive role modeling. Walt summarizes Joanne's childhood as "just way too many stepfathers, some of them abusive." In many ways Joanne's mother epitomized female dependence. Everyone knowing her background marvels at Joanne's ability to transcend it to be a caring person and an integral part of a stable family. But Joanne had found her media; she had her family, her work, and her play. Each served as a voice of her self-reliant self (for one can be both self-reliant and a member of a family or team), although in her sewing room she allowed her fabrications to express her. She sewed even more after the diagnosis of polymyositis, even when she was profoundly depressed and bothered by "horrible dreams of creepy, crawly critters over me" and too sick to keep food down. Sewing sustained her: "Did do a good bit of hand quilting; still too wobbly to go downstairs [to her sewing room]." Two days later: "Spent some time in sewing room—great feeling" [Diary 2]. There are numerous notes like these.

The materialism of contemporary American culture can protect and nurture, but it also degrades with its hierarchies and competitiveness (Rollins, 1985). The 19th century exaggerated the divergence of men's and women's activities, and wives became more dependent upon their husbands. The home was idealized as loving and the workplace as ruthless (Cancian, 1985). While 19th-century Victorianism polarized the sexes, the past century did much in the West to liberate individuals from the confines of sex-assigned traits (Heilbrun, 1993). The word *androgyny* (not to be confused with *hermaphroditism*) comes from the ancient Greek *andro* (male) and *gyn* (female). Women can be as self-reliant as men, men as tender as any stereotype of women. Both are educating themselves about equality. Social change is never even or without contradictions, however, and conventional definitions of *masculine* and *feminine* remain embedded in culture. Even today women shy away from collective anger at the patriarchy (Heilbrun, 1988). Nursing as a discipline is a prime example of such avoidance (Kavanagh, 2003). But in dealing with Joanne's situation, she and Walt displayed an impressive androgyny.

Quilting Woman: The Gendered Self

Women and suffering are old companions. Although our view keeps us from seeing existence in its totality, women's health cannot be isolated from self, family, and society. Sickness is not understandable apart from personal lifeways and the social setting in which it occurs (Cassell, 1991a). Compared with men's, women's symptoms are more likely to be bothersome than life threatening. Women tend to accumulate more nonfatal problems, more years of sickness and dysfunction, and more years of life than men, whose lives are often characterized by relative freedom from ill health or disability but then abbreviated by fatal disease when it does strike (Verbrugge, 1990). In short, women's experience of daily symptoms, chronic conditions, and disability due to health problems exceeds men's in each age group, yet their mortality rates are strikingly lower than men's.

Why do women experience more sickness than men? Any interpretation is complex. One medical anthropologist closely examining the question found that when women talk about their sickness, they talk about their experiences with home, family, work, and "life's lesions"—aspects of living embedded in existential conditions, contradictions, and the exigencies of everyday life (Finkler, 1994). To isolate life's lesions requires a contextualized examination of a life and, even then, looking at the totality of human sickness. Joanne's illness narrative (Kleinman, 1988) shapes 20 years of living with suffering and pain. Life's lesions are not fatal; they grind at the body, mind, and spirit with shifting symptomatologies that are linked closely with daily experience. Resting on the assumption that to be human is to simultaneously embody and interact with our physical and social worlds, illness narratives and life's lesions are not an analog to psychosomatic illness, which is lodged in the Cartesian separation of mind and body and rooted in psychological distress, not the lived world; instead, they are the embedding of humans in day-to-day experience.

A Few More Inches—The Fat Quarter: Weighing In

Fat is a three-letter word larded with meaning.
Kulick & Meneley, 2005, p. 1

In the West fear of fat has been around for a century, during which America, preoccupied with slimness, has grown ever heavier. In the

1970s Joanne and her friends, like many American women, worried about their weight. "We all did. We obsessed over it. We tried every kind of exercise and diet plan." I was shown photographs: Joanne was stylish and svelte—far slimmer than I ever knew her. By the summer of 1986 Joanne was finally in physical therapy

to rebuild and strengthen neck and shoulders; it hurts GOOD. But big time mental response to Chris seeing me saying "What's wrong with Mom?" He hadn't seen steroid swelling and poor posture problems before he left for the summer. . . . Bloated face and neck. [Diary 1]

There were also new symptoms. "Is it weather? Drugs or glucose related? I'm scared and concerned. . . . Steroids alone aren't doing enough. . . . Weight 164. I hate these steroids." Later:

[V]arious tests to stimulate the deltoids show they are dead so we'll work around them. I can handle that; just let's do something. Also started exercising in a pool—the water feels wonderful. Walt assists and hangs on because I'm so fat my brain doesn't know how to swim. . . . Walt can only do so much—he is truly an angel and without him I'd be nowhere and I know I don't show appreciation enough. I worry about him and his weight and me and my weight. [Diary 1]

Joanne, Ski, Carol, and Mary were together for dinner when Joanne told them the diagnosis. She described polymyositis as progressive, neuromuscular, and so on, but it wasn't until Joanne compared polymyositis to multiple sclerosis that they "got it—we could relate to that." Janet, like Mary, Carol, Clayton (Joanne's friend since high school), and even Chris after not seeing Joanne for several months, was shocked and "hardly recognized her." Clayton walked right by her at a game. Chris came home from college and found "something had changed; the disease got far worse." Joanne had become heavy; she was so sick as to be unrecognizable.

Filling the Empty Block: Wholeness

Everything is permitted in the imagination.
                    Levitt, 2003, p. xvi

To lose one's muscles is to disintegrate, to feel not whole. At best we are always becoming whole, but never completely whole, and always disintegrating as we go. Peeled away like an onion, we search for wholeness, only to find nothing left to peel. Giving up the ideal of wholeness and having disintegrated sufficiently to be touched by life, one is empty. It is a spiritual emptiness, an attitude of nonattachment, an openness to letting go (Moore, 2002) that is sometimes valuable and at other times threatening. People caught up in the collective unconsciousness of the time may not feel the struggle for meaning, but that often changes with serious illness. People have an instinct for transcendence (Moore, 2002). For some there is religion or reclamation in art; for Joanne it was working and sewing. Whatever the medium of expression, it is both paramount and mysterious. Isak Dinesen described the relationship between her art and her life as constituting "a pair of locked caskets, each containing the key to the other" (Thurman, 1982, p. 182). In January 1990 Joanne listed her goals:

to be able to shampoo my own hair, to be able to put on a fashionable jacket, to be able to bathe myself (especially underarms), to wear hair piled on top of my head, to train [my] dog, to save $100 month, to maintain my job, and [to] complete the sampler quilt before Christmas. [Diary 1]

Soon there were notes about having to give up the extra strain of "doggie training" and "backing out of the [nurses' association] stuff." Quilting continued, and she bought her Berninas: "Maybe I'll sell quilts. . . . You know what's sad, except for my men [Joanne's collective term for Walt, Skip, and Chris], there is no one who will get excited with me about this major purchase and happening" [Diary 1]. (No wonder Joanne and I liked each other when we finally met.) Work was increasingly stressful, Joanne wrote, "but I won't give in. I'm staying excited and positive about crafts. Will be a Master of Crafts soon. Learned smocking, tatting, appliqué sew and 'no sew' so far this summer. [Also] doing a lot of strategizing with Ski about work" [Diary 1]. And Joanne set a new goal: "to DANCE at Skip and Kristin's wedding." On the day after "THE" wedding, she reported: "Everything was wonderful" [Diary 1].

Pathos and tragedy are no substitute for reflection. In the intersubjective medium of social transactions in local moral worlds that we call experience, people search for the right teacher, the best book, the perfect community—but it takes a lot of energy and may leave little room for reflection and emptiness. Some people spot their potential shaman in recovery from serious illness or some disaster, but how suffering is linked to spirituality is a mystery although few doubt that it is. From Zen we learn that we never understand anything fully, from Taoism we find strength in yielding and accept the inaccuracy of our conception of the meaning of things. Christian mystics teach contentment in unknowing and risking the darkness (Moore, 2002). While lack of belief is associated with emptiness and ineffectuality, however, belief can be demanding, anxiety generating, self-satisfying, and potentially painful when confused with allegiance to an organization. Over the years Joanne reconciled herself with the religion of her youth. It helped a great deal, but living in a society that focuses on information and operates from anxiety also requires approaches that offer calm and joy. Anxiety comes from weakness in imagination, but Joanne had plenty of that as well as purpose. During the three and a half decades Walt worked for the federal government Joanne had half a dozen different nursing jobs. Her life was a patchwork of jobs in different areas of nursing plus new symptoms and more falls.

Funny handwriting? Broke right arm upper humerus on Tuesday 6/23 leaving work. Five stitches in eyebrow—embarrassed. Now I'm tied up to myself. It's hell. Dr. said I'll heal but will take longer and my greatest problem is to fall again and do more damage.

7/13 saw Karen to gain insight why I'm hating this injury so much. [Diary 1]

Soon Joanne broke her leg. Walt, her cobeing in this world (Heidegger, 2001), tried to break Joanne's fall, which she could not do herself without upper arm muscles: "We took care of each other."

The Nursing Quilt

I realized the depth of Joanne's attachment (she referred to it as being stitched) to both nursing and quilting when she talked me into making a quilt block for a project by the state nurses' association. Jung (1977) saw the crisis of modern life as the loss of an appreciation for the sacred and holy; for Joanne, nursing was both secular and sacred. Nursing is in large part about authority, science, and doing, but in the imaginative refining of the emotions and life's complexities, spiritual depth has many images. The Pueblo Indians center their religion around the kiva, in which the goal is to be open to being guided (Waters, 1969). Irish funeral processions often intentionally wander, taking the long route from church to cemetery. Why shouldn't Joanne find what she needed in nursing, even though she could no longer do the clinical work she loved? A face-to-face encounter with all five senses, nursing is hands-on. Nurses have a professional responsibility for human needs and existence. Within limits, they help lend compassion in unpretentious presence between people, emerging in the meeting between suffering and love. I made my square, and Joanne submitted it with hers. I thought about those squares after Joanne died. Around 1993, when she noticed increasing weakness in her upper legs, Joanne decided (based on an interest that went back at least to being close to a Jewish roommate and her mother during nursing school) that integrating cultural diversity and cultural competence into nursing was her life's mission. Her quilt square depicted cross-cultural nursing. Joanne made me a pot holder in the same design: the earth surrounded by appliquéd hands of many shades. I asked Walt one day what Joanne's favorite design was, and he described the one on my pot holder.

Moore (2002) recounts the story of a Sufi master who set himself up at a crossroads. He lit a bright lamp and, some distance away, a candle. Then he sat by the candle and read his book. People asked why he didn't read by the bright lamp. He explained that the lamp attracted all the moths, who ignored the candle and left him to read in peace. I wondered if Joanne was the moth going after the brightness with her quilts and crafts but decided I had it wrong. She loved human diversity and was intrigued by her observations in the clinics and by the stories of Walt's missionary aunt and uncle, Betty and William. She thrived on learning all she could and was interested in alternative healing methods, although she seems to have given herself permission to employ them only peripherally. Perhaps if cross-cultural nursing had had more clearly defined applications she would not have moved from job to job seeking a forum for another expression of her creativity and caring.

Joanne loved nursing. She was a nurse for more than 40 years, beginning as a hospital diploma graduate and eventually earning a baccalaureate and a master's degree, the latter more than a decade after being diagnosed with polymyositis. Occupational cohesiveness and networks provide both logical solutions to practical problems and emotional support (Kavanagh, 1989); most of Joanne's closest friends both worked and went to school with her. After working all week the women went to school most of the weekend. Janet told stories of five carpooling nurses supporting each other. They taught Joanne to drink Bailey's Irish Cream: "She was never much of a drinker, but she learned to like that well enough."

Over time, Joanne worked in maternity, emergency, and shock trauma; helped establish emergency response facilities and walk in health centers; managed clinical support services; and taught nursing. Finally,

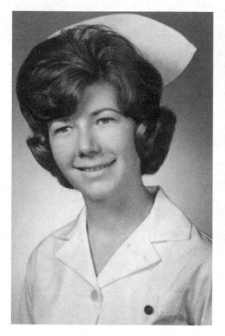
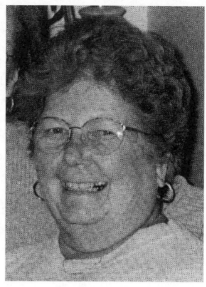

Left: Joanne, 1963
Above: Joanne, 2003

she worked in utilization review. Known as an excellent supervisor, a "get-in-there-with-you" person, "Joanne tended to get along with others." Even when the polymyositis was so intrusive that Walt had to transport her, Joanne would "not give up working because it meant giving in to the disease." Some of her closest friends believe that it was "doing what she really loved—nursing—that did her in." They describe her as driven, whether healthy or ill. Joanne planned *not* to retire. "She said they were not good planners and needed the income," Janet said, "but what Joanne meant was she was not going to retire because it meant giving in to the disease. Quality living meant doing things. It was many years before quality of life meant cutting back. . . . I tried hard to talk her into not working. If she would rest a little . . ."

Nursing practice changed substantially during Joanne's four decades. Most recently, healthcare reform has resulted in increasing workloads (sicker patients, more technology, and more paperwork), time compression, and increased dependence on minimally trained labor—all manifesting values of economics and efficiency rather than care per se. Joanne welcomed the increased cultural diversity she met in nursing but not the compromises she observed in patient care. In the transformed hospital organization there is little of the consultation and camaraderie that Joanne and her colleagues valued, laments Carol, a nurse-executive.

In the early 1970s, when mortalities in shock trauma were more common than they are today, Joanne and her colleagues openly discussed "the meaning of it all." As trauma medicine advanced, Joanne, Carol, Ski, and Mary took care of many young people who died. They developed a rhythm in their work and great respect for each other. Joanne and her colleagues "were closer than sisters; we talked about everything together. . . . We all grew up then," Carol says, "and we grew up together." Many of the policies and procedures used in trauma care today were developed by this team. Although they used known techniques, there were few trauma protocols except for patients known to be terminal, leading to innumerable conversations about the ethics and meaning of suffering and of dying.

Many of their patients faced severe posttrauma disabilities, yet the head of the trauma facility insisted that families not be allowed in to be with patients. The nurses circumvented that dictum, and Mary, as nurse-manager, made sure a nurse accompanied any physician talking with a family. Too often the nurses saw families dissolving over the trauma sustained by one of their members. Joanne helped mediate the family acceptance movement and the development of support groups. She also developed a puppet educational project to teach children about safety. Carol said, "She loved nursing and she loved using nursing differently."

In her eulogy for Joanne, Ski talked about Joanne's desire to leave a legacy. Walt thought about the family and I thought about quilts, but Ski was referring to nursing:

She always wanted to make a difference. Nursing had such an important impact on people's lives and it gave her a way to keep on fighting. . . . Joanne wanted all the information she could get and she wanted it straight. On the other hand, she would not pay attention to the really negative parts. We talked about so much of this back in Shock Trauma and since, the "what if."

Having seen and worked with people in dire need and mortal peril surely influenced Joanne's management of her own situation. I wondered whether being a nurse might have implied a responsibility to be "tougher than real life" or that others were worse off than she was, rendering her own situation inconsequential. It is often said that nurses learn how to take better care of others than of themselves. How does working with others who are desperately ill affect one's ability to meet one's personal needs? In her diaries Joanne tended to retreat into medical jargon when her emotions erupted. She consistently juxtaposed biomedical observations with her own visceral responses, but she seldom dealt on paper with the pain caused when the ragged edges of those realities either grated together or left gaping holes.

Creating a Pattern of Quilt Blocks: Arranging

When life gives you scraps, make a quilt.
Refrigerator magnet

To move along without a plan or goal is to be empty and generous, saturated with mystery (Moore, 2002)—but frustrated, if one is a skilled woman with things one wants to do. Joanne was not about to let polymyositis define or confine her, although sometimes she was powerless to prevent just that. The Romantics are said to have dealt successfully with death by transcending it: they allowed their artistic impulses to outshine and dwarf illness, thereby preventing it from being reduced to a pathological condition (Croce, 1994–1995). I'd like to ask Joanne how she saw herself conducting her last score of years now that I understand more fully what she did. It was like her quilting: "She never talked much about quilting, she just did it," just as she did many things, most of them related to giving. When Skip and Kristen (an elementary school teacher) were busy with two small children and expecting a third, Joanne and Walt started taking dinner over to the family one evening each week, a pattern they continued long after Devon arrived.

Joanne was honest about her condition, but she simply never brought it up or discussed the experience in depth. Consequently, her friends "did not look much at the disease but only at Joanne"; they fell into step when Joanne didn't talk about her feelings. Even her grandson Connor talks about remembering "the whole person Grandma Jo was." Mary said, "She was taking care of all of us while we were minimizing attention to her condition because she let us. Perhaps her creative outlets let her do that." The trade-off was that Joanne closed down potential avenues of support, but control was so important to her that she left no evidence of regretting the exchange. Throughout the interviews people communicated that they really respected Joanne; they were awed by her ability to live around the disease, and no one talked about feeling sorry for her, even when she was most debilitated. That is a significant constituent of Joanne's legacy.

Everyone also acknowledges that Joanne had a stubborn streak. She loved the scent of patchouli and wore it every day, even though many people don't find it pleasant. She had an aversion to wearing an emergency call button, despite her proclivity for falling and not being able to get up again. When Chris and Kathleen were planning their wedding, Kathleen's mother pointed out to Joanne that she did not think it appropriate for the groom's mother to wear the same flowers as the bride carried. Joanne retorted, "I'm paying for the flowers, and I will wear any flowers I like." She liked the bride's white gardenias, so she wore them too. Skip and Kristen shared the group photo: everyone is in black or white except Joanne, who is smiling in scarlet. Chris says, "My mother's relationship with polymyositis was really one of anger. She had to put up with it, but she never accepted it or gave in to it for a moment. It's just that she felt she was a burden, and was angry about that." And when she rebelled, it was in living color.

Joanne feared that people thought she was malingering or hypochondriacal; her symptoms were unusual, didn't show, came and went, and were not explainable, so she minimized and marginalized them. Nurses are accustomed to maintaining confidentiality, and Joanne did exactly that. The more I talked with people, the more clear it became that each person in her personal realm thought Joanne was sharing "her real pain" with someone else. Sometimes she provided explanations, such as when Skip, a physical education teacher and lifeguard, questioned why she could not do a full-range muscular workout. But when it came to living, she did it with all the aesthetic knowing associated with suffering (Cassell, 1991b). She did not talk about her condition and neatly misled her friends into believing that she was in therapy to discuss the deeper issues. She did indeed maintain contact with Karen, a nurse-therapist Joanne respected and admired. But Karen, going back over her records, was amazed at Joanne's skillful maneuvering away from discussion of living with a chronic, debilitating disease. Karen wrote:

Of all the chronically ill patients I ever treated (hundreds), she was by far the most adamantly opposed to being defined in any way with her disability. It wasn't denial; it was simply a position she maintained to approach accomplishing what I think she most needed—staying a productive person, who largely defined herself by her work and family. . . . She sewed out her frustrations.

I revisited Joanne's utter insistence that we NOT focus on her illness. She clearly said that was not what defined her and that she had done all the mental stuff related to it that she cared to at the time, and she was with me to talk about her issues with her Mom.

Joanne simply set boundaries—her chronicity was taboo. Karen continues:

One of my longest-living Non-Hodgkin's Lymphoma patients REFUSED to read one work or investigate one thing about the disease, and lived 2+ years longer than every expert gave her, including all of us, her medical friends/colleagues. We read everything and had her in the grave instantly; if she ever read what we did, she would have died much sooner, I am convinced. Again, positive denial and the differing needs for information—Joanne was very informed, but just didn't dwell.

Joanne worked with her friend Marie in the late 1970s. They remained close over the years, and their relationship intensified a few years ago when Marie was diagnosed with an autoimmune syndrome and learned firsthand the frustrations of not knowing what was happening or why. Marie says both she and Joanne were resolute about putting forth that healthy presence. Yet even with Marie there was "a point at which you stopped asking questions," because "Joanne did *not* talk about having poly." Marie believes that Joanne probably could have helped herself by getting more rest, but Joanne simply "wasn't going down." When Marie was diagnosed, Joanne said, "You don't deserve that. It's unfair." Marie replied, "*You* say that to *me*?"

Why didn't Joanne share her experience more? No one knows why. Perhaps because of her childhood, which was difficult, she learned not to trust others with her deeper dilemmas. Perhaps, being a woman of her era, she was not comfortable sharing bewildering personal information. Perhaps when a disease is too amorphous to describe with any certainty, the risk of being misunderstood is simply too great. Perhaps being a nurse meant she could not act in any way that might be construed as minimizing others' plights. Perhaps Joanne believed she could become the person she presented herself as. In any case, her choices seem to reflect a closure upon herself and her own reality that felt both significant and correct to her (Nancy, 1997).

For a seriously ill clinician there is particular agony when caregivers withdraw from treating the ill colleague as an equal. In volume 1 of this series there is a story of a nurse for whom loss of identity as a critical care nurse was one of the most painful aspects of her increasingly poor health (Kavanagh, 2002). Did Joanne read that story? If she did, she might have recognized her pattern of not talking about her health problems as insurance against being rejected by others who were so much a part of her private and professional life.

Joanne knew that insisting that others' lives be changed often does more to declare their inadequacies than to improve lives. Her self-reliant being resisted being a burden, surely a legacy of the rugged individualism that fueled American history and, later, its androgyny. Kathleen described Joanne as "someone who rejected traditional gender roles—a proud woman. . . . I'd never been around women that age who could do so much!" Joanne appreciated help when it was given, but she was loath to ask for it. Kathleen described feeling good about their choice of a home without steps and about small considerations such as giving Joanne a towel to put on her chest, since she could not lift her head and often spilled food. In reality we are better at imagining how burdensome we are than we are at actually asking and being open to the response. To Joanne it was a "package deal"—"<u>That</u> is me; that's who I am." She was living a life no one has any idea how to live, but she left few doubts about her intent to do it her way.

A Time to Stitch, a Stitch in Time: Producing and Creating

The universe moved from a self-unfolding phenomenon to one that was created.

Diekelmann, 2005, p. 7

Life is a collage of difficult tasks. Composing a life is like making a quilt: "[T]he materials are known, the hands skillful in tasks familiar from thousands of performances, the fit of the completed whole in the common life is understood" (Bateson, 1990, p. 1). Joanne was a nurse through and through. Being a nurse appealed to her; Walt says it is the only thing she ever wanted to be (not the only thing she did, but the only thing she wanted to *be*). She was a nurse, and that was often not easy for her. There is a kind of clear darkness in her living and caring: harrowing periods of insecurity juxtaposed with a deep bond with people unlike Joanne herself.

Perhaps she was a complex, compelling person because of her struggle with an inner driving force, being in the world *and* thrown into a world of suffering and meaning (Heidegger, 1927/1962a).

Nursing's materialistic methods of learning leave one to reconcile living on the edge of understanding with working in a system of applied knowledge implemented in life-and-death situations (Kavanagh, 2003). In the academic world we learn to worry about the validity of thoughts rather than to trust our intuition and imagination. As nurses we are taught not to own our uncertainty but to believe that correct actions are linked to positive outcomes. We make life-and-death decisions and depend on ideology to ensure their "correctness." We are not taught the ancient spiritual traditions of the senses or much about worlds other than the physical. There are books for developing skills and for crafting souls. Nursing is about the former; we grapple with experience to develop the latter.

Creativity is a gift given to those who are receptive to receiving it. By using and adding to the gift we are brought closer to whole (Metzger, 1992). In our culture a sharp distinction is made between creativity and standardization. Scattered throughout Joanne's diaries among the lab results and health concerns are numerous notes: "finished cross-stitch coasters," "worked on quilt," "spent time sewing," "prepared fabric for Lynn's quilt," "no procedures today; goal is complete some craft projects" [Diary 1]. It is our birthright to create—the urge to do so is inherent in human nature. Much has been written about anger being the consequence of repressing creativity and individuality as well as about whether art respects or disrespects the suffering of those portrayed. Art is among the most visible means of bringing attention to suffering (Spelman, 1997). When the artist is the sufferer, creating is both respectful and a medium of healthy expression.

Being creative requires giving ourselves permission to do the work we want and need to do (Levitt, 2003). Joanne took sewing courses when her sons were small. Later, friends such as Marie introduced her to new challenges, including quilting. Joanne sewed what she had imagined and what she had not, for as creations evolve one never really knows exactly how they will be. There is a willingness to risk that brings the moment and the work to life in a way that did not previously exist. Free and expressive exploration instills identity in each unique creation. Quilts exude presence and the making of memories. Those that Joanne made for "the boys" when they went to college in the early 1980s were her first. Skip's was used so long that it "wore totally out."

Sewing and quilting also engage solitude and concentration. Immersion in one's passion is integral to finding ways to dull the awareness of disease and disability. Only the courageous grant themselves permission to make room enough for that part of themselves (Levitt, 2003). Imagination creates a sacred space, a temporarily real world that is not fully lost with the end of play. Joanne literally made a place for her "play"; Walt nurtured it and kept its boxes of fabric stocked, spending "many a day in a fabric shop." Joanne's quilts overflowed into other people's lives. Her favorite was whichever one she was working on at the time. There was order and security in the ritual of creating, presenting holiday gifts, and gathering at quilt shows. Such play was recognized by Plato as both sacred and indispensable for the well-being of the community:

God alone is worthy of supreme seriousness, but man is made God's plaything, and that is the best part of him. . . . What, then, is the right way of living? Life must be lived as a play, playing certain games, making sacrifices, singing and dancing, and then a man will be able to propitiate the gods, and defend himself against his enemies, and win in the contest. (Plato *Laws* 7.796, cited in Huizinga, 1967, pp. 18–19)

Joanne loved play of all kinds, and she loved to dance. She and Walt did the slow dances, and she and Clayton swung through the fast ones. Clayton says their 25th high-school reunion in 1985 was the last time they danced. The diagnosis came around that time, and Joanne stopped attending reunions. She could no longer dance, but she could still play.

Art is not limited to specific forms of high culture or great profundity. Art celebrates play as craft celebrates art. The play element in culture was in full swing in the 18th century and has been on the wane since, with aesthetic concerns giving way to science, which is played with firmer rules and applied more seriously. To the scientific eye the world does not have personality (Moore, 2002); to the artist's eye it is a work of mystery and character. Quilting, neither frivolous nor strictly rule bound, progressed to being art from the salvaging of old fabrics to create needed bed coverings. Like many artful endeavors it takes faith and calm patience. An actor's stage, a painter's canvas, a quilter's cutting board—each is an empty space where the imagination makes contact with the irony of living a serious life while knowing neither the end nor the meaning of it all (Moore, 2002). There is a dramatic clarity in producing something beautiful from ordinary pieces and small actions. Hand-pieced crafts are idealized in a world in which the signs of the hand and imagination together are ever scarcer. We are seduced by convenience but awed by artful work in which the senses meet spirit and inspiration.

The Joy of Patches: Piecing Together Play and Sacrifice

Animals also play, so play is older than human culture. All play is significant; it means something beyond physiological phenomena or psychological reflexes. Play is both a natural part of being and part of its mystery. It is a mystery why we suffer and how we should respond to tragedy and why someone facing devastating loss and disease is also expected not to make jokes. People expect cheerfulness and patience in a disabled person's character but not that the person have a good time (Mairs, 1996). Joseph Campbell (1970) cautioned that there is delusion in taking our views too seriously. Myths and delusions are among many examples of humankind's creativity; stories and play are natural correlates. Humor takes on deeper, darker meanings at times, but it has the power to make the mundane memorable. Joanne loved jokes. She would call Clayton and tell him she needed a joke for some special person or occasion. He had a ready repertoire—not that it much mattered, he chuckles, because she often either mixed up the story or forgot the punch line. "But how she'd laugh!"

Some people collapse in the face of adversity; others find meaning in everyday challenge. It is tempting to assume that everyone with physical limitations is plagued with low spirits and to think that they "must be jollied out of them" (Mairs, 1996, p. 103). Despondency and desperation are not essential responses to pain and debility, which may alter who one is without making a being less human or independent in spirit. Joanne coped. Skip changed steps to small risers, and Walt had a chairlift installed, got a lift for the toilet, and put in bathroom rails. Joanne loved Skip's wedding at the beach, with the groom and his men in formal tuxedo jackets and beach shorts and the rehearsal dinner a barbecue. Kristen said, "She loved stories about the children and thought almost everything they did was funny." Joanne simply enjoyed games and people playing. She loved "yard sale-ing" with her friend Millie or her daughter-in-law Kristen, and she made colorful shorts for the students in Chris's drum corps (he teaches music in an elementary school where he has developed an African program and Afro-Caribbean and Brazilian themes). Instead of "jams," these were "jellies," created in the zaniest fabrics Joanne could find. They might have animals on them, or fruit, and several sets had concentric circles on the bottom. Joanne, who had played

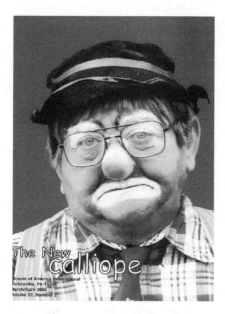

Wally, 2005 (*New Calliope* 22[2], cover)

the trombone in her high-school band, never got to do most of the traveling she wanted to, but "she loved travel and music," Chris says, "and she loved my drums. They made lots of noise." Today the hard work of making a playful spirit—of seeing humor and joy in the everyday—is found at home and at work, in the ordinary (Bender, 1996; Moore, 2002).

Clowning is a comfortable form of humor. It causes people to think about things in new ways and makes them laugh, clearing worry from their minds. There is no need to decide whether laughing is appropriate; the clowns give permission, and one just laughs, usually at them doing everyday things in an exaggerated way. The pianist sits to play and finds the seat too far away, so he pulls the seat up to the piano; the clown gets up, walks around and pushes the piano toward the seat, then walks back to sit down again. How similar that seems to some of the strategies Joanne developed to accomplish simple goals when her physical limitations interfered. Clowns help us laugh at ourselves (Ward, 1988), and Joanne did that when her failing muscles intercepted grace. Clowns are extreme, not trapped in neutral states. They just get on with solving the problem in the most absurd way possible (Ward, 1988).

Walt is known internationally in the world of clowning, and Joanne loved traveling with him to events and conventions. His tramp character, Wally, is similar to an Auguste (the colorful character with baggy trousers, painted face, and a red nose), but with a beard. The tramp is drawn to the elegance and knowing of the more priggish whiteface clown but is a figure of pathos, stirring melancholy emotions and allowing us to laugh at him as he bungles skills and reminds us of what we often take for granted (Ward, 1988). His suffering leads us to new consciousness. "It's good for your health to be a clown, you know. . . . Why do parents want their children to work in offices and not be clowns? It's all wrong" (Fellini, 1976, p. 73).

What is the *fun* of playing? Play is voluntary; like caring, it cannot be authentically compelled. Play stands outside ordinary life while being part of it. Whatever the rules of the game, they are essential (break them, and the game is over), yet the contrast between play and seriousness is always fluid (Huizinga, 1967). How like the quilt, with an intricate design yet never exact and perfect, for what in life ever is? The spirit of imagination is as present in the clown as in the quilt. Both provide a sense that life is bigger than we fully understand and remind us that we are surrounded by the mystery of unrecognized potential. To make someone laugh—I doubt anyone could hear Joanne laugh without smiling, and she laughed often and heartily—is to make a moment special, something that someone would love, as was sewing up a storm in what was known to her familiars as "the real Joanne's fabric store" and making quilts. Mairs (1994) points out that seeking other forms of expression for our deepest self is neither denial nor irresponsibility. Such immersion dissolves the usual thoughts and feelings in the endless realm of spirit and imagination as we create something new and partake in a sacred joy. When Joanne was not working, she was usually sewing.

Stacks of Fabric and the Art of Matching: Hope and Relating

We probably never appreciate the here and now until it is challenged (Lindbergh, 1955), and, however belatedly, we learn we must take care of it. Hall (2004) challenges the culture of healthcare in its counsel that ignoring the consequences of a diagnosis is denial and engaging fully with life in the face of illness creates "false hope." Humans' understandings of themselves come from society's beliefs about them (Mead, 1964). When those understandings substitute stark reality, information, and technology for hope, one is left bereft. Hope is hope, and it need not be blatantly realistic to be helpful. Hope need not be for cure; it can be for healing, a sense of well-being. When we don't fear darkness, we find treasures in that darkness (Siegel, 2004b).

Self-care is vital to our sense of ethical justice and our capacity for kindness toward others (Diller, 1999). It means learning to trust, love, and rely on ourselves and others, learning the significance of our own strength, to give all that we have, to forgive ourselves and others, and to accept meaning in our lives in whatever form it presents itself (Hall, 2004). If the self is a series of contingent, ever-changing momentary and elusive experiences, believing we still contribute, bringing care to people, and making them happy remain purposeful and meaningful.

In the barrage of self-talk that accompanies being alone with new experiences, the self is "less like an object than like a space occupied by a jostling crowd" (DuPrau, 1992, p. 68) with the singular subject of the self. Self-talk manifests and reinforces our beliefs about ourselves. If this multiplicity of internal voices is demeaning, self-regard is undermined and disrespected. If it addresses the self with respect and understanding, it can provide a receptive personal space for openness and honesty. Self-talk affects actions and decisions in the sense of self-fulfilling prophecies: when one feels useful and contributing, one *is* useful and contributing. On the other hand, self-disparaging self-talk is common, especially over issues of power (Diller, 1999); attitude can change what we do *for* someone into what we do *to* them. People presume that pain should be eliminated, most often by leaving the scene. Rarely do others maintain the closeness they had when they find out that someone is seriously ill (Hall, 2004).

To be caring in behavior we seek compassion. There is a chance that this transcendence might bring forth a consciousness rather than simple *Dasein* (Renaut, 1997). To Heidegger a transcendent imagination is necessary because, even in the dimension of spontaneity, the human mind is limited in capacity. It sketches out an image of objectivity and places it before itself in the expectation of perception. Understanding depends on imagination, which introduces a dimension of receptivity precisely where the mind is active. Respect appears to Heidegger as that moment of receptivity with regard to moral law that constitutes the practical subject by conferring upon it a dimension of openness and thus transcendence.

In many traditions respect applies to persons, not things. Although myths of early peoples suggest a divinity that can be represented in feminine as well as masculine form, patriarchy dominates in the Judeo-Christian and Islamic traditions almost to the exclusion of the feminine or any androgynous interpretation (Campbell, 1970). Heidegger (1962b) shows that dependence does not disappear; it is at the level of intuition or, perhaps, understanding and reason. Did Joanne know at some level that as a woman it is sometimes things made or done with one's own hands that bring respect? Employing a substitute to represent one's self is a form of justice. It carries a concern tied to the desire to meet people's needs (Lerner, 1980). Quilts are inherently concretely understandable, and they embody the potential to meet myriad personal needs.

Seeing the Whole Quilt: Making Sense of It All

Life is licking honey off a thorn.

Furst, 2003

What does it mean to be a person who suffers? The body grasps the world and moves with intention in that meaningful world (Merleau-Ponty, 1962). Some say suffering is valuable because we learn from it, but that suggests steady progress toward a self. Some claim a more romantic view of suffering as bringing us to our humanity (Moore, 2002). Still others explore the chakras, the gifts of the earth, survival, self-esteem, health, determination, rational thought, or higher consciousness (Myss, 2004). Rabbi Harold Kushner (1989) initially assumed that most people were going on with their lives while at any given moment a small sliver of humanity was afflicted and suffered. Instead, he has learned, there is a lot of hurting out there—multitudes of "life's lesions" (Finkler, 1994)—and that organized religion is inadequate to ease all of the pain all of the time, and even that people who try to help often make things worse. Kushner concluded that a warm hug and some patient listening mend far more hearts than platitudes. Lerner (1980) adds the caution of perspective, using the example of health professionals who don't see persons experiencing misery but only objects to be treated or cured. It is not a question of whose side God was on in the concentration camps but whom the suffering serves (Soelle, 1975). The significance of death and suffering is in learning not to fear tomorrow.

We live in a time of rebellious particularisms—ethnic, racial, political, sexual—against the totalizing ideologies that dominated preceding decades (Laclau, 1996). In healthcare, in addition to individual experience and the social symbolism of sickness, there is the body politic (Scheper-Hughes & Lock, 1987). Yet, as absolute subjectivity collapses before postmodernism, so does the possibility of an absolute object, so we live as *bricoleurs* in a plural world, making decisions within incomplete systems of rules (Laclau, 1996). No matter the philosophical turnings, however, that which is the result of the action of people can be changed. Joanne faced what we all must, in some form and at some time, and she did it with a zest for living that those involved with this memoir marvel at and admire. At the same time, we wonder what might have made things easier for Joanne, what healthcare personnel might have done differently, and how we as her friends might have diminished her suffering.

Hall (2004) frankly separates the "diagnosed" from others "not-diagnosed-yet"; "nobody is dying more than anybody else. We are all living as long as we live" (pp. 15, 20). She discusses turning fear into courage through a deep listening to the basic essentials of living, a striving to transform illness into exploration of one's strengths focused both on survival and on acquiring health. A life-threatening diagnosis lands us in a "beclouded, depressed, terrified, and uncanny" (Hall, 2004, p. 1) liminality that becomes the enemy. One goes to biomedicine to cure disease, not necessarily to seek healing or health.

"There is a great deal of suffering in life. It is unbelievable what people can endure." The words are Janet's, but others among Joanne's friends and family said similar things. Illness can bring a sense of futility, loss of control and of everything we know, and a sense of being alienated, alone inside ourselves. People respond in various ways when the body—always taken for granted—cannot be counted on to sustain life in a dependable, acceptable manner. They cope and crumble, find places of adjustment, or want to "cut, burn, or poison the part of the body that is troublesome and without another thought, keep traveling along their same path" (Hall, 2004, p. 3). Dwelling in unattached "humanness, without resorting to time-filling activity, is one of the scariest things one can imagine" (Hall, 2004, p. 5). You learn that help lies within you and all around you; wisdom, healing power, and life lessons are available. Some find these in prayer or use meditation as a way of listening to their being; some use imaging to explore their inner seeds of healing. But keeping busy is helpful only if there is personal meaning in it.

"Surviving starts out as a state of mind and a state of mental and physical readiness to live life to the fullest" (Hall, 2004, p. 9). Joanne's body did not survive, but part of her does. Survivors have a sense of meaningfulness and purpose in life (Moore, 1992). Joanne had purpose and made a difference. Her caring made a profound impact on innumerable lives: patients, family, friends, even her beloved dogs and Emmy Lou, the calico cat that still inhabits Joanne's sewing room. And for those privileged to be part of her life, her sewing and crafts left a tangible legacy of reminders and comfort, a sense of life grounded and anchored. Like her work, Joanne's sewing was a spiritual practice, and the creative person engaged in her life-enhancing work is neither exhausted nor disinterested. Creative work is play; the creator loses track of time and distress while she is wrapped up in a creative trance, and she can't be sick or in dire pain when she is so busy that she loses track of time. It is both clearing and release—that nearness that gathers everything (Heidegger, 1927/1962a, 1977). Everyone needs a special corner of the universe where she can take time for herself and let the waves of life flow through her (Siegel, 2004a). I treasure imagining Joanne in "the real Joanne's fabric store," accessible to her with her chairlift, allowing temporality to claim her (Diekelmann, 2005) as she sewed away "with Neil Diamond cranked up high." It was both Joanne's caring for herself and her being with others in the making of quilts that would stand in for her when she was no longer physically present, creating a provenance of meaning that is "never other than *we*" (Nancy, 2000, p. 27). Perhaps Joanne's greatest legacy was her sheer humanness, her not being all that different from the rest of us. She leaves a legacy that assures us that, since she did it, we have at least a model to consider.

Quilts stand on their own, much like van Gogh's painting of "a pair of peasant shoes and nothing more" (Heidegger, 1977, p. 157), while speaking with a clarity etched by experience itself. During her last several years Joanne signed her e-mails to me "Namasté" ("the divine in me honors the divine in you"). No one I asked knew why she used that salutation, but it was typical of her subtlety. Joanne captured her spirit in her art, just as Aphrodite is said to have stirred a statue to life by placing a butterfly on it. Where that spirit is present, life goes on. There are many caring arts: the pragmatic—getting down to sitting level to converse eye to eye with someone in a wheelchair; the considerate—not asking questions more personal than you would be comfortable answering yourself; the empathetic—not offering pity. People are not taught how to find happiness; with positive messages so rare, they are taught to drift into doubt, guilt, blame, or shame. "Encouragement [is] the helium of life" (Siegel, 1998, p. 26). Joanne, as much a giver as a doer, set out to make the lives of those around her different from the one she grew up with.

How might intervention in Joanne's journey have made a difference? If Joanne had made her self-talk about her relationship with polymyositis or disability better known, others could have responded with language that was caring, cooperative, respectful, and honest. Would that have helped? Caring listening means starting where the other is, respecting that, and then moving on. Healthcare, traditionally a function of the family, is being reclaimed by many people who operate out of paradigms different from those generally espoused by health professionals (McGuire,

1988). The current resurgence of interest in and popularity of alternative and complementary approaches to healing suggests a cultural shift in underlying beliefs about health and healing in the United States (Engebretson, 1994). Some of Joanne's friends doubt that Joanne had great faith in biomedicine, but she was not seriously into alternative approaches either. Joanne dabbled in complementary remedies such as aromatherapy because they made her feel good; they were healing and pleasurable, not curative.

Joanne and her friends, as experienced nurses, were and are not without doubts about the allopathic biomedical paradigm. They know that even "side effects" can be lethal, as ultimately occurred in Joanne's case. On the other hand, while "alternative medicines are time-proven," as Marie put it, the culture of science inhibits their utilization. When "you use biomedicine and you feel better than you did, you invest physically, psychologically, and financially in it." Joanne was prescribed huge doses of pharmaceuticals; she had great difficulty dealing with them both physically and intellectually—but she complied.

Joanne was a nurse, and "[n]ursing is a noble profession but too often a terrible job" (Chambliss, 1996, p. 1). The moral commitment to the welfare of the "whole person" gets buried under medical directives and financial and administrative imperatives. As Marie pointed out, "You have to trust somebody, but you are confused and desperate. Collaboration sounds so ideal, but no one really shares whatever it is you are going through." Nursing is in the throes of a paradigm shift, but nurses question whether the profession has the courage to make the change toward a caring paradigm involving the whole human being—one of body, mind, and spirit—with dignity, which for nurses often involves sharing the suffering of others (Eriksson, 1994).

Being Sewn as a Quilt: About Being Human

When the joints ache
When the hips break
When the eyes grow dim
Then I remember the great life I've had
And then I don't feel so bad.

Julie Andrews[5]

Walt still sometimes hears Joanne call from the other end of the house when no one is there, especially when he can't find something and

she would have told him where it was—"probably in no uncertain terms."
Joanne's friends think that Walt was so involved in Joanne's physical care
that losing her "may have been even harder for him than it would be for
someone to lose a spouse who was not so wholly dependent upon him for
actual personal care." Joanne loved the beach and the ocean. Joanne's
"men" and some of her friends tell stories about being there with her.
They would go way out on the sand with Joanne in a chair with big wheels
and sit there talking, "solving the problems of the world." Sometimes
they had to solicit help to move Joanne's chair through the sand.

It was Joanne's choice that her cremains be set into a memorial reef.
These foundations for coral reefs are "environmentally positive alternatives to cremation ash scattering" and involve "mixing a loved one's cre-
mated remains into liquid concrete to form a designed reef module."[6]
Walt, Skip, and Chris journeyed to Florida for the casting. Walt wrote:

The ashes of each [person] were placed in a bucket and stirred into a watery solution that included a substance that promotes fauna growth. Then came the
concrete from a truck into a metal mold that, when finished, will weigh close to
350 lbs. We watched the ashes being put into the buckets and noticed that all had
a little dust flying around EXCEPT you know who, who came out of the pouch in
a large lump. Chris said MOM had to have it her way. Probably true. After pour-
ing [the ashes] into the mold we were allowed to put our finger prints into the
soft concrete and Skip wrote MOM. When we looked at it upside down, it said
WOW. Had to come from her.

Being human refers to the existence of certain rhythms and limits to
experience (birth, life-cycle change, moral development, death, bereavement), while the intersubjective experience of suffering is a shared and
defining characteristic of humans in all societies (Kleinman, 1995). There
are contingent forms of suffering, such as acute serious illness, and rou-
tinized forms, such as chronic illness or experiences of deprivation or
oppression. There is suffering resulting from extreme conditions (e.g.,
surviving trauma) and cultural meanings (punishment or salvation). A
phenomenological approach to suffering asks us to sacrifice our hubris
and adopt an attitude of humanity, becoming acquainted with the world
around us and giving up anxieties for living with greater regard for community and the natural world (Moore, 2002). Suffering teaches us to depend on each other and to connect with the world. "Joanne always valued
time with people," Carol says, but after the diagnosis of polymyositis those
relationships became even more valuable to her. Even seven-year-old

Devon, the youngest of Joanne and Walt's grandsons, says, "She was always busy, but she always had time to play with you." She simply worked around the disease and through it; relationships were sacrosanct.

Suffering is the human condition; honoring the humanity of others involves a willingness to consider their meanings of suffering. It is through suffering that crucial differences among humans are articulated, and the experiences of suffering of some can be put to good use by others. Our experiences are so completely integrated that the self is constituted of visceral processes as much as expressed through them (Kleinman, 1995). Suffering is an equalizer in the human ability to benefit others with experiences. How we represent suffering and learn from it also leads to commodifying it. The human appetite for experiencing anguish poetically and vicariously can cause us to pay too little attention to other ways of understanding.

Human beings find their plans and actions resisted by various aspects of the life course, social relations, and biophysical process. From those forms of resistance emerge what is shared in our human condition: loss, oppression, pain, and suffering. Human conditions are also shaped by responses to the forms of resistance: grief, rage, fear, humiliation, and transcendent responses, such as endurance, aspiration, humor, and irony (Scheler, 1971). These are elaborated by systems of meaning and individual inclination so that human conditions contain great divergence (Kleinman, 1995). For most people, in Marie's words, being human means that

you just don't know where it's going to go, what's going to happen. You have a great family, a great husband, a great life—and suddenly you are frail. . . . It's overwhelming, but you also change over time, slowly and subtly; it's not like a sudden, catastrophic accident. The changes lure you into dealing with the increments. You make adjustments, you push aside the big picture.

In the past people spent the best times of their lives telling each other stories because they helped make experiences more meaningful. Ours is also a time in which relating personal narrative can be healing and therapeutic (Atkinson, 1995). Stories about family members carry important messages that give a family definition and provide it with esteem and ideals to live up to. As adults, most of our growth is psychospiritual; when we deal with experiences of intimacy and creativity, life crises and peak experiences, we become more fully conscious of our lives. Thus story is a tool toward wholeness, for gathering parts and putting them together, quiltlike, makes meaning. Making our stories sacred means consciously acknowledging the experience of personal suffering, experiencing symbolic death, attaining greater inner freedom, and entering into a sort of rebirth (Atkinson, 1995). Stories are rites of passage even when they are part myth, for "[w]here we had thought to travel outward, we shall come to the center of our own existence; where we had thought to be alone, we shall be with all the world" (Campbell, 1949, p. 25). I began this inquiry wanting to know how someone bears suffering, uncertainty, and living with a severely compromised existence. Asked what Joanne taught them about suffering and being human, her friends and family offered, "You could see in her eyes the joy she felt when she laughed and you laughed with her" and "She taught us to laugh to work through adversity." Joanne was both "the consummate nurse" and "a glass-half-full person; if there was a bright side, she would find it." "She taught us how to give of yourself—that we have more to give than we think we do, and you have only yourself to give. It is about sharing your being." Crafting neither travel guide for still unknown territory nor fairy tales about releasing spirit, our job is not to look for the end but to see the end (Moore, 2002).

Notes

1. Joanne's diaries are designated in this manuscript simply as [Diary 1] and [Diary 2]. All underlining, boldface, and capitalization are in the original.

2. Suffering is a phenomenon that affects the whole person; an individual experiences suffering when the meaning of pain, loss, or distress is a threat to the self (Kahn & Steeves, 1986).

3. I thank Clayton Cieslak; Marie Cooley; Carol Curran; Mary Kellogg; Karen Kleeman; Millie Krainski; Chris, Kathleen, Kristen, Skip, and Walt Lee (as well as grandsons Brendon, Connor, and Devon Lee); Ski Lower; and Janet Rogers for the many hours of conversation we spent together in this inquiry. My greatest gratitude goes to Joanne Lee, who even in her absence nurtures my own understanding and creativity. I also thank the "Writing Women" at Mount Saint Agnes Theological Center for Women (Baltimore, MD) and in particular Diane Caplin, PhD, and Irene Morin for their encouragement and critique.

4. The sources for the biomedical information in this section include the Web sites listed in the cited references, all retrieved on May 15, 2005. Additionally, see Dalakas & Hohlfeld (2003); Masteglia, Phillipos, & Zilko (1997); and Plotz (1995).

5. To commemorate her 69th birthday actress/vocalist Julie Andrews performed at Manhattan's Radio City Music Hall to benefit the AARP. One of her musical numbers was "My Favorite Things" from the movie *The Sound of Music* with the lyrics changed for her older audience.

6. These quotations are from the company's information packet: Eternal Reefs, Inc., P.O. Box 2473, Decatur, GA, 30031.

References

Albrecht, G. L., & Verbrugge, L. M. (2000). The global emergence of disability. In G. L. Albrecht, K. Fitzpatrick, & S. C. Scrimshaw (Eds.), *Handbook of social studies in health and medicine* (pp. 293–307). Thousand Oaks, CA: Sage.

Arendt, H. (1959). *The human condition.* Garden City, NJ: Doubleday.

Arendt, H. (1977). *On revolution.* New York: Penguin.

Atkinson, R. (1995). *The gift of stories: Practical and spiritual applications of autobiography, life stories, and personal mythmaking.* Westport, CT: Bergin & Garvey.

Bachelard, G. (1969). *The poetics of space* (M. Joles, Trans.). Boston: Beacon Press.

Bateson, M. C. (1990). *Composing a life: Life as a work in progress — the improvisations of five extraordinary women.* New York: Penguin.

Baylor College of Medicine. (2005, January 28). Polymyositis. Retrieved May 15, 2005, from http://www.bcm.edu/neurology/research/nmus/nmus3a1.html

Bellah, R., Madsen, R., Sullivan, W., Swindler, A., & Tipton, S. (1985). *Habits of the heart: Individualism and commitment in American life.* Berkeley: University of California Press.

Bender, S. (1996). *Everyday sacred: A woman's journey home.* San Francisco: HarperSanFrancisco.

Better Health Channel. (2003, September 15). Polymyositis. Retrieved May 15, 2005, from http://www.betterhealth.vic.gov.au/bhcv2/bhcarticles.nsf/pages/polymyositis

Book of common prayer. (1928 version). New York: T. Cranmer.

Borland, K. (1991). "That's not what I said": Interpretive conflict in oral narrative research. In S. B. Gluck & D. Patai (Eds.), *Women's words, women's words, women's words: The feminist practice of oral history* (pp. 63–75). New York: Routledge.

Buber, M. (1958). *I and thou* (2nd ed., R. G. Smith, Trans.). New York: Scribner.

Campbell, J. (1949). *The hero with a thousand faces.* Princeton, NJ: Princeton University Press.

Campbell, J. (1970). *The masks of god, Vol. 4: Creative mythology and Occidental mythology.* New York: Viking Press.

Cancian, F. M. (1985). Gender politics: Love and power in the private and public spheres. In A. S. Rossi (Ed.), *Gender and the life course* (pp. 253–264). New York: Aldine.

Cassell, E. J. (1991a). *The nature of suffering and the goals of medicine.* New York: Oxford University Press.

Cassell, E. J. (1991b, May–June). Recognizing suffering. *Hastings Center Report,* 24–31.

Chambliss, D. F. (1996). *Beyond caring: Hospitals, nurses, and the social organization of ethics.* Chicago: University of Chicago Press.

Croce, A. (1994, December 26). Discussing the undiscussable. *New Yorker,* p. 54.

Cruikshank, J. (1992). *Life lived like a story: Life stories of three Yukon Native elders.* Lincoln: University of Nebraska Press.

Dalakas, M. C., & Hohlfeld, R. (2003, September 20). Polymyositis and dermatomyositis. *Lancet, 362*(9388), 971–982.

Davis, A. J. (1981). Compassion, suffering, morality: Ethical dilemmas in caring. *Nursing Law & Ethics, 2*(5), 1–2, 6, 8.

Detrixhe, S. (2004). *Zen and the art of quilting: Exploring memory and meaning in patchwork.* Avon, MA: Adams Media.

Diekelmann, J. (2005). The retrieval of method: The method of retrieval. In P. M. Ironside (Ed.), *Beyond method: Philosophical conversations in healthcare research and scholarship* (pp. 3–57). Madison: University of Wisconsin Press.

Diekelmann, N. (1991). The emancipatory power of the narrative. In *Curriculum revolution: Community building and activism* (pp. 41–62). New York: National League for Nursing.

Diller, A. (1999). The ethical education of self-talk. In M. S. Katz, N. Noddings, & K. A. Strike (Eds.), *Justice and caring: The search for common ground in education* (pp. 74–92). New York: Teachers College Press.

DuPrau, J. (1992). *The earth house.* New York: Penguin.

Engebretson, J. C. (1994). Voices of healing: Elements of caring. In D. A. Gaut & A. Boykin (Eds.), *Caring as healing: Renewal through hope* (pp. 38–47). New York: National League for Nursing.

Eriksson, K. (1994). Theories of caring as health. In D. A. Gaut & A. Boykin (Eds.), *Caring as healing: Renewal through hope* (pp. 3–20). New York: National League for Nursing.

Fellini, F. (1976). *Fellini on Fellini* (I. Quiqley, Trans.). New York: Delacoste Press.

Finkler, K. (1994). *Women in pain: Gender and morbidity in Mexico.* Philadelphia: University of Pennsylvania Press.

Frank, G. (2000). *Venus on wheels: Two decades of dialogue on disability, biography, and being female in America.* Berkeley: University of California Press.

Furst, A. (2003). *Kingdom of shadows* [cassette recording]. Recorded Books.

Hall, B. A. (2004). *Surviving and thriving after a life threatening diagnosis.* Bloomington, IN: First Books Library.

Hampl, P. (1999). *I could tell you stories.* New York: Norton.

Hauerwas, S. (1979). Reflections on suffering, death, and medicine. *Social Science & Medicine, 6,* 229–237.

Heidegger, M. (1962a). *Being and time* (J. Macquarrie & E. Robinson, Trans.). New York: Harper & Row. (Original work published 1927)

Heidegger, M. (1962b). *Kant and the problem of metaphysics* (M. Heim, Trans.). Bloomington: Indiana University Press.

Heidegger, M. (1968). *What is called thinking?* (F. D. Wieck & J. C. Gray, Trans.). New York: Harper & Row.

Heidegger, M. (1977). *Basic writings* (D. F. Krell, Ed.). New York: Harper & Row.

Heidegger, M. (2001). *Zollikon seminars* (F. Mays & R. Askay, Trans.). Evanston, IL: Northwestern University Press.

Heilbrun, C. G. (1988). *Writing a woman's life.* New York: Norton.

Heilbrun, C. G. (1993). *Toward a recognition of androgyny.* New York: Norton.

Huizinga, J. (1967). *Homo ludens: A study of the play element in culture.* Boston: Beacon Press.

James, A., Hockey, J., & Dawson, A. (1997). Introduction: The road from Santa Fe. In A. James, J. Hockey, & A. Dawson (Eds.), *After writing culture: Epistemology and praxis in contemporary anthropology* (pp. 1–15). New York: Routledge.

Jung, C. G. (1977). *C. G. Jung speaking* (W. McGuire & R. F. C. Hull, Eds.). Bollingen Series XCVII. Princeton, NJ: Princeton University Press.

Kahn, D. L., & Steeves, R. H. (1986). The experience of suffering: Conceptual clarification and theoretical definition. *Journal of Advanced Nursing, 11,* 623–631.

Kaufmann, S. R. (1988). Toward a phenomenology of boundaries in medicine: Chronic illness experience in the case of stroke. *Medical Anthropology Quarterly, 2,* 338–354.

Kavanagh, K. H. (1989). Nurses' networks: Obstacles and challenge. *Archives of Psychiatric Nursing, 3*(4), 226–233.

Kavanagh, K. H. (2002). Neither here nor there: The story of health professionals' experience with getting care and needing caring. In N. L. Diekelmann (Ed.), *First do no harm: Power, oppression, and violence in healthcare* (pp. 49–117). Madison: University of Wisconsin Press.

Kavanagh, K. H. (2003). Mirrors: A cultural and historical interpretation of nursing's pedagogies. In N. L. Diekelmann (Ed.), *Teaching the practitioners of care: New pedagogies for the health professions* (pp. 59–153). Madison: University of Wisconsin Press.

Kavanagh, K. H. (2005). Representing: Interpretive scholarship's consummate challenge. In P. M. Ironside (Ed.), *Beyond method: Philosophical conversations in healthcare research and scholarship* (pp. 58–110). Madison: University of Wisconsin Press.

Kleinman, A. (1988). *The illness narratives: Suffering, healing, and the human condition.* New York: Basic Books.

Kleinman, A. (1995). *Writing at the margin: Discourse between anthropology and medicine.* Berkeley: University of California Press.

Kulick, D., & Meneley, A. (2005). *Fat: The anthropology of an obsession.* New York: Jeremy P. Tarcher/Penguin.

Kushner, H. S. (1989). *When bad things happen to good people.* New York: Schocken Books.

Laclau, E. (1996). *Emancipation(s).* London: Verso.

Lerner, M. J. (1980). *Belief in a just world: A fundamental delusion.* New York: Plenum Press.

Levitt, P. (2003). *Fingerpainting on the moon: Writing and creativity as a path to freedom.* New York: Harmony Books.

Lindbergh, A. M. (1955). *Gift from the sea.* New York: Pantheon.

Mairs, N. (1993). *Ordinary time: Cycles in marriage, faith, and renewal.* Boston: Beacon Press.

Mairs, N. (1994). *Voice lessons: On becoming a (woman) writer.* Boston: Beacon Press.

Mairs, N. (1996). *Waist-high in the world: A life among the non-disabled.* Boston: Beacon Press.

Masteglia, F. L., Phillipos, B. A., & Zilko, P. (1997, June). Treatment of inflammatory myopathies. *Muscle & Nerve, 20,* 651–657.

Mayo Foundation for Medical Education and Research. (2005, July 14). Polymyositis. Retrieved May 15, 2005, from http://www.cnn.com/HEALTH/library/DS/00334.html

McGuire, M. B. (1988). *Ritual healing in suburban America: Sociological research.* New Brunswick, NJ: Rutgers University Press.

Mead, G. H. (1964). *On social psychology: Selected papers.* Chicago: University of Chicago Press.

Mead, M. (1972). *Twentieth-century faith: Hope and survival.* New York: Harper & Row.

Merck & Co., Inc. (2005). Polymyositis and dermatomyositis. In *The Merck manual of diagnosis and therapy.* Retrieved May 15, 2005, from http://www.merck.com/mrk shared/mmanual/section5/chapter50/50i.jsp

Merleau-Ponty, M. (1962). *Phenomenology of perception* (C. Smith, Trans.). London: Routledge.

Metzger, D. (1992). *Writing for your life: A guide and companion to the inner worlds.* San Francisco: HarperSanFrancisco.

Moore, T. (1992). *Care of the soul.* New York: HarperCollins.

Moore, T. (2002). *The soul's religion: Cultivating a profoundly spiritual way of life.* New York: HarperCollins.

Myss, C. (2004). *Invisible acts of power: Personal choices that create miracles.* New York: Free Press.

Nancy, J.-L. (1997). *The gravity of thought* (F. Raffoul & G. Recco, Trans.). Atlantic Highlands, NJ: Humanities Press.

Nancy, J.-L. (2000). *Being singular plural* (R. D. Richardson & A. E. O'Byrne, Trans.). Stanford: Stanford University Press.

National Institute of Neurological Disorders and Stroke. (2005, February 9). NINDS Polymyositis Information Page. Retrieved May 15, 2005, from http://www.ninds.nih .gov/disorders/polymyositis/polymyositis_pr.htm

Pappu, R., & Seetharaman, M. (2005). Polymyositis. Retrieved May 15, 2005, from http://www.emedicine.com/med/topic3441.htm

Phillips, M. J. (1990). Damaged goods: Oral narratives of the experience of disability in American culture. *Social Science and Medicine, 30,* 849–857.

Plotz, P. H., et al. (1995). Myositis: Immunologic contributions to understanding cause, pathogenesis, and therapy. *Annals of Internal Medicine, 122,* 715–724.

Renaut, A. (1997). *The era of the individual: A contribution to a history of subjectivity* (M. B. DeBevoise & F. Philip, Trans.). Princeton, NJ: Princeton University Press.

Richard, I. A. (1957). The aesthetic response as an organization of attitudes. In E. V. Vivas & M. Kreiger (Eds.), *The problems of aesthetics.* New York: Rinehart.

Rollins, J. (1985). *Between women: Domestics and their employers.* Philadelphia: Temple University Press.

Scheler, M. (1971). *Man's place in nature* (H. Meyerhoff, Trans.). New York: Noonday.

Scheper-Hughes, N., & Lock, M. (1987). The mindful body: A prolegomenon to future work in medical anthropology. *Medical Anthropology Quarterly, 1*(1), 6–41.

Schwarz, M. T. (1997). *Molded in the image of Changing Woman: Navajo views on the human body and personhood.* Tucson: University of Arizona Press.

See, C. (2002). *Making a literary life: Advice for writers and other dreamers.* New York: Random House.

Siegel, B. S. (1998). *Prescriptions for living: Inspirational lessons for a joyful, loving life.* New York: HarperCollins.

Siegel, B. S. (2004a). *Meditations for difficult times* [CD]. Carlsbad, CA: Hay House.

Siegel, B. S. (2004b). *Meditations for overcoming life's stresses and strains. Stress and the inner self: Self and blood pressure* [CD]. Carlsbad, CA: Hay House.

Silko, L. M. (1981). *Storyteller.* New York: Arcade.

Soelle, D. (1975). *Suffering* (E. R. Kalin, Trans.). Philadelphia: Fortress Press.

Spelman, E. V. (1997). *Fruits of sorrow: Framing our attention to suffering.* Boston: Beacon Press.

Spitzer, D. L. (2004). In visible bodies: Minority women, nurses, times, and the new economy of care. *Medical Anthropology Quarterly, 18*(4), 490–508.

Steward, E. C., & Bennett, M. J. (1991). *American cultural patterns: A cross-cultural perspective.* Yarmouth, ME: Intercultural Press.

Tedlock, B. (2000). Ethnography and ethnographic representation. In N. K. Denzin & Y. S. Lincoln (Eds.), *Handbook of qualitative research* (2nd ed., pp. 455–486). Thousand Oaks, CA: Sage.

Teitel, A. D. (2005, October 13). Polymyositis—adult. In *MedlinePlus medical encyclopedia.* Retrieved May 15, 2005, from http://www.nlm.nih.gov/medlineplus/ency/article/000428.htm

Thurman, J. (1982). *Isak Dinesen: The life of a storyteller.* New York: St. Martin's Press.

Verbrugge, L. M. (1990). Pathways of health and death. In R. D. Apple (Ed.), *Women, health, and medicine in America: A historical handbook* (pp. 41–79). New York: Garland.

Wallman, S. (1997). Appropriate anthropology and the risky inspiration of "Capability" Brown: Representations of what, by whom, and to what end? In A. James, J. Hockey, & A. Dawson (Eds.), *After writing culture: Epistemology and praxis in contemporary anthropology* (pp. 244–263). New York: Routledge.

Ward, R. (1988). The importance of being foolish. In J. Durant & J. Miller (Eds.), *Laughing matters: A serious look at humour* (pp. 109–120). New York: John Wiley & Sons.

Waters, F. (1969). *Book of the Hopi.* New York: Ballantine.

Watson, J. (1988). *Nursing: Human science and human care: A theory of nursing.* Norwalk, CT: Appleton-Century-Crofts.

Wuthnow, R. (1991). *Acts of compassion: Caring for others and helping ourselves.* Princeton, NJ: Princeton University Press.

Younger, J. B. (1995). The alienation of the sufferer. *Advances in Nursing Science, 17*(4), 53–72.

Zinsser, W. (2004). *Writing about your life: A journey into the past.* New York: Marlowe.

2

The Gift of Suffering

INGRID HARRIS

What really raises one's indignation against suffering is not suffering intrinsically, but the senselessness of suffering.

Nietzsche, n.d.

In this paper I aim to focus attention on suffering in a way that seeks to be useful to the healthcare professional. I argue that suffering is a gift to both sufferer and healer and that the way the gift becomes present to them is through their interaction in what well-known phenomenologist Calvin Schrag calls a "fitting response" to the call of the other in the visage of the neighbor.

Lorraine M. Wright (2005) argues that suffering is at the heart of nursing. She maintains that although reducing or diminishing suffering is the essence of nursing clinical practice, there still exists a lack of attention to suffering by the healthcare professional and the healthcare delivery system. About eight years earlier, Ira R. Byock, hospice medical director of Partners in Home Care in Missoula, Montana, and chair of the Academy of Hospice Physicians Ethics Committee, expressed concern about the lack of material available on the topic of suffering for geriatric medicine in particular and for medicine in general. He observed that most physicians get no formal education in the phenomenology of human suffering and very little training regarding the terminal phase of illness. Empirical experience, he argued, typically accumulates during practice, when opportunities for formal study and thoughtful reflection are scarce. Meanwhile, education remains focused on cure, life prolongation, and restoration of function, which, while important, do not address the relief of suffering.

Despite voiced acceptance of "whole person care," Byock argues, the Cartesian separation of mind and body continues to dominate clinical training. Suffering affects not just the body but the mind and the spirit as well. How each of these dimensions is treated in a clinical setting has far-reaching repercussions for patient and healer alike. At the time when Byock was writing, suffering was understood mostly in terms of physical pain, and training in the theory and practice of controlling pain and other sources of distress remained absent from general medical and nursing curricula. The coming to awareness of the perceptual world was hampered by this manner of thinking. Byock (1996) suggests that for the patient to benefit optimally and for clinicians to feel confident in their care, the approach to a suffering patient must be preceded by thoughtful preparation. This is more and more often the way that healthcare professionals are proceeding today, and much literature is now available on the topic of suffering.

Suffering is universal, and it is something we talk and write about at length and often. According to recent work of Black and Rubenstein (2004), the definition of suffering is connected to the culture in which it is defined, to the ethos of the society, and to the way an individual communicates suffering within that society. They argue that suffering is a form of social communication. As a lived experience, suffering is laden with social connotations and marked by symbols that are recognized and shared throughout the culture. Black and Rubenstein (2004) apply this to discussing the themes of suffering that they discovered in elderly patients. They found that collective interpretations of suffering create its value as well as a rejection of its value—acceptable, unacceptable, a cultural exemplar, or even an "outrage" in a given society.

Following Heidegger's understanding of the meaning and truth of being as an ever-coming-to-presence, Schrag (2002) takes up the appeal to responsibility, where we find ourselves "thrust into another space, a space of an 'ethic,' or more precisely a 'protoethic,' that is in some manner otherwise than Being" (p. 78). For Schrag, ethics is prior to ontology. Before being, the call to the ethical is the call to responsibility (Schrag, 2002). This of course implies that the ethical quality (responsibility) of the multifaceted relationship between people is a determinant of the sort of outcome (being) that might be anticipated. This relationship is largely language based, but obviously the physical dimension of caring plays a feature role as well.

What Is Suffering?

We all know what suffering is—no human life is without suffering of some kind. When we try to define it, however, as with many philosophical enquiries, just what suffering is becomes unclear. What is clear is that, whatever suffering is, it has several dimensions. These dimensional threads that make up the experience of suffering are not entirely separated but rather are interwoven with each other.[1] Grief, for example, not only has spiritual, emotional, and psychological dimensions but can also be felt physically as a suffocating, stomach-wrenching sickness of heart. In fact, the question of suffering is primarily a question about pain of a spiritual nature and only secondarily about physical pain. This is not to downplay the significance of physical pain, for there may be no suffering that does not have a physical dimension. Moral suffering has a physical, or somatic, element that is often reflected in the state of the entire organism. As Dorothee Soelle (1975) notes, "The word suffering expresses first the duration and intensity of a pain, and then the multidimensionality that roots the suffering in the physical and social sphere" (p. 16). The "social sphere" means that suffering is always an interdependent phenomenon. Suffering has an ineradicable social dimension that is experienced not only physically but also morally.

The forms of moral suffering are more varied than the forms of physical suffering. Unfortunately, the varieties of moral suffering seem less identified and less reachable by therapy as it now stands than do the forms of physical suffering. Some types of moral suffering lie hidden within actions abhorrent to society. W. H. J. Martens, director of the W. Kahn Institute of Theoretical Psychiatry and Neuroscience and advisor of the Forensic Psychiatry Hospital in the Netherlands, for example, has recently stressed the extreme importance of recognizing hidden suffering, loneliness, and lack of self-esteem as risk factors for violent criminal behavior in psychopaths. He argues that the current picture of the psychopath is incomplete when emotional suffering and loneliness are ignored. Suffering lies at the root of antisocial behavior in such cases and plays its role in less extreme cases as well. When these aspects are taken into consideration, our idea of the psychopath reaches beyond the heartless and sees him or her as more human (Martens, 2002). This gives us hope that we may yet find ways to prevent and mitigate the sort of suffering that manifests itself in such horrific actions.

Suffering is unavoidable. It brings us face to face with the fact that we are not in control of very much at all. At various times most of us have something painful, distressing, or injurious imposed upon us, for example, grief, judgment, disaster, hardship, sorrow, care, wrong, injury, loss, shame, guilt, disgrace—or illness. We use *suffering* to talk about our psychological, emotional, social, and spiritual distress as well as about the world-destroying capacity of physical pain. Elaine Scarry (1985) discusses in great detail how suffering breaks down the world of the sufferer by disconnecting the sufferer from everything except the pain, especially in extreme cases.

Suffering may be defined as having to endure, undergo, or submit to an evil of some sort, for example, banishment or widowhood. Suffering evokes compassion and respect for someone who bears it with dignity— and it intimidates as well. At the center of suffering "there is always an experience of evil, which causes the individual to suffer. . . . Man suffers on account of evil, which is a certain lack, limitation or distortion of good" (John Paul II, 1984, II:7). Martens's example of the psychopath illustrates how what is good can get distorted into what we call evil. Perhaps it is this sense of evil that gives us a clue as to why no way of dealing with suffering can be effective without involving a faith of some kind. I suggest that this sense of evil, from a phenomenological point of view, is a shutting down of possible ways of being in the world, an emptying, a loss of something valuable to human life.

The sense of evil, or of something being "not right," awry, or terribly wrong, in suffering is universal; why else would everything that is sentient attempt to avoid suffering? Which particular beliefs are at issue, whether religious or nonreligious, is not the point. This is not an argument in support of some religious perspective on suffering as "the answer." Mainly, religious language assists in the discourse that the individual carries on with herself and with others. The metaphors of religion provide individuals with a vocabulary to express their suffering and to find meaning therein.[2] A particular set of beliefs gives the individual a framework within which to articulate the nature of her suffering and to make sense of it. Wright (2005) writes: "[F]indings across studies demonstrate the possible influence of spiritual and religious dimensions of life for health and well-being in the context of serious illness" (p. 82).[3]

In this paper what is important is the universal or what we shall, following Schrag (2002, p.40), call "transversal"—meaning(s) that a belief structure contributes to help us deal with suffering. Although spiritual and religious dimensions influence the course of healing, this is not to say that certain particular dogmas or rites add anything to the completeness and depth of the reality of suffering expressed (see Soelle, 1975, p. 76). The point is that, at the very least, faith of one sort or another is required even to bring suffering to expression. This is first of all a point about communication, whether with oneself or with another.

Jacques Derrida has pointed out that a fundamental faith is required in the very act of speaking or listening, a faith that transcends any given religion. One cannot address the other, speak to the other, without an act of faith. When I address the other I request that the other believe me. Even when lying we are addressing the other and asking for her trust, his belief that we are telling the truth.

This "Trust me, I am speaking to you" is of the order of faith, a faith that cannot be reduced to a theoretical statement, to a determinative judgment; it is the opening of the address to the other. So this faith is not religious, strictly speaking; at least, it cannot be totally determined by a given religion (as cited in Caputo, 2004, p. 216). Faith is an opening up to the world, an invitation to the other to enter into being with us, to create new ways of being in the world. No single belief system—all views to the contrary notwithstanding—can provide us with *the* total and definitively final answer to the mystery of human suffering.

Methodology

Suffering has not come to our attention in this way previously because, as Byock points out, it was hampered by the prejudices arising from objectivist thinking. It is outside the scope of this paper to articulate in detail the philosophical principles that are nonetheless presupposed by the approach taken here. The interested practitioner would benefit from reading G. B. Madison's "On Suffering" (2005), which pursues a radical enquiry into the meaning of suffering in human life as opposed to taking the standard technocratic approach to the question. He argues that understanding some basic philosophical principles is prerequisite to a satisfactory understanding of suffering and hence to a satisfactory manner of dealing with it in oneself as well as in others.

Madison also undertakes a critique of the mechanistic–materialist approach to human life because it can find no meaning in suffering. It treats suffering only as something to be cured of as opposed to something to be learned from, leaving one living much like a machine that needs repairs and, when finally irreparable, simply gets thrown on the junk heap (or into the recycling system). Madison suggests that, overall, science has a rather tragic view of human life. All is destined eventually to come to naught, and there is nothing in the universe of science that suggests any purpose for humanity. From a reductionist perspective—the scientific way of proceeding as a matter of fact—the whole cosmic drama is, in the final analysis, futile and devoid of meaning. Madison (2005) writes:

[A]ny thoroughgoing or radical (in the etymological sense of the word) critique of the modern technocratic mindset must also, at some point, seek to get at its root causes and must seek, not just to rectify this or that aspect of it, but must attempt also to call into question its underlying presuppositions, for it is a basic fact in human affairs that bad theories (and the unwholesome practices they promote) can ultimately be countered only by means of better theories or ways of viewing things. (p. 2)

The basic question that needs to be addressed in Madison's view is, "What does it mean to be human?" He devotes an entire chapter to the implications that philosophical principles and arguments against the mechanistic approach have for healthcare practitioners in particular. His own critique of technoscientism is set within a wider historical–cultural–philosophical context. He reflects on a number of fundamental issues whose relevance to the topic of suffering, although perhaps not at first evident, is nevertheless of crucial importance for achieving a proper understanding of what it means to be human and thus for dealing with suffering in an appropriately humane way, in accordance with the principles of humanness.

Madison argues that the essential restorative function of the art of medicine is today being eclipsed by the science-inspired view of medicine as "disease theory." He argues against three intertwined and mutually reinforcing trends: the medicalization of life, the industrialization of healthcare, and the politicization of medicine, which jointly promote a "disease-centric" view of medicine while at the same time corroding the theory and practice of medicine. Madison does not oppose *healthcare* to *medicine,* because the distinction is redolent of the old mind–body dualism, but uses the terms in a generally interchangeable fashion. In opposing healthcare to medicine nurses are reacting to what he maintains is in fact an inappropriate understanding of medicine to begin with.

All of these considerations are crucially important because suffering crosses the boundary between body as subject and body as object, and it crosses dimensions between mind and body, soul and spirit. Hence, in sum, a purely rationalistic or scientistic (objects in *partes extra partes* relationships) vocabulary is inadequate to our aims in this enquiry, as is obviously a purely intellectualist or subjectivistic vocabulary.

In this paper I depart from the position on first-person knowledge defended by Jack Petranker (2003). Petranker, following Maurice Merleau-Ponty, Michael Polanyi, William James, Edmund Husserl, Martin Heidegger, and Tarthang Tulku, provides important resources for first-person knowledge that may be useful to the health practitioner using the intersubjective approach to suffering and healing. I make use of one of Petranker's methodologies in discussing various belief systems, namely, that of switching back and forth between stories—seeing what happens when we inhabit one, then another. I then seek commonalities, the common ground of transversality from one story to the next.

An existential–phenomenological–hermeneutical approach to considering the concept of the "gift" in association with that of suffering and the closely associated notion of forgiveness guides the overall investigation. The notion of the gift has come under considerable scrutiny. Views as to its nature differ radically between extremes such as those that make the gift ultimately impossible (e.g., by authors such as Jacques Derrida and Emmanuel Levinas) and that of the gift as a coming to presence in everyday affairs (of the kingdom of God) (Schrag, 2002).[4]

The focus in this paper is on first-person knowledge. First-person knowledge focuses on the individual. Scarry (1985) warns us that to bypass the voice of the individual is to bypass the bodily event, the patient, and the person in pain. The first-person knowledge of intense suffering isolates us from others. The healer cannot feel the pain that makes life hell for the one who suffers. As isolated as he is in his pain, however, the individual cannot be healed in isolation from others.

On the one hand, isolation is part of the pain of suffering. Healing, on the other hand, is an intersubjective activity in which sufferer and healer work together to bring the pain to expression as part of the healing process. In this approach we are collaborators with each other in consummate reciprocity. According to Merleau-Ponty (1992), our perspectives merge into each other, and we coexist through a common world. The terms of expression may serve as well to ground sufferer, healer, and others in our common humanity—or not. When compassion, concern, or understanding is lacking, the expression of suffering can serve to isolate us even further from each other. I suggest that this isolation results from a shutting down of certain important ways of human being in the world (see Merleau-Ponty, 1992, p. 142).

My investigation attempts to increase our understanding of the structures and dynamics of suffering with regard to how those structures and processes can be transformed (i.e., opened up) by compassion and forgiveness. I deploy a phenomenological paradigm of causality that crosses over from the language of the subject and the lived body to the language of the object and the body as object and back again, just as we do in everyday life.[5]

Moral Suffering

One significant and common form of moral suffering is loss of dignity. Dignity requires that at least two people play their parts well, and the number of those involved expands, as a third party is required to evaluate the second person's attribution of the first person's dignity. For instance, too often with disabled people caregivers address questions to their companions and refer to the disabled in the third person: "Where would she like to sit?" Here there is no dialogue with the sufferer. As Merleau-Ponty (1992) writes, the other's gaze transforms me into an object if I am observed as if I am an insect. The objectification by the other's gaze is felt as unbearable because it takes the place of possible communication.

Disabled people can suffer a shutting down of perhaps the most important way for humans to be in the world, that of interacting as an I with another I. This happens when they are treated in this instance as an object rather than as a subject, with the result that they can become isolated by and from the very enquiry that could bring them into a space of caring. They are further alienated in their suffering. Such treatment is demeaning and reinforces the perception that disability reduces personal and social worth (Toombs, 2004). In this situation the caregiver does not play his or her part well, does not manifest a "fitting response" (more about that later) to the given situation.

Arthur W. Frank (2004) writes that care that takes dignity seriously is a dialogue. The dialogue that conveys dignity is an intersubjective relationship rather than something that inheres in individuals taken as having a separate existence. It makes an appearance between subjects, involving both sufferer and witness together. Dignity can also be seen to be a result of the individual's way of acting (see Radley, 2004). It is, from one point of view, a subjective experience brought about by the action upon oneself of the objective world of the other. A loss of dignity brings about a closing down of a way of being that becomes a vicious circle—comprising loss of dignity, further suffering, and an increase in pity from others—out of which sufferers feel the need to break free. One way this break can be achieved is through sufferers (subjectively) reclaiming their subjectivity by exposing the objectivity of their suffering in a way that shows others how they live with illness—an action that can give rise to (subjective) respect on the part of others for those who suffer. As we can see, this interplay of the subjective and objective sides of experience is constantly involved in everyday activity; this example illustrates the intersubjectivity of everyday dialogue and action. It also begins to give us a clue as to how, when sufferer and healer interact in a manner that illustrates a fitting response, a transformation of the worlds of both healer and sufferer can take place.

In this interaction (subjective) pity is not simply supplanted by (subjective and objective) dignity but transformed by it (see Radley, 2004). Even by, at the very least, talking about occasions or states of indignity, sufferers can demonstrate how they have overcome these and can regain or maintain their dignity. In all cases, bringing pain (subjective) to expression (objective) is an activity that opens up possibilities for finding meaning for that suffering (see Toombs, 2004). When it is imbued with meaning, a new way of being emerges, and suffering becomes easier to bear. The meaning (subjective and objective) eases the (subjective) pain. Such openings up serve to bring sufferers together with each other, creating solidarity and hence diminishing alienation. This may go some way toward understanding how self-help groups work—by creating a new meaning for a shared sort of suffering, people help each other as well as themselves, reducing their alienation in the process.

The importance of seeking meaning is double-edged, since it is all too often that negative instead of positive meanings for seeking relief from suffering are taken up. Negative, destructive meanings close down our ways of being in the world. They prevent healing and distort attempts on the part of the psyche and the body to regain wholeness, resulting in, for example, the victim complex, the martyr complex (what Soelle calls Christian Masochism), along with such things as rage and murderous impulses, such as Martens observes in the psychopath. Cognitive psychology teaches that negative meanings serve to bring about depression and depression-related ailments, anxiety, and phobias. Toxic meanings, learned in childhood and formed into habitual ways of being over time, result in forms of moral suffering that are only lately being taken seriously and coming under close investigation. Various books on cognitive therapy, for example, show how toxic meanings operate and how they can be transformed.

In my investigation I attempt to identify structures or principles of meaning that transcend individual cultures and systems of thinking, that may count as causes or at least catalysts of healing. At the very least I endeavor to find reliable ways to overcome fear and to gain strength from suffering.

The Mystery of Suffering

What do mortals get from all the toil and strain with which they toil under the sun? . . . For all their days are full of pain and their work is a vexation.

Eccles. 1:3, 2:3, New English Bible, 1972

"Man [*sic*], in his suffering," is an "intangible mystery" (John Paul II, 1984, I:4). Indeed, suffering makes us a mystery to ourselves as well as to others. Extreme suffering isolates us from others and destroys our ability to communicate. Feelings for others die, and we no longer care about anyone else (Soelle, 1975). Soelle (1975) writes of existential pain that uses our own thinking and feeling against us. Our thoughts and emotions (subjective) become toxic, and our world (subjective) empties of positive meanings and fills with images and feelings of sorrow and death. In the extreme of physical pain, language is "shattered" (Scarry, 1985, p. 5). The most important way of being in the world is lost. In this breakdown of language that occurs through suffering the other becomes most alien, most irrevocably Other (Scarry, 1985, p. 6). Nancy Johnston (2003) speaks of the "turning" brought about by adversity as making the self bereft, bewildered, insubstantial, and unrecognizable.

Extreme suffering, in breaking down the most human way of being in the world, that is, language, also breaks down one's personal identity as a human being. We lose our way, losing both inner and outer points of reference, and the stories that we tell ourselves about ourselves no longer make sense to us. Scarry (1985) observes: "Physical pain is not only itself resistant to language but also actively destroys language, deconstructing it into the prelanguage of cries and groans. To hear those cries is to witness the shattering of language" (p. 172). The self itself becomes lost to us, absorbed into that bitter eternity. Scarry's view agrees with Soelle's (1975) that suffering can take away even the consciousness of the cause for which one is suffering, leaving the person an empty shell. Suffering can take away from us what it is to be human, that is, the ability to communicate with others and with ourselves.

There is yet hope. Merleau-Ponty (1992) writes:

The natural world is the horizon of all horizons, the style of all possible styles, which guarantees for my experience a given, not a willed, unity underlying all the disruptions of my personal and historical life. Its counterpart within me is the given, general and pre-personal existence of my sensory functions in which we have discovered the definition of the body. (p. 330)

When all identity is lost, there is yet the natural world, from which we may hope to invent linguistic structures that will reach and accommodate this area of experience normally so inaccessible to language (Scarry, 1985). As Heidegger points out, in breakdown of meaning there is the possibility of meaning arriving as "potential that is hidden in the very experience of meaninglessness" (cited in Johnston, 2003, p. 80).

Inventing new linguistic structures is a project laden with practical and ethical consequence for those who hope to deal with suffering in its many forms. Even under normal circumstances our lives slip away from us on all sides and are circumscribed by impersonal zones. Nonetheless, as Merleau-Ponty (1992) observes, "there is no experience without speech, as the purely lived-through has no part in the discursive life of man [sic]" (p. 337). The primary meaning of discourse is found in the text of experience that it is trying to communicate (Merleau-Ponty, 1992). To have an identity, then, one must be able to tell a story about the self's experience to oneself and others. The sort of story one tells of one's suffering—and is told about oneself—determines what sort of identity comes into being. The quality of the healer–sufferer relationship, therefore, has repercussions for the sort of identity that will emerge from the healing process. All the facets of personal interaction become the loci for ethical action, that is, "fitting response" in the storytelling that goes into creating a new way of being in the world, into creating a new self for the sufferer.

There is also the immense difficulty involved in listening to stories about suffering (see Wright, 2005), and there is no doubt a natural aversion to taking on and coping with such a burden, even for those who have chosen the healing professions. Nonetheless, as Innis, Bikaunieks, Petryshen, Zellermeyer, and Ciccarelli (2004) argue, if pain is to be relieved, healthcare providers need to ask patients to describe their pain experiences.

Since suffering constitutes an assault on one's identity and since it turns our own thoughts and emotions against us, how one speaks or acts toward a suffering person has greater impact than otherwise would be the case, depending on the degree of that suffering. It matters to a far greater degree than it would ordinarily whether the sufferer is met with empathy, caring, and understanding along with a willingness to listen to the expression of his or her pain.

The person becomes entirely vulnerable, and the identity that emerges from the process is what is at stake in our dealings with him or her. The fact that pain and other forms of suffering, such as isolation, are used effectively in torture and brainwashing stands as testimony to the critical relationship between the healer and the sufferer. Wright (2005) observes that suffering begs for explanation and that a lack of understanding about that suffering "seems to invite us to suffer more" (p. 125). It closes the door that the sufferer is attempting to open to a new way of being by speaking of his or her suffering.

To put it another way, lack of understanding stops the sufferer from integrating new meaning into his or her life story, an integration that is fundamental to the development of personal unity and coherence. The suffering in one's life must be written into the plotline of one's personal story so that the unforeseen episode not only fits with or bridges what has gone before but also blends into and harmonizes with the plotlines of projected future episodes. Imaginative projections of the future can be dismal and defeating, unrealistic and unachievable, or they can be constructive, liberating images. At the end of the day Merleau-Ponty (1992) once again gives us hope in his view of the world as "the inexhaustible reservoir from which things are drawn" (p. 344).

Suffering and Speaking

Wright (2005) argues that talking is healing, both mentally and physically, especially talking about suffering from illness. Scarry (1985) also reveals a fundamental relationship between expressing and eliminating pain. She argues that implicit in the work of Amnesty International, as in medical work itself, is the assumption that an individual must verbally express pain as a necessary prelude to the collective task of diminishing pain. In all the areas in which language is still accessible to us in our suffering, we must try to find ways to express and identify that suffering.

Soelle (1975) argues that it is not sufficient to have someone else speak on one's behalf. No other can express the pain (subjective) in a way that brings the desired healing (subjective and objective). Sufferers must find their own ways to speak about their afflictions, lest they be destroyed by it or swallowed up by apathy. Indeed, if one has no dialogue partner or has one who is mute, resignation is the inevitable result. The sufferer is deprived of a way of being, and no other is created to replace it. Instead of finding what authentically matters, one withdraws farther into the ontological abyss, where there is little or no hope of deliverance, no recourse to unifying metanarratives or beliefs, a place where little is expected of life except more of the same.

The paths that lead to the experience of nothingness are diverse, but the experience of annihilation that results from unremitting suffering is transversal. There is, however, hope for relief in the intersubjective development of the vocabulary for articulating pain that has in fact originated from the very ones who suffer. Wright (2005) describes ill people as "wounded storytellers," the "suffering others" (p. 157) who need to tell stories to make sense of their suffering and thereby be healed. Families in her practice often remark about the healing effect that storytelling has upon their lives.

Change in suffering is possible, but the quality of change to the suppliant and his or her world depends upon who is the individual's dialogue partner. Healing depends upon the quality of the person, upon his or her attitude, upon the quality of meanings (ways of being) found together, regardless of the particulars of diverse cultural icons and practices. How an individual person (e.g., a nurse or a doctor) interacts with the sufferer is of primary importance in finding ways to bring suffering to expression and hence to begin to relieve it.

The importance of the individual is illustrated in an article by Kristine Williams, Susan Kemper, and Mary Lee Hummert (2004) in which they argue that therapeutic communication is a critical tool for nurses who provide healthcare to older adults. They suggest that the power of social interaction is demonstrated by the fact that older adults live longer and respond better to healthcare interventions when they have social support and relate closely with care providers. From the other side of the balance, Farouk Mookadam (2004) and Heather Arther (2004) find that a low "social safety network" is equivalent to many of the classic risk factors such as elevated cholesterol level, tobacco use, and hypertension. Therefore, the absence of social interaction is to be considered a risk factor.

The manner of interaction between healer and sufferer can actually be damaging to the sufferer. For example, too many healthcare providers use what Williams and colleagues call "elderspeak," a manner of patronizing talk that demeans the elderly client and takes away his or her dignity. Health professionals, as well as the rest of us, bear a burden of moral responsibility to try to change speech patterns that include elderspeak so as to avoid increasing the burden of suffering in being old. Mary Brown (cited in Todd, 2004, p. 37) talks about how everything we do matters; how we talk and we interact make a difference in the lives of others as well as in our own.

Suffering and Personal Responsibility

Spiritual and emotional, mental, and physical suffering must all be considered when dealing, for example, with the interwoven dimensions of suffering that accompany old age:

> Until now, others praised and honored one,
> But having changed,
> One becomes an object of ridicule even by children.
> One's own sons scorn one, and one's good fortune decreases.
> The body does not experience warmth;
> And the mouth does not experience delicious taste;
> One's speech is not taken to be true,
> And one comes to the point of mentally praying for death.
> (Lhundrub, 1991, pp. 41–42)

One loses many important ways of being as one ages until the end of all ways of being in the world arrives. Praying for death offers no solution, however, when one considers the suffering involved while undergoing the pangs of conditions from which one knows one will not recover. "Frightened by the messenger of death, one remembers one's own sins. . . . [P]owerless to carry all the wealth and prosperity one has collected[,] . . . one must go alone to some unknown, empty region" (Lhundrub, 1991, p. 43). One must travel alone.

This reality brings us to the ethical responsibility of the sufferer in his or her suffering. It seems there is no escape from suffering. In the Buddhist view life as a whole is suffering. This is the first of the Four Noble Truths. Nonetheless, for Buddhists there is hope. The second Noble Truth is that we can come to know the cause of suffering. Once we know the cause, we can hope at least to diminish the effect.

For Buddhists the cause of suffering is attachment, exemplified in the various *klesas*, that is, negative, destructive emotions. For the Nyingma teacher Longchenpa (circa 1308–1364), regarded as perhaps the most accomplished master within the Tibetan tradition, suffering involves a loss of pure awareness; it is a condition made up of cupidity, aversion, and delusion (Longchenpa, 1975). As another author writes, "[W]hen one depends on phenomena of the Desire Realm, one does not know satisfaction. No matter what one gets in terms of place, food, clothing, and so forth, more attachment is generated: something further is desired" (Lodro, 1992, p. 332). Hence, there is more suffering. Does this mean a life sentence of imprisonment or banishment?

No, it does not. Within each suffering individual there spontaneously emerges a characteristic struggle to get rid of the suffering, a struggle that all human beings have in common. Longchenpa (1975) makes clear that nothing is ever purely an object, since there is always a cognitive side to being; our awareness is present as a "sheer lunacy" that he terms "affinity with being" (p. 52). This affinity with being, the desire to open new ways of being in the world, is in fact the cause of our disgust with suffering and frustration, of the desire for liberation, and of the struggle to get away from suffering and frustration when they are experienced. This awareness is described as the "power of the wholesomeness of the absoluteness of Being since time without beginning" (Longchenpa, 1975, p. 53). The presence within each human being of the challenge to find new meanings, new selves, new ways of being in the world is one's affinity with being. In other words, our very desire to be rid of suffering and frustration is the work of the wholesomeness of being itself.

Lhundrub (1991) provides detailed instructions on contemplating impermanence to liberate oneself from the suffering caused by attachment to conditions that are continuously changing. In general Buddhism teaches that letting go of attachment to what has been is the pathway to ending suffering. Soelle (1975) also notes that it is the personal ego's attachment to things (such as our selves) that lies at the root of everything that can injure the self, such as pain, care, disconsolateness, fear, and despair. Merleau-Ponty (1992) reminds us that we never manage to seize our *now* with apodictic certainty in any case—that in fact we are never even quite at one with ourselves.

Letting go is allowing change (becoming) to occur, trusting that change will occur; it is letting be, no matter what that becoming is.[6] This is not the passivity that can accompany the recognition of terminal illness.[7] On the contrary, letting go requires willing and enduring, loving even the suffering. Letting go is also the ability to forgive, to allow the pain that others have caused to loosen and be swept away by life's cleansing current. Letting go brings release for the self; letting go of the self brings release for the spirit. The great Tibetan Buddhist saint Milarepa recounts the lesson of letting go in his song about a storm that blew everything out of his hands and snatched even his meager clothing. So long as he struggled to retain his clothing and the wood he was carrying he suffered; when he let go he became free of the suffering associated with this struggle. Letting go allows us to live in the present without being burdened by the wrongs of the past and without overmuch anxiety about what the future may bring. Letting go opens us to new possibilities of meaning, new ways of being in the world.

This Buddhist viewpoint is also found in Christianity. In Paul's letter to the Corinthians he argues that "in weakness power reaches perfection" and that "when I am powerless, it is then that I am strong" (2 Cor. 12:7–10, New English Bible, 1972). The well-known hermeneuticist Richard Kearney (2001) describes letting go in terms of powerlessness, in a way that gives profound religious significance to the powerlessness that is characteristic of suffering. By choosing to be a player rather than an emperor of creation, the deity chooses powerlessness.

This choice expresses itself as self-emptying, *kenosis*, that is, letting go. The deity empowers human powerlessness by giving away power, by making possible our good actions and us, so that we may supplement and coaccomplish creation. To be made in God's image is, paradoxically, to be powerless, but with the possibility of receiving power from the deity to overcome our powerlessness by responding to the call of creation toward authentic being (Kearney, 2001)—the authentic being of compassion, forgiveness, and recognition of others. Letting go, then, is the letting go of what is "ours" in order to open ourselves to something greater and more meaningful.

Johnston (2003) writes of the self-emptying as an "element of surrender and emptiness to this outward and inward reaching that clears out the clutter, and turns down the din, in order to hear and connect with others and oneself" (p. 113). She cites Marcel's use of *disponibilité* as an availability that fetches back possibilities in the form of a new responsiveness to life.

The previous Roman Catholic pontiff also emphasized this idea when he wrote of how Jesus manifested his power in his weakness and all his messianic greatness in humiliation. The words Jesus uttered during his agony were, for John Paul II, proof of this greatness, especially his asking his Father to forgive the perpetrators, who "know not what they do." These words have the power of a supreme example. "Suffering is also an invitation to manifest the moral greatness of man, his spiritual maturity" (John Paul II, 1984, V:22).[8]

Suffering and Compassion

To suffer with dignity and without rancor allows the individual to transcend the everyday meaning of his or her life. Resoluteness in the face of suffering, resoluteness that may or may not be religiously oriented, enables one to confront oneself squarely and without self-deception and seems to give rise to a sense of integrity and a coherent life plotline.

At the heart of the experience of resoluteness is the supreme gift of suffering, namely, compassion, which is, as Karen Armstrong (1993) maintains, found at the heart of all true religions. She later reemphasizes this position: "All the world religions insist that no spirituality is valid unless it results in practical compassion" (Armstrong, 2000, p. 13).

Suffering is universal. Through our own suffering we come to understand the suffering of others. Spiritual growth occurs through one's compassionate involvement with the suffering of the other. When we in our turn see concern in the faces of others and express our pain to the best of our ability, our own pain will be related to the pains of the people among whom we live. Our isolation will be broken open.

Healthcare workers have the most extensive opportunity to help others learn about the gift of suffering. However, Walton, Craig, Derwinski-Robinson, and Weinart (2004) reveal that healthcare workers are not always empathetic to the multiple needs of suffering. People with fibromyalgia, for example, often express anger toward healthcare providers who do not treat their disease as anything but a psychological problem. Imagine the feelings of those whose psychological illnesses are treated as "just" psychological problems. The spiritual suffering of loneliness and isolation would be only the beginning.

Others who are more fortunate find that, despite episodes of severe loneliness, they nonetheless feel an overwhelming sense of the transcendent presence of divinity, friends, community, and nature. Some say that they received more emotional support from and had more intimate connection to the divine than before they became ill. Participants felt loved by the divine as well as by friends. These connections gave them strength and hope to endure their chronic illness (see Walton et al., 2004). As Soelle (1975) observes, serving the pain of divinity by your own pain leads suffering out of its private little corner and achieves human solidarity. To put the point another way, although suffering closes off ways of being in the world, those who are fortunate are able to find new and expanded ways of being in the world that offer more or deeper meaning than hitherto has been the case.

Is there some commonality among those "fortunate" ones from which (hopefully) everyone can draw benefit? Polly Young-Eisendrath (1996, p. 91) argues that letting go of the self-defined boundaries that we call our self allows us to become part of something greater, part of a larger context (see also Walton et al., 2004). This retrieval of meaning, then, involves relinquishment. Fetching back life's possibilities necessitates a letting go. It requires accepting the trial as part of oneself while expectantly hoping that it will be absorbed and transmuted by the creative process that is life itself.

From the witnessing of suffering, a larger context emerges, with a feeling of pity, compassion, or love for others for which methods of cultivation are crucial features of Buddhist practice (see, e.g., Lhundrub, 1991). When we stop to reflect upon what our brothers and sisters are suffering, we experience compassion. This experience translates meaning from an individual level to a transversal one (see Young-Eisendrath,

1996). In other words, we can come to a broader understanding of who we are through suffering. This wider context is crucial to moving from suffering to creative purpose. Just as ideas spring forth that we had no inkling we had when we are deeply engaged in conversation, so new identities can emerge in the intersubjective activity that is the healing process.

For the witness, what is most important is the opportunity to "encounter pain within a context of meaning and to find that one's compassion (one's suffering-with) has power" (Young-Eisendrath, 1996, p. 98). Compassion sustains the belief that the world is good and in order. Compassion opens new ways of being. Young-Eisendrath (1996) suggests that alleviating someone's suffering permits us to recognize what she calls a "transcendent coherence." Compassion is powerful because it is itself a connection to the larger context of others and the universe. In whatever state one finds oneself thrown into, compassion transforms all of one's actions into spiritual practice (Lhundrub, 1991) that binds us to others, making a coherent whole out of what had otherwise been a chaos of meaninglessness.

Without compassion hope is impossible. One becomes de-energized, and apathy takes over. Young-Eisendrath (1996) remarks: "To engage in compassion relieves suffering and makes pain tolerable. . . . True compassion [the desire to destroy the suffering of others] is a powerful antidote to our own suffering because it counteracts alienation" (pp. 58–59), which is a major part of suffering.

Compassion keeps us engaged. Johnston (2003) argues that remaining engaged with others becomes more and more problematic where there is no mutual concern, since there is no engagement, and where there is no engagement, abandonment is inevitable. This indicates the importance of the role of healthcare professionals, who remain engaged even when they cannot fully alleviate much of the isolation and helplessness of suffering—the spiritual and social as well as the physical. When all else fails, these forms of suffering can still be relieved by the experience of compassion from others. One is "called" by it to overcome the blindness and deafness to others that pain engenders, to find new ways of caring and belonging.

Young-Eisendrath (1996) explores how resilience can be learned using a mixture of Jungian analysis and Buddhist practice. She recommends some kind of practice or belief that returns one again and again to compassion and connection with others. It is the power of faith in something beyond oneself and the practice of connecting with the transcendent that bring resilience to life's inevitable pain, loss, and even death. One such practice, for example, is Tonglen, a Tibetan Buddhist meditation practice (way of being in the world) in which one "breathes in" the pain and suffering of others and "breathes out" peace and compassion (see Chödrön, 1999). The practice lifts one out of paralyzing concern with one's own ego into a larger context.

The benefit of compassion is unquestionable. Turning outward to a larger context, one assents, lets go of one's aversion, of one's attachment. In letting go of prior ways of being one becomes open to new ways that, one can then hope, will present themselves in the course of healing. In Christian terms the assent turns the cup of suffering into the cup of strengthening. Soelle (1975) suggests that we use the traditional practice of acceptance of suffering to confront our readiness and capacity for its transforming power.

Letting go releases one from the past self and permits a new self to be formed. Suffering then becomes not a gift from outside but a change within, whereby apathy becomes calmness, and independence, invulnerability, and serenity are present more than in any other life situation (Soelle, 1975). Johnston (2003) tells us about Nadine, whose father was struggling with a stroke and dementia. One day, while changing his diaper, she came to realize that something had been given to her by giving to him. This realization put everything into perspective and made Nadine's own struggles worthwhile.

John Paul II observed that perseverance in bearing whatever disturbs and causes harm unleashes hope, which is another prerequisite for healing.[9] Hope maintains the conviction that suffering will not get the better of one, that it will not deprive one of human dignity, which is linked to one's awareness of the meaning of life. The Dalai Lama concurs that the patient endurance of suffering breeds dignity.

Suffering that calls us to transcend the narrow existence of self-centeredness and to reach out—this applies to both sufferers and those who are called to help—can transform the sorrow of suffering. The practice of offering up suffering for one's own sins or for those of others gives suffering a deep significance. It expands the self's suffering into the suffering of a Bodhisattva or of Christ on the cross. Giving suffering such a meaning transcends its isolation, bringing what begins as stark immanence into a relational context through language and in other social ways, such as ritual and music. Once again a new way of being is born.

Peace of mind is found in overcoming the sense of the uselessness of suffering, a feeling that is sometimes very strongly rooted in human suffering. This feeling not only consumes the person interiorly but also seems to make him or her a burden to others. The person feels condemned to receive help and assistance from others and at the same time seems useless to himself or herself.

Roman Catholic doctrine maintains that discovery of the salvific meaning of suffering in union with Christ transforms this depressing feeling (John Paul II, 1984, VI:27). John Paul II observed that suffering makes us particularly susceptible to the salvific power of God, pointing out yet another commonality between Buddhism and Christianity.[10] This transversal played itself out in the life of Milarepa (Evans-Wentz, 1971). Suffering in his youth from the greed and acquisitiveness of his aunt and other members of his extended family, Milarepa wound his way through anger and resentment to the extreme of murder by black magic. He made others suffer until, by way of enduring much suffering and despair himself in the search for emancipation under the great guru Marpa, Milarepa reached compassion, forgiveness, and the freedom he sought.[11]

Milarepa's story and songs foreground suffering as a catalyst to producing change both negative and positive—and the role of attitude and action in playing out whether the result will be spiritual maturity or not. Rabbi Blech (2003) writes in the same vein in discussing the death of one's child as a moment filled with spiritual potential. One can respond to the call positively or negatively, in accordance with free will. He argues that to learn something that improves the quality of one's life after a tragedy allows us to see how we can emerge from darkness into light. Responding positively turns an otherwise meaningless calamity into a meaningful message. To respond positively is to open oneself to new ways of being in the world while letting go of the way that has been closed by circumstances. To respond negatively is, in Johnston's (2003) words, to dwell resignedly, to experience suffering as a "humiliating conquest in which one has suffered defeat. In defeat, the self closes in on itself, slips its moorings and drifts languidly without a sense of destination" (p. 107).

Nonhatred

To choose positive attitudes and actions decreases suffering in the world, both for oneself and for others. One guaranteed way of mitigating suffering in the world is to refrain from creating it oneself. The Buddhists make a positive virtue of the cause of that restraint—an absence of hatred. Nonhatred is absence of the intention to torment sentient beings, to quarrel with frustrating situations, or to inflict suffering on those who are the cause of frustration.

It is not easy to refrain in some circumstances. The Taoist litany of evildoers goes on for numerous pages (Lao Tse, 1973). Reading it makes it easy to see how living so as to refrain from such behaviors indeed counts as a positive virtue.[12] For Buddhists, nonhatred functions by providing a basis of not getting involved with evil behavior (Ye-Shes Rgyal-Mtshan, 1975). This is easy to understand when one considers the motivations for evil behaviors aroused by anger, resentment, and hostility. As a counterforce, loving-kindness is associated with nonhatred, its function being not to be malicious (Ye-Shes Rgyal-Mtshan, 1975).

This absence of hatred can require heroic efforts to maintain, as becomes evident in a study of the psychology of evil that clearly demonstrates how difficult it is to resist going along with evil in certain situations, for example, in jails and concentration camps. The study illustrates "the relative ease with which ordinary, 'good' men and women can be induced into behaving in 'evil' ways by turning on or off one or another social situational variable" (Zimbardo, 2004, p. 22). However, Victor Frankl (1946/1984) remembered heroes in concentration camps who would somehow transcend the malevolence-inducing conditions in which they found themselves and make a practice of helping others, giving up even their last piece of bread.

There are conditions under which people easily become less than human, and it takes nothing less than heroism to overcome them and maintain one's humanity. Milarepa represents such a hero, having learned how to maintain a compassionate heart even in the midst of the most severe suffering and persecution (Evans-Wentz, 1971). Compassion involves hope, the awakening to the possibilities for being that are present in the situation. One's existential situation can be transcended if it is accepted in the sign of the eternal, that is, not as a deterministic hell of what is likely and probable, given one's deficiencies and obstacles.

This is a task we all share as human beings, since it is not easy to avoid the machinations of villains. As the Taoists pointed out in their litany, evildoers are insidious and deceptive and seek success through the degradation of others (Lao Tse, 1973). Socrates observed that we are fortunate if we can find a spot sheltered from the storms of inhumanity that swirl around us. We may be content if we may keep ourselves free from iniquity through this life and depart from it with fair hope, serene and well content when the end comes (Hamilton & Cairns, 1961). Of course, the kind of contentment of which Socrates speaks (Hamilton & Cairns, 1961), which was available in pagan and Stoic times, is much more elusive these days, when we are prone to recognize our complicity in all the evils of the world. Nonetheless, the message still has value. The practice of the absence of hatred can serve to mitigate some of the life-guilt that a Christian heritage has bequeathed to us by helping us to abstain from producing more suffering than that to which our survival and our human finitude condemn us.

Forgiveness

Arising out of compassion, forgiveness—properly defined—is central to healing suffering. Forgiveness is an important practice for both healer and sufferer. Forgiveness from others heals the sufferer of her alienation and guilt; forgiveness of others heals the sufferer of his attachment, freeing him from corrosive emotions and toxic imaginings. As, for example, Graeme Cunningham puts it, recovering from addiction—a terrible sort of suffering—"is a process of forgiveness. You forgive yourself in the context of forgiving other people" (cited in Todd, 2004, p. 16). He saw his chance to recover as a gift, an opportunity to change, to be reliable and predicable as a physician, which he was unable to be when in the hellfire of alcoholism.

There is an ancient practice in Christianity, one that perhaps traces back to Egyptian funerary practices, that illustrates the central importance of forgiveness in giving meaning to life as a whole. This is the practice of the sin eater: someone who is otherwise shunned but when death approaches is called to take upon himself or herself the burden of the dying one's sins, granting absolution outside the church's stranglehold on salvation.

The sin eater played a role in Protestant communities, filling the vacuum left by departure of the Catholic sacraments of confession and absolution. Eating bread and salt (representing body and blood) that had been laid on the chest of the dying person, the sin eater thereby absorbed the dying one's earthly malfeasance, leaving him or her free from sin and ready to enter paradise. The sin eater heard the confessions of those who were dying or who wanted some other kind of reconciliation.

In his or her own way the sin eater brought ultimate meaning to the death of those whom the authorities had rejected, much as Jesus did by forgiving the thief during their final hours together. That such a practice was perpetuated, even though suppressed and rendered taboo, indicates the crucial role of forgiveness in mitigating the suffering of death or alienation. Gary D. Schmidt's (1996) novel characterizes the sin eater as a man with a gift. When people baked bread with their sin in it and left it on the windowsill, the sin eater came by and took it away, and people felt healed. Sometimes they would just talk to him and so were able to leave whatever they needed to leave and not have to carry it any farther. "He gave them the chance to let go of their hurt. And for that he lived alone on the edge of a Welsh marsh most of his life" (Schmidt, 1996, p. 91). Buddhists also make links between repentance, confession, and remission of sins, seeing the process as the shortest path to rapid expiation of all evils done.

As I suggest above, healing is an intersubjective activity in which sufferer and healer each plays a role in bringing the pain to expression. Clearly, forgiveness is an intersubjective process that plays a crucial role in healing spiritual suffering. Empirical evidence is mounting in recent psychological studies on the process of forgiveness, which Kaminer, Stein, Mbanga, and Zungu-Dirwayi (2000) define as a

voluntary choice or decision by the injured person to forgo anger, revenge, or justice in response to the injurious act. Forgiveness is thus an active choice rather than a passive remission of angry or vengeful feelings over time. Forgiveness is frequently likened to the cancellation of a debt; while both parties acknowledge that the offender owes the forgiver a debt, the forgiver nevertheless releases the offender from this debt. (p. 345)

Kaminer and colleagues (2000) provide an operational definition of forgiveness as forgoing one's right to feel anger and resentment toward the offender. Instead one feels compassion, benevolence, and love for the offender, even while both recognize that the offender has no right to these. Just as important as their positive identification of forgiveness is how they define the negative, that is, what forgiveness is not—namely, simple pardon, excusing, or condoning of the behavior of the offender. None of the latter has the healing effect of true forgiveness. Kaminer and colleagues outline various categories of models of forgiveness and suggest that future models should integrate existing ones, given that each contributes to the understanding of the complex and multifaceted process of forgiveness and that each has limitations. What is needed is a model that overcomes the limits of each of its components while providing a framework general enough to "capture universal forgiveness processes" (Kaminer et al., 2000, p. 355).

From the opposing point of view, it might be argued that revenge plays an equal if not more important role than forgiveness in healing suffering. Michael McCullough, a psychologist at the University of Miami, maintains that there is a "gene" for revenge. He argues that this need requires being fed, just as hunger for food requires being satisfied in order for health to be maintained. It is obvious that the desire for revenge is a powerful motivation (Carey, 2004). It has a strong allure, generating vicious and hurtful thoughts, tempting one into its path with the promise of satisfaction and closure. Nonetheless, revenge seeking and revenge taking do not mitigate suffering but rather increase it. Karen Armstrong (2000), for example, suggests that premillennialism is a fantasy of revenge:

[T]he elect imagined themselves gazing down upon the sufferings of those who had jeered at their beliefs, ignored, ridiculed, and marginalized their faith, and now, too late, realized their error. . . . Like many concrete depictions of mythical events, the scene looks a little absurd, but the reality it purports to present is cruel, divisive, and tragic. (p. 139)

As the Buddhists point out, the "closure" that revenge appears to offer is an illusion, simply reinforcing and exacerbating ill will between the parties involved.

Here we find ourselves confronted once again with the example of the Christos and of so many others, such as St. Francis and Milarepa, who reached beyond the self's desire for compensation for wrong toward the spirit of compassion, which freely forgives without being blind to what evil has been wrought. With eyes wide open, the spirit of compassion lets go of the self in forgiveness, making evident the transcendent coherence that gives meaning to life as a whole. Without faith in the transcendent—something beyond the immanent, the here and now—the closest one can come to coherence is in the closure granted by justice; on this path, however, no greater spiritual maturity is achieved.[13]

Fitting Response

For atheistic Buddhism as well as monotheistic Catholicism, the wellspring of meaning is love. To contemplate the sufferings of a Christ or a

Bodhisattva (one who vows to remain until the end of time to save sentient beings) gives rise to compassion. This is the most extraordinary gift of suffering. It is evident from what has been said so far that compassion and forgiveness are keys to alleviating suffering, especially spiritual, mental, and emotional suffering. This is transversal; the particulars of how compassion and forgiveness are applied are subject to the singularities of the case and its time and place. Like other universal goods (such as freedom), compassion and forgiveness are to be felt globally and acted upon locally—and presently—in what Calvin Schrag (2002) calls a "fitting response that keeps the gift as its measure" (p. 125).

Schrag (2002) argues that any ethic of rights and duties finds its initiating catalyst in an "ethic of care that has caritas as its content and measure—a caring that expects no return" (p. 126). Schrag (2002) describes this caring as a gift of love, the asymmetrical dimension in all justice and democracy that is the future as what is possible. Compassion is a love devoid of any expectation of repayment; it is the source of the gift in an economic transcendence.

Schrag's view is very different from that of Derrida. For Derrida, the gift, in order to count as a gift, must be metaphysically pure (see, e.g., Derrida, 1992, p. 29); that is, it must be absolutely free of all exchange relations and of all recompense as well as thought of recompense, even of recognition of the gift as a gift.[14] Derrida's notion of the gift and its requirements is transcendental (as opposed to empirical). Derrida's postmodern scruples regarding the notion of the gift take it out of the realm of human possibility, so there can never be a true gift in the here and now of everyday life. There can never be a true (i.e., pure) gift to God or to anyone else. For Derrida (1992) there is a "structural disproportion" between the finite and mortal, on the one hand, and the goodness of the infinite gift of love, on the other. This disproportion inevitably transforms the experience of responsibility into guilt, that is, suffering. One never has been and never can be up to this level of goodness.

As Schrag (2004) writes, "It was Jacques Derrida who, in his book, *Given Time: Counterfeit Money*, radicalized Mauss's economics of the gift and Nietzsche's ethics of the gift to the juncture at which they congeal into an aporia of gift-giving as an impossibility" (p. 196). For Derrida, the moment a gift is given it succumbs to an interplay of exchange relations, making an impossibility of gift giving and gift receiving (see Schrag, 2004). Any "politics of friendship" based upon it will always come up short. For Merleau-Ponty (1992), any such notion of the gift would be like that of a love or a will unaware of itself, and hence an unloving love and an unwilling will "as an unconscious thought would be an unthinking one" (p. 378).

Schrag's view contrasts markedly with that of Derrida. For Schrag, the gift is not some utopian dream. He is a realist who declares that self-sacrifice and self-interest are never entirely separated (Schrag 2002). Nonetheless, in spite of the less than perfect metaphysical purity of the gifts of compassion and forgiveness, they are gifts both in being given and in being received. They testify to what transcends both ownership and moral intent (Schrag, 2004). They testify to the transcendent coherence that makes life as a whole meaningful. The future as what is possible is preenacted through our own fitting response in the present, in our everyday communicative practice. A moment in which we manifest compassion and forgive others as we do ourselves is a moment when we make reality and find ourselves in the act (see Merleau-Ponty, 1992, p. 383). It is the ultimate gift, that of the kingdom continually coming to presence.

Suffering and Imagination

It is evident from what has been said so far that whatever we as individuals suffer from, we help make it so by the meaning we ascribe to it. Wright (2005) observes that the meanings we harbor about our suffering can increase or decrease that suffering. In other words, we bear the responsibility for interpretation—an activity that Gary Madison argues makes use of the imagination. As Madison (1990) asserts, language is human thought; moreover, imagination is "essentially linguistic" (p. 184) in character. Things first come into being in words and language.

From this point of view we can readily see how important the imagination is in regard to suffering, since it is imperative for healing that suffering be expressed, and most commonly this is done linguistically. When we think imaginatively, we see things otherwise than we did previously. Things get integrated into a new semantic context. Imagined meanings are ways in which we relate to or take up an existential attitude toward things; new meanings are new ways of relating to things (Madison, 1990).

New meanings are new ways of being in the world. The main work of the linguistic imagination is to bring together disparate semantic fields, which has the effect of altering how we think of, categorize, and interpret things (Madison,, 1990). It is in the imagination that we begin to make ourselves into who or what we will become. We are free in this making, since we always have the possibility to yet become "otherwise than what we merely are" (Madison, 1990, p. 191).

Imagination gives us the gift of freedom in our suffering. Imagination opens the prison gates of the deterministic hell into which we may find ourselves thrown as a result of strict cause-and-effect relationships. Imagination provides us with alternatives, other possible ways that things may be. When, on the one hand, we accept a system of thought as a totalistic view, we become bound. Rejecting such totalization, on the other hand, means that we are free to ask different questions, to get different answers, ones that reveal different dimensions in the world.

Experience of suffering can, like other experiences, give rise to an infinite number of possible expressions; hence, any experience can always be expressed further (Madison, 1982). The imagination is involved in this interpretation and reinterpretation. Madison (1982) argues that the imagination is the means whereby we understand reality; it plays a central role in our having the kind of world that we do at any given time. We play an active role in determining the meaning of events for ourselves and for others. This is true of our everyday lives and events and importantly so of our suffering.

Elaine Scarry reveals how worlds are unmade by pain. Sufficiently intense pain—such as from torture—obliterates "all psychological content, whether painful, pleasurable, or neutral" (Scarry, 1985, p. 34). Suffering takes on the character of a natural event, a senseless and alien fate. Pain brings the unmaking of the world because, of all events, pain is the only one to have no object, and, having no object, it cannot easily be objectified in any material or verbal form. Its power to create madness is one way that we acknowledge its power over all aspects of self and the world. Intense pain shuts down all other ways of being in the world.

For Scarry, worlds are remade by the imagination. To be present when the person who is in pain "rediscovers speech and so regains his powers of self-objectification is almost to be present at the birth, or rebirth, of language" (Scarry, 1985, p. 172). Imagination brings the making of the world. It opens new ways of being. This activity of creation has an identifiable structure (Scarry, 1985) in which there is a relationship between physical pain and imagining. Expressing the pain eases it. The crest of the pain moves along with a form of activity. Suffering is not merely tolerated, it is "worked through." How we imagine in suffering, how we speak of it to ourselves and to others, determines how a new world gets made, how the process of healing takes place. Talking about suffering opens our world to our fellow human beings and allows their world to affect ours.

Many of those who have suffered testify to the efficacy of putting the suffering in the context of a larger picture, for example, of participating in a cause that is greater than the individuals working for it. This allows us to transcend the ego-centered concerns that bind us to that very suffering, once again opening new ways of being in the world. Such participation in a larger context requires the function of the imagination in the creation of a story.

There is also a shadow to this brightness. One of the larger contexts that suffering too often gets put into is that of suffering as recompense or punishment for wrongdoing. To imagine this is the case is one method of satisfying the "revenge gene" (see Carey, 2004). As one author writes in the *New York Times,*

Revenge can be a very good deterrent to bad behavior, and bring feelings of completeness and fulfillment. Dr. Michael McCullough, a psychologist at the University of Miami, was quoted as saying "The best way to understand revenge is not as some disease or moral failing or crime but as a deeply human and sometimes very functional behavior." (Carey, 2004)

The doctrine of karma also satisfies this desire for revenge, at least insofar as it applies to others. To believe that one's enemy is feeling just retribution when circumstances turn against him or her can indeed "bring feelings of completeness and fulfillment." The story is not so pleasant when the shoe is on the other foot. Karma, as elucidated in some instances, makes us responsible (in some lifetime) for everything that happens to us, including where and when we are born—as indeed does Jean-Paul Sartre's view of human freedom.

This brings us to another *locus communis* (common ground) between Christianity and Buddhism. Although both speak in terms of a complex involvement, a fundamental intertwinedness, between suffering and sin, both also reach beyond either harsh and personal or harsh and impersonal justice, as recompense for sin, toward compassion and forgiveness as their ultimate source of meaning. There are indeed some cases of suffering that seem to cry out to be interpreted as punishment, but there are many more where the opposite is the case, where it makes little or horrible sense to do so. The point here is that we use imagination to tell either sort of story, and its role in increasing and in easing suffering must not be overlooked. All too many times we are indeed the cause of our own suffering when the closing down of a certain way of being in the world has come about because of our own actions. To become mired in this revelation, however, is to lose sight of the possibilities for new ways of being that are offered by the imagination.

Because there is an infinite number of possible ways to interpret any event, it is possible to change one's interpretation of one's own or another's suffering. Scarry writes that pain becomes a state only once it is brought into relation with the objectifying power of the imagination. Through that relation pain can be "transformed from a wholly passive and helpless occurrence into a self-modifying and, when most successful, self-eliminating one" (Scarry, 1985, p. 164). Acceptance of the suffering requires such a transformation and fulfills it as well. It is the first change that must occur in order to allow the birth of a positive attitude and hence the self-modifying and self-eliminating process of pain.

Janis Abrahms Spring (2004) writes in detail about the process of acceptance as an alternative to forgiveness when, for whatever reason, forgiveness is not possible. Acceptance requires nothing of the offender yet is a healing gift one may give oneself when the offender cannot or will not engage in the healing process (Spring, 2004). Spring (2004) writes:

We don't have to love or even like the person, but we can see him fairly and choose to get along, if that's in our best interest. We can be ourselves in his presence and accept that he'll never be anyone other than who he is. We can even give him a chance to do better and earn genuine forgiveness if he chooses to rise to the challenge. (p. 5)

Spring's text challenges the extreme views on forgiveness that require us to be lofty and even saintly in order to heal. She argues that this is not necessary—that making such an effort often leads to "robotic" gestures of goodwill—while also recognizing that refusing to forgive leaves one stewing in one's own "hostile juices." She proposes a down-to-earth vision of forgiveness, "one that is human and attainable" (Spring, 2004, p. 8), making it the job of the offender to earn forgiveness in order to be forgiven and, equally importantly, to forgive him or herself.

In any case, there must be change in oneself. Change is always difficult, but it is especially so in suffering, which renders one feeling utterly
helpless. Soelle (1975) points out that the consciousness of one's powerlessness is a fundamental element in suffering. To be without power is to
be unable to change either oneself or one's situation. In order for healing
to occur we must activate forces that enable us to overcome the feeling
that we are without power (Soelle, 1975, p. 11). A prerequisite for the
work of making anew is the conviction that we live in a world that can be
changed, that we are not completely powerless. If we live with a static
worldview, then our attitude toward suffering cannot get beyond resignation. "Only where change itself is comprehended as an essential human
value and acknowledged by society, only there can the passive attitude toward suffering change" (Soelle, 1975, p. 70). Taking change as an "essential human value" means that we value it as ontologically basic to human
being-in-the-world and allow ourselves to be open to the creative action
of change. The value of change is the possibility for creative action such
as a "fitting response."

Change and the Fitting Response

I have argued above that the quality of the healer is a significant factor in bringing into being a new identity through suffering. We have seen
that compassion and forgiveness are able to produce positive benefits to
the person who suffers as well as to the one who heals. I have also argued
that faith of some kind is necessary to bringing about a wholesome healing process. Above all, faith in the very possibility of healing, that is, of
change of condition, is required to bring forth an attitude that transcends
mere passive resignation. Faith in change—and that change can be positive, whether physically, mentally, or spiritually—is required in order for
a positive outcome to occur.

Schrag's notion of the fitting response is useful in understanding how
this change can come about by means of the relationship between healer
and sufferer. The fitting response illuminates the ethical dimension of the
healer–sufferer relationship. It makes use of the theological concept of
the "kingdom" as the goal of action, but the idea need not be taken in a
religious sense. Rather, it can supply an ideal type of the relationship and

action toward which sufferer and healer can strive and within which optimal healing/growth can occur.

In this context ethics is not subsumed under ontology. To put it differently, the call to responsibility is announced before the call to being (whether identity or relationship) and influences the manner in which one becomes what one will become in the course of the relationship. Schrag (2002) writes: "The space of ethics lies beyond the ontological quest. I experience the ethical demand in confronting the other; more precisely stated, the call to ethical responsibility surges up when the other confronts me" (p. 80).

This ethical move beyond ontology opens the self to responsibility, since the transcendence is ethical in character. Subjectivity takes on the character of responsibility. The subject is not an autonomous ethical subject, asserting its rights and privileges as an independent moral entity, but is transvalued into a responsibility to and for the other (Schrag, 2002). This is a personal identity that is not extracted from its social milieu but is interdependent with it in an intersubjective relationship. With the notion of the fitting response Schrag provides a new perspective on the coming to presence of self and other in the ethical relationship.

The fact that identity has a narrative structure means that temporality is constitutive of the self. The ethical subject is present to itself in both its memories and its hopes. The past and future are constitutive of selfhood, the past holding previous decisions and the future the horizon of self-actualization that marks out the region of existential possibilities, the possible ways of being in the world.

In this context the asymmetrical quality of the gift becomes the proper content for a viable morality (Schrag, 2002). The asymmetrical dimension of the gift allows the incarnation of an ethical and moral relationship. On the one hand, Levinas and Kierkegaard agree that the deity is wholly other, "related to the finite only under the conditions of an asymmetry which no Hegelian dialectic of reciprocity is able to penetrate" (cited in Schrag, 2002, p. 113). On the other hand, as we have seen above, healer and sufferer give to each other in a relationship that is asymmetrical but nonetheless reciprocal.[15]

I have argued above that suffering is a gift to both healer and sufferer. Healer and sufferer both receive something from the suffering, something unique to each that is unable to require compensation.[16] Although the nurse or doctor is gainfully employed in his or her profession, there is nonetheless in this ethical dimension (one among many that coexist) an asymmetrical caring (caritas) that expects no return.

As Schrag (2002) observes, acknowledgment or gratitude as attestation also issues from an economic region. In other words, acknowledgment and gratitude (Derrida's arguments to the contrary notwithstanding) transcend the realm of production and exchange. Schrag (2002) writes:

The central point that needs to be underscored and reemphasized is that the gift is outside of, external to, independent of, and in a quite robust sense otherwise than the economy of interactions within our personal and social existence. . . . This transcendence of the gift, in its concrete expression of a love devoid of any expectation of repayment is an economic transcendence. It is otherwise than the nomos, both implicit and explicit, that governs the commerce of human interactions, which remain beholden to the authorities and established mores of civil society. (pp. 111–112)[17]

On the part of the sufferer, his or her active involvement in (care about) the healing process and his or her gratitude/acknowledgment—as well as the gift of compassion that is a side effect, if you like, of the very witnessing of suffering—are gifts to the healer for which no return is expected. The ethical relationship between healer and sufferer is itself a gift of life that tempers and transfigures the configurations of reciprocal exchange relations that remain beholden to the constraints of laws of distribution, for example, consideration of professional fees.

Schrag's (2002) hermeneutics of acknowledgment is able to disclose the dynamics of the gift as "ceaselessly centrifugal, always proceeding outward, never returning to the center—lest it lose its dynamics of giving without expectation of return" (p. 119). In fact, a gift becomes genuine—in Schrag's (2002) view, an "event yearning for fulfillment and oriented toward actualization" (p. 126)—only when there is an acknowledgment and response on the part of the receiver of the gift. Acknowledgment in this view is a fitting response to a gift and not—as authors such as Derrida have argued—a return that somehow comes back to the giver, nullifying the gift itself. In the case of the healer–sufferer relationship, acknowledgment comes in many forms, such as cooperation, effort, listening, willingness to follow prescriptions, kindness, gentleness, openness, and so on—ethical actions that result in a change in ways of being in the world of both parties to the relationship. This is the kind of giving, the sort of action that creates and sustains transcendent coherence for both healer and sufferer. This is a notion of the gift that leaps the unbridgeable asymmetry between the divine and the human into the fallible, finite way of being in the world.

Conclusion

Suffering is a gift that awaits transformation by sufferer and healer alike. Since the body is inescapably linked with phenomena, a transformation of the worlds of both healer and sufferer can take place when they interact in a manner that illustrates a fitting response. The quality of the healer, then, is a significant factor in bringing into being a new identity through giving meaning to suffering.

Healers as well as sufferers each have something unique and precious to gain from as well as give to the intersubjectivity that is involved in the healer–patient relationship. We are not spectators; we are involved—in mutually implicative and mutually motivating actions. The intersubjective gifts of compassion, forgiveness, and acknowledgment give to healthcare professionals an exceptional opportunity to work together with sufferers in bringing about ethical action in the form of a fitting response to suffering.

We have seen that the importance of the phenomenological approach to suffering is to get beyond the "objective" suffering, which is essentially meaningless, to reach and cocreate meaning for the suffering in a fitting response to it. Healthcare workers have the most extensive opportunity to help others learn about the gift of suffering. Indeed, the individual healthcare professional is of primary importance in finding ways to bring suffering to expression and hence to begin to relieve it. Each fitting response creates a new meaning for a particular suffering, a wider and more transcendent meaning, one that can then ripple out and eventually affect the whole of society.

Notes

1. In the Old Testament, Psalm 22 is a paradigmatic expression of this entwining, as are Psalms 88 and 116.
2. On the importance of metaphor in religion see Armstrong (1993).

3. Evidence suggestive of a role for religious or spiritual involvement in health and healing may be found in Levin (2003).

4. The theological concept of the kingdom as the goal of action need not be taken in a religious sense. Rather, it may supply an ideal type of the fitting response.

5. For a full discussion of this paradigm see Harris (2004).

6. See Todd (2004), where Doug Dane speaks of letting go as the key to faith: "Resenting everyone and everything for the rest of his life guaranteed the rest of his life would be as lousy as the beginning. So he sorted. The memories of pain and exploitation he threw away. Cut the chains and hurled them like rusty anchors off his sleek new sailboat" (pp. 67–69).

7. To find out that one's condition cannot be cured is to experience the most elemental loss of control (see Toombs, 2004).

8. John Paul II echoes St. Paul's call to "come to the unity of the faith and of the knowledge of the Son of God, to maturity, to the measure of the full stature of Christ" (Eph. 4:11–13, *New English Bible*).

9. "[A]lthough the world of suffering exists 'in dispersion,' at the same time it contains within itself a singular challenge to communion and solidarity" (John Paul II, 1984, II:8). Christians share in the unending sacrifice of Christ on the cross. Each person in his or her suffering becomes a sharer in the redemptive suffering of Christ; that is, he or she becomes the Christos. In his letter to the Romans St. Paul argues that, in return for the sacrificial offering of suffering, one will receive the gift of compassion.

10. John Paul II concurs that "suffering cannot be transformed and changed by a grace from outside, but from within" (1984, VI:26). St. Paul spells this out to his congregation (Rom. 5:1–5, *New English Bible*) when he speaks of boasting in our suffering, in the knowledge that suffering produces endurance, endurance produces character, and character produces hope.

11. In one of his songs Milarepa brought about the cure of a *dakini* (the spirit of a place) who had become malignant because of villagers burning brush in her territory.

12. Taoists have bequeathed a litany of the sorts of evil persons one might encounter in the world:

> They impede and obstruct the professions and crafts. They vilify and disparage the holy and the wise. They ridicule and scorn reason and virtue. They shoot the flying, chase the running, expose the hiding, surprise nestlings, close up entrance holes, upset nests, injure the pregnant, and break the egg. They wish others to incur loss. (Lao Tse, 1973, p. 56)

13. See Merleau-Ponty (1992): "When I say things are transcendent, this means that I do not possess them, that I do not circumambulate them; they are transcendent to the extent that I am ignorant of what they are, and blindly assert their bare existence" (p. 369).

14. See, for example, Derrida (1992), when he asks where goodness exists beyond all calculation and answers that it is a goodness that forgets itself, that the movement must be a movement of the gift that renounces itself in order to be a gift of infinite love.

15. See Schrag (2002): "The lesson to be learned from the suggestive notion of asymmetrical reciprocity is that living in civil society with its moral demands requires a task of mediation without identity, convergence without coincidence, acknowledging the presence of an asymmetrical gift within an economy of reciprocity" (p. 127).

16. It should be noted that Schrag (2002) is a realist on this point, recognizing that "self-sacrifice issues from motivations that are never wholly liberated from self-interest" (p. 131).

17. See Schrag (2002) on nomos: a "system of laws and criteria for quantification that governs the distribution of signifiers within a predicate calculus" (p. 114).

References

Armstrong, K. (1993). *A history of God: The 4000-year quest of Judaism, Christianity and Islam.* New York: Knopf.

Armstrong, K. (2000). *The battle for God.* New York: Knopf.

Arther, H. M. (2004). Social support and its relationship to morbidity and mortality after acute myocardial infarction: Systematic overview. *Archives of Internal Medicine, 164,* 1514–1518.

Black, H. K., & Rubinstein, R. L. (2004). Themes of suffering in later life. *Journals of Gerontology: Series B, Psychological Sciences and Social Sciences* 59b(1), S17–S24.

Blech, B. (2003). *If God is good, why is the world so bad?* Deerfield Beach, FL: Simcha Press.

Byock, I. (1996). The nature of suffering and the nature of opportunity at the end of life. *Geriatric Medicine, 12,* 237–252.

Caputo, J. (2004). Good will and the hermeneutics of friendship: Gadamer, Derrida, and Madison. *Symposium, 8,* 213–226.

Carey, B. (2004, July 27). Payback time: Why revenge tastes so sweet [Electronic version]. *New York Times.* Retrieved April 23, 2005, from http://www.nytimes.com/2004/07/27/health/psychology/27reve.html?ex=1248667200&en=0232e8cf9bd1bcf1&ei=5090&partner=rssuserland

Chödrön, P. (1999). *Conversation on the meaning of suffering and the mystery of joy* [Video]. Boulder, CO: Sounds True.

Derrida, J. (1992). *The gift of death* (D. Willis, Trans.). Chicago: University of Chicago Press.

Evans-Wentz, W. Y. (1971). *Tibet's great yogi Milarepa.* New York: Oxford University Press.

Frank, A. W. (2004). Dignity, dialogue, and care. *Journal of Palliative Care, 20,* 207–211.

Frankl, V. E. (1984). *Man's search for meaning.* New York: Washington Square Press. (Original work published 1946)

Hamilton, E., & Cairns, H. (Eds.). (1961). *The collected dialogues of Plato including the letters.* Princeton, NJ: Princeton University Press.

Harris, I. (2004). Causal knowledge and causal emptiness. In J. Pertanker (Ed.), *A new kind of knowledge: Vocations, exhibitions, extensions, and excavations.* Berkeley, CA: Dharma.

Innis, J., Bikaunieks, N., Petryshen, P., Zellermeyer, V., & Ciccarelli, L. (2004). Patient satisfaction and pain management: An educational approach. *Journal of Nursing Care Quality, 19,* 322–328.

John Paul II. (1984). *Salvifici Doloris* [Electronic version]. Retrieved April 23, 2004, from http://www.vatican.va/holy_father/john_paul_ii/apost_letters/documents/hf_jp-ii_apl_11021984_salvifici-doloris_en.html

Johnston, N. (2003). Finding meaning in adversity [Abstract]. *Dissertation Abstracts International, 65* (01). (UMI No. AAT NQ86530)

Kaminer, D., Stein, D. J., Mbanga, I., & Zungu-Dirwayi, N. (2000). Forgiveness: Toward an integration of theoretical models. *Psychiatry, 63,* 344–356.

Kearney, R. (2001). *The God who may be.* Bloomington: Indiana University Press.

Lao Tse. (1973). *Treatise on response and retribution* (D. T. Suzuki & P. Carus, Trans.; P. Carus, Ed.). LaSalle, IL: Open Court.

Levin, J. (2003). Spiritual determinants of health and healing: An epidemiological perspective on salutogenic mechanisms. *Alternative Therapies in Health and Medicine,*
9(6), 48–57.

Lhundrub, N. K. (1991). *The beautiful ornament of the three visions* (L. Dagpa & J. Gold-
berg, Trans.). Ithaca, NY: Snow Lion.

Lodro, G. G. (1992). *Walking through walls: A presentation of Tibetan meditation* (J. Hopkins, Ed. & Trans.). Ithaca, NY: Snow Lion.

Longchenpa. (1975). *Kindly bent to ease us, Vol. I* (H. V. Guenther, Trans.). Berkeley, CA:
Dharma.

Madison, G. B. (1982). *Understanding: A phenomenological-pragmatic analysis.* Westport, CT: Greenwood Press.

Madison, G. B. (1990). The philosophical centrality of the imagination: A postmodern approach. In G. B. Madison, *The hermeneutics of postmodernity: Figures and themes*
(pp. 178–195). Bloomington: Indiana University Press.

Madison, G. B. (2005). *On suffering.* Unpublished manuscript.

Martens, W. H. J. (2002). The hidden suffering of the psychopath. *Psychiatric Times, 19,*
1–7.

Merleau-Ponty, M. (1992). *Phenomenology of perception.* London: Routledge.

Mookadam, F. (2004). Social support and its relationship to morbidity and mortality after
acute myocardial infarction: Systematic overview. *Archives of Internal Medicine, 164,*
1514–1518.

New English Bible with the Apocrypha. (1972). New York: Oxford University Press.

Nietzsche, W. F. (n.d.). *Scholar island* [Electronic version]. Retrieved November 28, 2005,
from http://www.scholarisland.org/suffering.htm

Petranker, J. (2003). Inhabiting conscious experience: Engaged objectivity in the first-
person study of consciousness. *Journal of Consciousness Studies, 10*(12), 3–23.

Radley, A. (2004). Pity, modernity and the spectacle of suffering. *Journal of Palliative
Care, 20,* 179–184.

Scarry, E. (1985). *The body in pain: The making and unmaking of the world.* Oxford: Oxford University Press.

Schmidt, G. (1996). *The sin eater.* New York: Penguin.

Schrag, C. O. (2002). *God as otherwise than being: Toward a semantics of the gift.* Evanston, IL: Northwestern University Press.

Schrag, C. O. (2004). Ethics of the gift: Acknowledgement and response. *Symposium, 8,*
195–212.

Soelle, D. (1975). *Suffering* (E. R. Kalin, Trans.). Philadelphia: Fortress Press.

Spring, J. A. (2004). *How can I forgive you?* New York: HarperCollins.

Todd, P. (2004). *A quiet courage: Inspiring stories from all of us.* Toronto: Thomas.

Toombs, S. K. (2004). Living and dying with dignity: Reflections on lived experience. *Journal of Palliative Care, 20,* 193–202.

Walton, J., Craig, C., Derwinski-Robinson, B., & Weinart, C. (2004). I am not alone: Spirituality of chronically ill rural dwellers. *Rehabilitation Nursing, 29,* 164–168.

Williams, K., Kemper, S., & Hummert, M. L. (2004). Enhancing communication with
older adults: Overcoming elderspeak. *Journal of Gerontological Nursing, 30*(10),
17–25.

Wright, L. M. (2005). *Spirituality, suffering, and illness.* Philadelphia: F.A. Davis.

Ye-Shes Rgyal-Mtshan. (1975). *Mind in Buddhist philosophy* (H. V. Guenther & L. S.
Kawamura, Trans.). Emeryville, CA: Dharma.

Young-Eisendrath, P. (1996). *The gifts of suffering: Finding insight, compassion, and renewal.* New York: Addison-Wesley.

Zimbardo, P. B. (2004). A situationist perspective on the psychology of evil: Understanding how good people are transformed into perpetrators. In A. Miller (Ed.), *The social psychology of good and evil: Understanding our capacity for kindness and cruelty.* New York: Guilford Press.

3

Finding Meaning in Adversity

NANCY E. JOHNSTON

Finding meaning and joy in one's circumstances, rather than being over-taken, diminished, and embittered by life's inevitable adversities, consti-tutes a universal human challenge. Yet knowledge about this subject is fragmentary and sparse. Although empirically based models have been proposed that address the basic human needs that are disrupted by ad-versity and posit ways of responding to these needs, the models remain largely theoretical. Sandler (2001) suggests that, in order for health pro-fessionals to understand how to assist people undergoing adversity and how to prevent long-lasting and damaging effects on the self, two key di-mensions must first be understood. These are the nature of adversity it-self and of the resources that people call upon to be resilient in the face of adversity. Such research, he remarks, is at the present time incomplete.

This hermeneutical, phenomenological study is an overture in the di-rection of illuminating the nature of adversity and how people construct meaning in the face of great trial, hardship, and tribulation. Being inter-pretive in approach, this study offers no claims about the frequency of the experiences, nor does it provide statistical correlations linking certain kinds of experiences and others that might be expected to follow from them. Rather, I interpret the experience of adversity and the meanings given to it based on the narratives of 20 people who either wrote about their experience of adversity or had conversations with me. My interpre-tation is further influenced by seven autobiographical accounts read to extend my understanding. Describing practices that people engaged to recover meaning, I offer a picture of their dynamically fluid experiences and self-understandings. Such unified knowledge is important for prac-titioners of care because understanding the indivisible and mutually constituting influences of personal meaning, action, and social practices offers new possibilities for thinking and acting.

Health professionals witness daily the extremities of human suffering. Given our presence at critical times in the lives of our patients, it is reasonable to ask how well we bear the burden of witnessing such suffering. Do we really understand how adversity jeopardizes the sense of meaning and direction in life? And, even if we do grasp the significance of the threats and losses that occur, can we remain compassionately available and emotionally engaged with people as they live through their overwhelming circumstances?

Mahoney (2005) argues that professional programs are not adequately preparing their graduates to engage skillfully and compassionately with their clients who are suffering. Maintaining that the evident supremacy of logical rationality over wisdom has corrupted the scientific spirit and left the academy spiritually impoverished, he demands a radical reorientation of the dominant discourses.[1] Addressing his own field in particular (psychology), he calls for educational approaches that engage with the human experience of suffering so that compassionate care can be restored. Speaking to a nursing audience, Rogers and Cowles (1997) note that "health care providers more often talk around the subject of suffering, enveloping it in a 'conspiracy of silence' common to the equally difficult subjects of death and dying" (p. 1048). They further note that there is a strong need for systematic inquiry focused on suffering as it is perceived by the persons experiencing it. Such research, they state, needs to extend beyond mere questions about whether the person is suffering to embrace a whole-person approach that illuminates threats to meaning and purpose in the context of the individual's whole being. I suggest that research and discourse need to go even farther if they are to be able to help health professionals overcome the tendency to care "at a distance." Not only must our discourses enable us to come to grips with suffering and help us to understand the threats to meaning and purpose that people experience during a time of adversity, but they also need to generate knowledge about how meaning comes to be restored in the face of great trial and hardship. Only with this knowledge can the possibility for thoughtful, helpful, compassionate, intimate engagement with those who suffer be pursued. Seeing the opportunities to cocreate new meanings involves imagining new possibilities that are specific to the situation at hand. It is this imagination for new possibilities that lies at the very heart of knowing how to respond fittingly. A fitting response requires imagination and alertness to the arrival of new possibilities in the midst of uncertainty, grief, and anguish, and it requires the ability to engage courageously with questions that have no easy answers. This study illuminates how people reconstruct meaning in a situation of adversity and sheds light on human and healthcare practices that both help and hinder the restoration of positive meanings. It contributes to our understanding of how to engage compassionately and helpfully with people during the times in their lives when they experience great suffering.

Coming into the Hermeneutic Circle

Approaching as Foregrounding Understanding

Adversity elicits vast existential questions: "Why did this happen to me?" "Is there any meaning in this apparently senseless occurrence?" These questions, commonly posed by patients, are questions we all come to ask ourselves in our own lives during times of great hardship and adversity. In this section I show how hermeneutical phenomenology not only encourages engagement with these kinds of questions but also enables inquiry to begin with the consideration of one's own experience. In this way researchers stand inside the phenomenon rather than trying to look at it "objectively" from the outside. When they bring their own experiences into the foreground, understandings are certainly not accepted unquestioningly but are situated and actively interrogated.

Gadamer (1960/1989) helps us to understand that bringing ourselves into the inquiry is, after all, only common sense. When we think about what really happens when we come to a study, we understand that we do not leave ourselves behind in some vain attempt to avoid bias. Rather, we can look for something, to begin with, only if we have some sense of what we are looking for. Moreover, we are always already in a position of understanding, since we use words to express ourselves, and the words we use are inherited meanings. All understanding, as human interpretation, is temporal and historical and thus subject to the influences of time and place. Thus no understanding or interpretation is ever final. This is because each interpretation arises within a particular time and a different place. Therefore, rather than attempting to deny foreknowledge of a phenomenon—which in any case cannot be denied—and rather than striving for "truth" through mathematical procedure, hermeneutics makes the scientific project secure by different means: by bringing what is already known into the foreground, where it can be questioned (Heidegger, 1996).[2]

As I began this study I considered what I already knew about adversity based on my own experiences, and I thought about how this knowledge could potentially both help and hinder this study. Pondering the importance of accessing my own experience of adversity to build bridges to the experiences of others rather than having my interpretations be a filter through which only congruent understandings flowed clarified my aims. These were to engage with people who volunteered for this study and to encourage them to share their experiences without reservation. Just as I aimed to get a sense of where my blind spots might reside in interpreting their experiences, I endeavored to uncover not only the content of what was revealed but also the context and that which the speaker could not or did not question.

By reliving times in my own life when I had suffered serious health challenges, anguish, personal danger, financial insecurity, career uncertainty, and bereavement, I came to understand adversity as a severe obstacle thwarting my will and desires. My illusions of security and unobstructed passage into the future that I projected, planned, and expected were shattered. Most significantly, I came to see that adversity called into question my self-understanding and what was important to me. Questions arose, such as "Who am I?" and "Will I have a future, and, if so, what kind of a future will I have?" These questions issued huge challenges for me not only to come to a new understanding of myself but to come to an acceptable self-understanding. My reflections also provided the awareness that, while I could grasp the dimensions of some forms of adversity because of my own experiences, there were huge expanses of human suffering of which I had no personal knowledge. Considering the relative ease of my own life, I needed to hold my understanding of adversity in openness so that I could be taught by the experiences of others.

Professional Perspectives

Moving from my own reflections on the nature of adversity, I examined ways the phenomenon had been characterized in the professional literature. Synthesizing knowledge from the stress, coping, and resilience literature, Wyman, Sandler, Wolchik, and Nelson (2000) propose that adversity can be understood in terms of its quality and ecology—as a relationship between individuals and their environment in which basic human needs are threatened. Sandler (2001) conceptualizes the relationship between adversity and resilience as two lenses through which the same phenomenon can be explored. Drawing on the research of Lazarus (1999), Skinner and Wellborn (1994), and Masten and Coatsworth (1998), Sandler conceptualizes adversity as a threat to individual goals, an obstruction to self-affirmation, and a barrier to meaningful role competency.

Summarizing the literature on resilience and adversity accumulated over a 20-year period, Richardson (2002) describes three "waves of thought." The first wave, based upon the work of authors such as Rutter (1985), Werner and Smith (1992), and Garmezy and Masten (1994), drew upon phenomenological descriptions of resilient individuals and support systems to offer a set of qualities and factors that help people grow in the wake of adversity.[3] The second wave of thought described the choices that people make (consciously or unconsciously) that result in the identification, fortification, and enrichment of protective factors, that is, factors that protect individuals from succumbing to destructive behaviors in the face of adversity (Richardson, Neiger, Jensen, & Kampfer, 1990). The third, postmodern, multidisciplinary wave of thought is characterized as a paradigm shift from a reductionistic, problem-oriented approach to one that sets out to explore personal and interpersonal gifts and strengths that can be accessed to grow through the suffering associated with adversity. This body of literature is still in its infancy.[4]

Noting the frequency with which the word *suffering* appears in relation to adversity and resilience, I next explored definitions of suffering. Rogers and Cowles (1997) point out that the Latin roots of the words *suffer* and *patient* are strikingly similar, both meaning "to bear." Using the method of concept analysis and drawing upon the thinking of authors such as Cassell (1982), Copp (1990a, 1990b, 1990c), Kahn and Steeves (1986, 1995), Gadow (1991), and others, Rogers and Cowles (1997) describe suffering in terms of its attributes as "an individualized, subjective and complex experience characterized primarily by a person's assigning to a situation or a perceived threat an intensely negative meaning. This meaning involves the loss, or perceived loss of one's integrity, autonomy, and actual humanity" (p. 1050).

Language as Understanding

Consistent with the hermeneutic notion that all concepts are inherited meanings that come to us through language, I undertook an etymological inquiry into the meanings that come to us through the word *adversity*, which revealed derivation from the Old French *adversité* and the Latin *adversitas*, connoting opposition from (*adversus:* turned against). Also interesting is the related word *advert*, borrowed again from the Old French *avertir* and from the Latin *advertere* (*ad:* to + *vertere:* to turn around toward) (*Oxford English Dictionary Online*, 2005). Thus the word connotes both disorientation and reorientation. Adversity can be understood to be a situation in which one is opposed, displaced, and turned. In the turning one encounters something else, something new, something that had until now escaped attention. The word reveals the potential of being turned around in relation to the being that one is—the coming to a new understanding of one's being and one's becoming (possibilities). In considering the turning brought on by adversity, I explored approaches to thinking and systems of thought that could inform my understanding of how personal coherence is preserved in a time of adversity through the reshaping of meaning.

Philosophical Thought, Personal Coherence, and the Reshaping of Meaning

Hermeneutical interpretive phenomenology is an approach to thinking about what it means to be human, and it is an approach that illuminates appropriate ways of getting at how humans understand themselves. The philosophers I was drawn to for this study—Kierkegaard (1849/1989), Heidegger (1953/1996), and Marcel (1960, 1963, 1967)—appealed to me because they expanded epistemological concerns about what it means to "know" to concerns of ontology, that is, how we come to be. Gadamer (1960/1989), whose thought is also extensively integrated into this study, emphasizes a different dimension that is still ontological in character: the basic way in which self-conscious, historically existing beings relate to the world. Agreeing that what makes humans human is their overriding interest in who they are and in being themselves truly and understandingly (Madison, 1988), these philosophers share a common interest in the modes of being and the processes by which the basic structures of being are made known. In illuminating modes of being Kierkegaard suggested that we exist only in the mode of becoming. Thus what we are most fundamentally is not anything that is determined or fixed but rather what we can become, that is, possibility (Madison, 1994). An important part of Kierkegaard's project was moving beyond objective and rational notions of arriving at certain truth to instead work out an approach to subjective truth in a life context that relies upon uncertainty to necessitate decision and to illuminate possibility. For Kierkegaard, uncertainty is not so much a defect of subjective truth as its essence.

If for Kierkegaard the meaning of being, or truth, is revealed in becoming and choosing in the face of uncertainty, then for Marcel the meaning of being is revealed in choosing to participate. To be a person, according to Marcel, is to be *with,* to be a part of—a contributor to, in relationship with—something larger. Marcel (1963) writes that being is revealed only in creative acts; that is, the presence of being is observable only by being read back out of human experience. Creative acts are generous acts that arise from and are simultaneously constituted by a self that is a self-in-communion. Self-in-communion, like the work of an artist, which comes to be only in the artistic process, acts to reveal the meaning of being through love, hope, and fidelity (Gallagher, 1975). Heidegger's understanding of hermeneutics is that it is an interpretation of *Dasein*'s being. *Dasein* is the German word for "being there," the human capacity to comprehend one's own existence; it is the openness, the "there being" in which meaning occurs or is disclosed (Grondin, 1990). Similar to Kierkegaard's (1849/1989) understanding of "interestedness" and Marcel's (1963) notion of participation as a mode of being, comprehending human existence for Heidegger (1953/1996) can be accomplished only in the company of and by understanding one's relationship with other entities in the world. Thus *Dasein*'s primary way of being in the world is one of concern; that is, who we are is constituted by the concerns that engage us in our world and is how we interpret ourselves in our practices and ways of engaging socially (Koch, 1995). It is in this practical, concerned engagement with the world that the meaning of being comes to be revealed.

In addition to exploring philosophic understandings as a way of coming to a deeper understanding of how meaning comes to be revealed, my search took me into the psychoanalytic literature. There I discovered, with reference to the work of Kohut (1977, 1984), Stern (1991), Stolorow and Atwood (1992), Stolorow (1994), Orange (2000), and Schafer (2004)—all practicing psychoanalysts—that existential and ontological thinking is reshaping the contours of psychoanalytic thought. This is particularly evident in writings over the last 10 to 15 years that have increasingly grappled with the restoration of personal coherence through the reshaping of meaning. Important concepts include empathy, attunement, and mutuality. Empathy is defined as emotional knowledge gained by participation in a shared reality, which comes from the analyst's attunement to the emotional reality shared with the patient in the intersubjective situation (Orange, 2000). Validating attunement constitutes a response that occurs at the interface of mutually interacting, affectively attuned subjectivities (Stolorow, Atwood, & Orange, 2002). Significantly, such thinking represents a departure from the conventional objectivist epistemologies, since it rejects the notion that it is possible to have privileged access to the essence of the patient's psychic reality and to the "objective truths" that the patient's psychic reality obscures. Thought that is related to the concept of intersubjectivity integrates the philosophical understandings of Heidegger and Gadamer that pertain to the nature of truth, experience, and self-knowledge. It does this by emphasizing the constitutive interplay between worlds of experience. This leads inevitably to a stance in which the healer joins the other in the process of making sense together. Implicit to practice based on this understanding is the building of a capacity for emotional understanding that is facilitated in an atmosphere in which the analyst "undergoes the situation" with the patient. Dialogical conversation unfolds as that which is triadic rather than dyadic, since the nature of understanding is neither the understanding of the analyst nor the understanding of the patient but rather a new understanding that arises out of a situation of mutuality, connection, and relatedness (Schafer, 2004). While such understandings were developed in relation to the practice of psychoanalysis, they offer rich insights into how the sense of the self's being coherent, resilient, and acceptable can be restored in the healing conversations that are offered practitioners of care from a variety of "helping" disciplines. But what, the question could well be asked, is the self?

Hermeneutical phenomenology, as a project devoted to overcoming the mind–body or objective–subjective split begun by Descartes, takes the position that the self is not a *what*. The self is not a thing that "can be conceptualized as some kind of essence which somehow underlies, supports, is the basis and cause—or else, the transcendental, overarching unity" (Madison, 1988, p. 9). Schafer (1981) writes that the story about the self is both a conversation and a narrative:

The story is that there is a self to tell something to, and someone else serving as an audience who is oneself or one's self. The self is a kind of telling about one's individuality. It is something one learns to conceptualize in one's capacity as agent; it is not a doer of actions. The inner world of experience is a kind of telling, not a place. (p. 31)

Having brought background understandings into the open for questioning and having characterized a philosophic lens that offered possibilities for seeing more deeply into "the heart of things," I was now ready to invite people to share their experiences of adversity with me.

Inviting Stories, Welcoming Narratives

Twenty people who endorsed living through an experience of adversity accepted the invitation to participate in this study either by engaging in a conversation or a series of conversations about their experience of adversity (13) or by writing a story of their experience of adversity (7).[5] Individuals who engaged in conversations or wrote stories about their experiences came by referral from colleagues, by self-referral, or as a result of my follow-up of newspaper stories in which individuals had left e-mail addresses. It is important to note that sharing a story about an experience of adversity—in which meaning typically breaks down and the world turns upside down—is not an experience that people are generally willing to share with an absolute stranger. Before asking people to sign consents and initiate formal participation in the study, I took care to introduce myself and to invite people to meet with me several times, if necessary, to establish a relationship. Initial introductory meetings took place in a variety of settings, including offices, coffee shops, waiting rooms, restaurants, parks, and individuals' homes.

All but 2 of the 22 people approached agreed to participate in the study. When interest in participation was confirmed, a letter explaining the study and a consent form approved by an ethics review board were provided, and consent was obtained. Anonymity was assured by agreeing to alter names and locations given in stories or conversations so that the identity of participants could not be reconstructed. In addition, participants were given the choice of withdrawing from the study or refusing permission for the use of their interview or text at any time.

Of the 20 people who participated, 12 were women and 8 were men. The ages of the participants ranged from the mid-30s to early 80s. Of the 12 women participating, 11 were of European extraction, and 1 was Asian. Of the 8 men participating, 1 man was African American, and the rest were European Canadian. Marital status included single, common law, married, divorced, and widowed. Employment status included individuals who were unemployed and receiving social assistance, homemakers, those employed outside the home, and retired persons.

Consistent with hermeneutical phenomenological approaches and in order to extend my thinking, I also read seven extant autobiographies pertinent to the lived experience of adversity. Autobiographies selected included stories of losing career aspirations and other hopes for the future because of a chronic disease (Goldstein, 2000), traumatic injury in a diving accident (Selder, Kachoyeanos, Baisch, & Gissler, 1997), surviving the collapse of the World Trade Center towers (Devito, 2001), losing an important relationship (Nouwen, 1996), and growing up in a dysfunctional family (Dane, 2002) as well as two stories of becoming ill and struggling with depression (Bentley Mays, 1995; Solomon, 2001).

The Interpretive Process

The interpretive process was accomplished in four phases. In the first phase I brought conversations, narratives, and autobiographies into a "whole text." As I read and reread the whole text I asked three main questions of it: How is adversity experienced? What practices are engaged by people to get through adversity? What changes in understandings emerge for those who have experienced adversity? During this phase I kept field notes, and I maintained them throughout all subsequent phases; I shall explain a little later the way in which the field notes were used.

In the second phase I read each transcribed conversation and written narrative provided by the participants as well as extended passages from the autobiographies separately and repeatedly. The purpose of reading separately and repeatedly was to try to bring out the intention of the author in an attempt to resolve a central existential *problematique*— dilemma or issue — brought on by an experience of adversity and to bring to the surface the questions raised by the text itself. With these aims in mind I interpreted each individual text, taking care to consider Madison's (1988) nine criteria for judging the adequacy of an interpretation.[6] When possible I supplemented interpretations with poetry that seemed to resonate with aspects of the person's experience. To strengthen the credibility of interpretations associated with each individual text I forwarded the interpretations, along with the original text, to a research committee composed of individuals skilled in hermeneutical interpretation.

During this phase of the interpretive process and following confirmation of my interpretations by the research committee I offered participants an opportunity to meet with me, to read my interpretations based on their conversations or stories, and to have a further conversation with me. It was at this phase of the research process that some of the most affirming feedback was given and recorded as field notes. All the participants who wrote stories were eager to meet with me. When asked whether the interpretations rang true with their experience, all confirmed that the interpretations were insightful and helpful. No participant expressed disagreement with any interpretation, and each participant expressed appreciation for the care that was taken in trying to understand the meaning of his or her experience. Some expressed appreciation for the poetry in particular. One participant remarked, "I really feel understood, and, what is more, I understand myself better." Another remarked, "No one [else] has ever taken this much care to try to understand what this experience was like for me."

In the third phase of the interpretive process I read across transcribed conversations, written narratives, extended autobiographical passages, and field notes, looking for strong consistencies and common threads of meaning and insights in relation to the three key questions. I recognized these strong consistencies and common threads as emergent themes.

Finally, in the fourth phase, I brought themes accompanied by substantiating excerpts or examples into dialogue with the philosophical understandings of Kierkegaard, Heidegger, Marcel, and Gadamer. At this phase of the interpretive process I aimed to present a unified picture of the meaning and experience of adversity, the existential challenges and issues that arose, the practices that people engaged in to recover meaning amid adversity, and the nature of the dynamically fluid understandings that people had of themselves as a result of their experiences.

Adversity as Turning, Dwelling, Calling

I came to understand the meanings that people gave to their experiences of living through adversity in terms of three overarching themes: adversity as turning, dwelling, and calling.

Adversity as Turning

Conversations, stories, and published autobiographical accounts illuminate adversity as a time of turning, in which one is turned away from that which is familiar, desired, and expected. This turning is experienced as the threatened or irrevocable closing down of possibilities. The turning involves loss, separation, and alienation; can occur abruptly or gradually; can arise as disquieting inner turmoil or an unbidden external event; and can be an experience of pain, perplexity, disruption, and departure. That which is familiar fades from view, and in its place the alien, ominous, and appalling loom.

TURNING AWAY FROM THE EVERYDAY AND
THE TAKEN-FOR-GRANTED

Sarah describes the familiarity and ease of life before her teenage daughter's gradual downhill slide:

We lived in nicer homes and took nicer vacations as the family finances expanded in an appropriate way. We had lots of friends who admired our drive and accomplishments. Life was unfolding as it should . . . [b]ut then things changed. It was little things at first, just irritations—typical teenage stuff, everyone said[,] . . . [then] small amounts of money missing, calls from the school that she was skipping classes, defiance at home, foul language, no respect for others' property, stealing the car, staying out all night, sleeping all day (at age 14)! . . . Ultimately she was expelled from several schools. There were drugs, alcohol, body piercing, tattoos, the clothing and language of a prostitute.

Katrina contrasts the lightness and luxury of life before the discovery of her husband's malignant lump with the radical challenges following it:

A car door slammed; I saw my husband emerging from a cab, paying the driver, and head bowed, he walked across the square. I bolted down the stairs with hope and dread, flung open the door, and stomach tightening, read the expression on his face. It could be serious, and probably was! My husband was a successful scriptwriter. . . . We enjoyed a wonderful social life—[a]ll of that changed with the appearance of a lump. Ironically enough, "the malignant lump" came during the time of great enjoyment, possibly the best time of our life.

Tom tells a story of immense, horrific, and catastrophic loss descending suddenly, out of the blue, in the prime of his life:

Some years ago, while vacationing . . . I went swimming. . . . I was jumping off a tree that hung over the bay. The first time I landed on my feet in shallow water, so when I climbed onto the tree again, I dove out further, toward what I thought was deeper water. . . . I hit a sandbar and fractured my sixth and seventh vertebrae. . . . I woke up in the intensive care with a severed spinal cord. . . . The nurses had to do everything for me: brush my teeth, bathe me, take care of all of my bodily functions. (Selder et al., 1997, p. 64)

We see in all of these excerpts the sense of adversity as a gradual or abrupt turning away from the expected. That which was formerly anticipated and relied upon is swept away, and a new set of concerns and priorities suddenly comes into view. Thus the "perfect family" is confronted with imperfection; health, ease, luxury, independence, career, family life, and social standing are all jeopardized. Important questions that arise in consideration of such evidently severe disruptions are, How did these individuals come to understand themselves? What existential dilemmas are posed?

Kierkegaard (1849/1989) suggests that the loss of being able to take the unfolding of life for granted has potentially far-reaching implications because the loss of the taken-for-granted is a loss of the state of immediacy that promotes a kind of unreflective, automatic finding of one's way around one's world, based on conventional notions of what one can and should do. Heidegger (1953/1996) illuminates a similar understanding of being caught up in the everyday. The more one comes to define oneself as self in relation to the conventional notions of respectability and success, the more one risks becoming estranged from the self, or, to put it another way, one risks becoming inconspicuous as a self to the self.

Adversity is experienced as a painful departure, a wrenching away from the everyday, a situation of profound shock in which very little can be taken for granted. This turning away from the everyday may hold within it the possibility for further reflection on the being that one is, given that one has been wrenched away from one's everyday preoccupations. Kierkegaard and Heidegger imply that there are hidden possibilities within adversity; however, the wrenching disjuncture does not offer the quick access to meaning guaranteed to be acceptable to the self, as related by participants in this study. Rather, access to acceptable meaning is most often gained only by way of a journey into alien, appalling, and ominous territory.

TURNING TOWARD THE ALIEN, APPALLING, AND OMINOUS

Sarah says of her feelings in relation to witnessing the deteriorating behavioral pattern of her daughter,

I felt as though I was living in a war zone, unable to relax, feeling a permanent sick feeling in the pit of my stomach. This was my beautiful, brilliant daughter! We no longer recognized our child anymore. It was as though she was now alien to us. My child had died and been replaced with a monster.

Harold tells of the time when his son committed suicide:

When my son committed suicide I was unable to make any sense of it at all. I went over and over in my mind what I might have done differently, how I should have understood how hopeless he was feeling and saved him but I didn't see it and I didn't take action and there was just this sense of terrible loss. Just a huge dark gaping hole.

With reference to these examples it has been shown that adversity constitutes a turning and that, as is characteristic of all turnings, there is a sense of departure, disappearance, and absence—the sense of being moved in a different direction, one that is not of one's choosing. The familiar fades from view, and, in its place, the fearsome and formidable loom. The etymological roots of the word *turning* reveal the sense of being whirled around an axis or center, of being reversed and inverted, or of being molded and shaped by being worked on a lathe. Other root meanings include the notion of a point where a road or path turns off and where one embarks on a tortuous course of deflection, deviation, and winding (*Oxford English Dictionary Online*, 2005).

In invoking the metaphor of the lathe to stand for adversity as a life experience that molds and shapes and imagining a piece of wood as a symbol for the human being who comes to be molded and shaped by adversity, the question arose as to whether there are ways of dwelling with adversity that are "lendings" of oneself to the coerciveness of experiences characteristic of adversity.[7] Considering the metaphor of the winding and tortuous path through unfamiliar territory, I wondered whether (and how) people are sustained along their journey and how (and whether) they find their way home. In pursuing these questions it was helpful to consider the turning as the context that calls forth a manner of dwelling.

Adversity as Dwelling

In the turning brought on by adversity life takes on the features of treacherous territory, sustained wandering, and homeless exile. The self comes to be experienced as bereft, betrayed, bewildered, ill equipped, insubstantial, and even unrecognizable. In the losing of one's way both inner and outer points of reference are simultaneously lost as the stories the self tells the self about the self no longer make sense to the self; the plotline has been lost.[8] Life careers madly off course in the turning, or, as if one were trying to find the way through a labyrinth, each rounding of a corner seems nothing more than a series of mirages, cul-de-sacs, and confinement. Thus it can be seen that the sheer inescapability of the situation necessitates simply dwelling with *what is.*

Dwelling with *what is* is an experience that has been variously described as a desert or wilderness experience—an experience of confrontation with danger and formidable struggle (Frank, 1995; Picard, 1991; Younger, 1995). The etymological roots of the word *dwell,* from the earliest Old English, include the idea of *duel*—of being stunned, led into error, hindered and delayed—while later understandings of the word encompass the notion of abiding and continuing for a time in a place, state, or condition, as well as letting things remain as they are or letting be (*Oxford English Dictionary Online,* 2005). Dwelling with *what is* as a hindering or as being held in position while being whirled on a lathe suggests captivity—a compulsory mode of existence, the sense of being confined and restricted to a realm of limited choices.

Exile is another form of compulsory mode of existence—the experience of being alienated, cut off, and banished from access to support and authentic engagement (Marcel, 1963). An abyss of confusion, chaos, and insatiable need is yet another expression for the experience of living through adversity (Nouwen, 1996). Lacking a purpose and particular goals to strive for, there is no (or only a vague sense of) destination and thus little that compels action and striving. Accordingly, desire and will are diminished. Moreover, since there is no desired end point, nothing has significance as a landmark along the way by which to judge one's movement. Movement loses the sense of progress and takes on the form of a vicious circle.

Dwelling in Captivity, Exile, and Finitude

Sarah tells us what it was like to be the wife of a well-known lawyer, to be in the courtroom when her daughter faced charges, and to endure the captivity and torture of inescapable shame: "Sometimes, I felt that . . . I was covered with a sticky coating of shame [and that] my eyes would always burn from crying, and that the lump in the back of my throat would never go away." Katrina offers a glimpse into adversity as exile. She tells what it was like to be cut off and banished from caring relationships by the demands of keeping up appearances in the face of her husband's serious illness and treatment for cancer: "By keeping our fear to ourselves and acting like we had everything under control, we were left entirely to ourselves without guidance or emotional support. I didn't know where to turn or what to do." Allison describes the loneliness and sense of exile that accompanied a failed relationship and the ending of her hopes and dreams following her live-in boyfriend's suicide:

The situation was that I had no idea of what to do. We were planning to be married and now I was pregnant with his kid, not able to work and he was dead. I didn't have many friends left. Nobody really wanted to help me. Needless to say, the future didn't look bright.

Interwoven throughout these stories is a sense of angst and groundlessness. What is angst, and how is it significant? Heidegger unfolds the possibility of meaning arriving as potential that is hidden in the very experience of meaninglessness. In angst there lies the possibility of a distinctive disclosure, since angst individualizes.

This individualizing fetches Da-sein back from its falling prey and reveals to it authenticity and inauthenticity as possibilities of its being. The fundamental possibilities of Da-sein, which are always my own, show themselves in Angst as they really are, undistorted by innerworldly beings to which Da-sein, initially and for the most part clings. (Heidegger, 1953/1996, p. 178)

By these statements Heidegger takes us a step farther in understanding how adversity holds the potential for the "they" self to become an individualized and authentic self. If the jolt out of the everyday and the taken-for-granted throws into question the meaning of life, then the angst associated with dwelling in meaninglessness draws me farther away from the banal concerns of mundane survival. As such, angst "individualizes"; that is, it reveals what really matters to me, thereby bringing me in touch with who I authentically am.

Anxiety, as an experience that necessitates meaning making, comes to presence most compellingly when finitude, or one's very being, is called into question. Thus it is in dwelling with the finite that a disquieting insight arrives—that one's plans and dreams may not, or now evidently will not, be realized.

Natalie relates how, in a situation in a foreign country that provided very limited access to crucial medical treatment, the meaning of her relationship with her husband presented itself clearly. This insight came in the face of the realization that her husband was seriously ill and might not survive:

I thought it possible that I could be taking him home to Canada, but that my infant son and I would be in passenger seats in the front of the plane and that Mark would be in a coffin, as freight, in the back of the plane. I thought about how empty my life would be without him. I thought about James [her infant son] growing up without a father and of never being able to have his father at his wedding. I thought of never being able to grow old together and [of not having] the comfort of uninterrupted companionship and shared memories. It was only then that I realized how much I loved him and needed him.

Joanne relates how her diagnosis of cancer enabled her to face her mortality and thus to see the importance of establishing different relationships with her grown children:

While my kids were growing up, life was difficult. My husband was abusive and there were often terrible fights. My kids were confused by all the fighting and they didn't know whose side to be on. After a while they grew up and just drifted away. . . . When I understood that my time was limited, I felt so bad about all that had been wasted. I wanted to make it up to them and I could see that I needed to change, but I was so worried that it might be too late!

These examples illuminate adversity as an encounter with finitude that introduces the possibility of seeing what is truly important. Yet, as the excerpts below reveal, dwelling with the finite does not necessarily call forth clarity about what is important. For some it discloses a malaise induced by the devastating assault. Allison, in relating her continuing experience of adversity almost three years after the suicide of her boy-friend, the father of her son, says:

A couple of weeks ago I got the news that my liver is not in good condition. In fact the Doctor told me that I had better make out my will. The news didn't come as a big shock to me. I have been drinking heavily for a long time. What do I think about the diagnosis [of advanced liver cirrhosis]? In a way I will be glad when my life is over. Other than my son and my mother, no one really cares whether I live or die. My mother is in a nursing home, and my son has severe learning disabilities. I don't have a clue of what will happen to him after I am gone.

Gloria relates dwelling with the death of her children not as an experience of abiding with finitude that calls forth meaning but as a landslide that has buried her alive:

My daughter had many, many health problems and she was intellectually handicapped as well. I coped with her health problems and her slowness but then she got cancer on top of everything else. For three years there was nothing else in my life but her. . . . When she died, I felt that I died too. I haven't been able to enjoy life at all since that time [10 years ago]. Two years ago my son was killed in a car accident. Many people said that I would go completely to pieces, but I didn't. I just felt pretty much the way I have felt for 10 years . . . numb.

The stories reveal that some individuals come to a clearer meaning of what is important to them and are even overtaken by an urgent need to take action in light of this understanding, whereas for others adversity is experienced as a near fatal blow that leaves them debilitated and apathetic. What is presented for understanding are ways of dwelling, some of which allow possibilities to appear, while others appear to close down possibilities.

Dwelling Resolutely and Dwelling Resignedly

As has been seen, an important dimension is the angst of dwelling in the twilight zone between the meaning that has been and the meaning yet to arrive. Thus "dwelling resolutely" demands the absorption and ultimately the integration of what has occurred. One is no longer the "who" that one was before the intrusion of adversity; life has changed fundamentally, and new meaning must be made of oneself in relation to the circumstances in which one now finds oneself immersed. Such an integration of meaning is fundamental to the development and restoration of personal unity and coherence. Thus this abrupt disjuncture or problematic episode brought on by adversity in one's life must be written into the plotline of the personal narrative.

Katrina gives us a glimpse of some of the difficulties encountered in coming to an acceptable self-understanding following the death of her husband:

I thought I would never get used to coming home from work and putting the key in the lock and feeling an almost physical blow in my stomach that my husband would not be on the other side. I felt angry with the Doctors; I thought they should have been able to do more. I found myself taking offense with people for little or no reason and would start an argument. I really thought I was going crazy. I didn't recognize or respect the person I had become.

Beth describes the loss of self that came with the loss of her job as a senior administrator:

I used to look at people as I traveled on the subway and I would think about how lucky they were. They looked like they were "in place." They had jobs they were heading to, and they knew what to expect from the day. I felt lost—like I was just drifting, going through the paces but without any sense it would make a difference to anyone

Heidegger (1953/1996) explains that resoluteness "does not escape from reality, but first discovers what is factically possible in such a way that it grasps it as it is possible as one's ownmost potentiality of being" (p. 275). Explaining further, he writes that resoluteness is seen when it "brings the self right into its being with things at hand, actually taking care of them and pushes it toward concerned being with others" (Heidegger, 1953/1996, p. 275). A turning away from concerned dwelling with others, on the other hand, seems to give rise to fragmentation, rigidity, constriction of the self, and a diminishment of meaning ("dwelling resignedly").

The stories from this study revealed that insight—as a seeing into the inner heart of things—arrives, but it is frequently insight gained at a price and without relief, since the possibility of regret and self-alienation has now been introduced. "Insight into the limited degrees to which the future is still open" (Gadamer, 1960/1989, p. 357) is reached, and with this insight comes the awareness that not all possibilities are open and that some possibilities will never return. Fissures and impassable crevasses may thus open up in the self between the person that one is, the person one has been, the person one wishes one had been, and the person one wishes to be in the future. For Marcel (1967) this period of resolute dwelling is a period of intense questioning about one's being and becoming—a time when one questions the meaning of one's life and the future to come. As an ontological dimension of becoming, this time is a necessary period of recollection, silent reflection, and concentration, and it necessarily precedes and calls forth the experiences of refuge, release, and awakening. Marcel (1967) opines that intense questioning about the meaning of one's life is an intentional, virtuous, and courageous act. It is an act that intends the attainment of unity and freedom—and it is an act that manifests courage and steadfastness in the unwavering pursuit of self-truth:

Recollection taken in its primary meaning of silent reflection or concentration of thought . . . is the act by which I recover my being as a unified whole, with this recovery or reprise assuming the aspect of a relaxation or a release. In the depths of recollection I take a stand with respect to my own life and in some way I withdraw from that life. . . . [In] this withdrawal I bear with me what I am and what my life perhaps is not. . . . Recollection is probably what is least spectacular in the soul. It does not consist in looking at anything; it is a reprise, an inner reflection, and, I would add, we may wonder if it is not the principle of unity. . . . The only approach to freedom is through the reflection of a subject on himself. Properly speaking, this reflection allows me to discover—not that I am free, or that freedom is an attribute with which I could be invested—but rather that I must become free—that is, my freedom must be won. . . . Recollection [may be understood] as a reestablishment of contact with an illuminating source. . . . Recollection bestows upon us certain resources for the exploration within ourselves . . . the direction of . . . plenitude, or the full life. . . . [This] is so . . . because recollection shields or protects us from all kinds of distractions that tend to estrange us from our true selves and to divert us from the unity which is at once both behind and before us. (Marcel, 1967, pp. 86–88)

This period of recollection and dwelling resolutely toward unity and freedom, shielded from distractions and stripped of illusions, unveils disquieting visions. These include the specter of absences and disappointments to be endured, lost dreams to be grieved, and expectations to be relinquished so that the choices that may remain can be vigorously grasped and pursued. Clearly, this movement toward unity and freedom is one that is excruciatingly painful and one that requires great courage to undertake. Nouwen (1996) writes of this movement back to the self as one in which pain is "brought home":

As long as your wounded part remains foreign to your adult self, your pain will injure you as well as others. You have to incorporate your pain into your self and let it bear fruit in your heart and the heart of others. (p. 88)

Resolute dwelling, then, is understood as a movement that is not around but through pain. It is a movement in which the self moves toward the self. Resigned dwelling, on the other hand, does not bring the pain "home" but instead turns away from suffering and in so doing conceals itself from itself. In resolute dwelling the self stands out to itself in all of its starkness, and life opens from within life toward itself. In resigned dwelling the self camouflages itself from itself, becoming more and more inconspicuous to itself as a self, and life, rather than being replenished, closes down and is diminished.

This "life-giving" movement of the self back to the self is given various names by the philosophers consulted for this study. Risser (1997) explains that this movement is called recollection by Marcel, repetition by Kierkegaard, and retrieval, or *Wiederholung* (the opening of life that occurs by retrieving—literally, fetching back—possibilities in life), by Heidegger. In his exegesis of Heidegger's use of Kierkegaard's notion of repetition and Heidegger's own concept of retrieval, Risser (1997) says that resolve is manifested as repetition and retrieval:

Dasein takes over its past through repetition by fetching back time and again its possibilities. In its fullest sense, in retrieval/repetition Dasein comes toward its authentic potentiality for Being when it comes back to itself, when it comes back to that which it has been all along. (p. 34)

An important aspect of attaining refuge, relaxation, and release in a time of adversity is found in the capacity to open oneself fully in solitude to the sadness of loss. This is a time to treasure that which was lost, to mourn that which will never be, and to be able to let go. Marcel (1967) helps us to understand the meaning of drawing apart by clarifying the meaning of solitude:

It does not in fact mean isolation, for isolation is a lack, a deprivation[,] whereas solitude is a fullness. . . . Solitude is as essential to fraternity as silence is to music. We should remember that fraternity is perhaps above all a form of respect, and that there is not respect without distance, which in this case means that every human being must have access to an interior space without which he [*sic*] withers like a plant or a tree. (p. 157)

Thus solitude is understood as stillness—space and silence that distance and shield from distraction and demand. Solitude offers refuge—sanctuary for the safe outpouring of grief. Solitude as sanctuary suggests the housing of the holy, mysterious, sacred, and illuminating. It is a place of awesome beholding, of seeing into and beyond. Beth describes her need for stillness and silence following the loss of a job:

I found that I needed some time to myself away from everyone just so I could cry and be sad and think about my future. I didn't want to listen to friends' well-intentioned reassurance that I had lots of talent and prospects and that soon I'd have another job. I'd given a lot and I'd lost a lot and I didn't really know what I wanted to do in the future. I didn't want any of that to be glossed over.

David describes the time when civil war erupted in his country and he and his family were forced to move:

I had poured my whole self into making a life for myself and my family in Cuba. When we had to leave, I was devastated and didn't know where to go or what to do. I spent hours and hours by myself just walking and thinking and praying and waiting for some sense of direction.

Rilke (1934) powerfully expresses the release of perplexity paralysis and sadness through being alone in the stillness, silence, and sanctuary of solitude:

The more still, more patient and more open we are when we are sad, so much the deeper and so much the more unswervingly does the new go into us, so much the better do we make it ours, so much the more will it be our destiny, and when on some later day it "happens" (that is, steps forth out of us to others), we shall feel in our inmost selves akin and near to it. And that is necessary. It is necessary—and toward this our development will move gradually—that nothing strange should befall us, but only that which has long belonged to us. (pp. 64–65)

Thus we have seen that dwelling resolutely involves a return to the self (recollection) and a relinquishment of that which has passed (grieving). There is, however, an additional movement that is futural in its orientation: hope. A close look at hope, Marcel (1963) reminds us, does not reveal simply a capacity for naive optimism. Rather, it is an arduous and difficult "dwelling toward" that anticipates the renewal and refreshment that have not yet arrived, and in its anticipation it actually appropriates the rejuvenation it seeks. Nouwen (1996, p. 50) describes this as dwelling in the "not yet." Hope requires patience, and patience requires hope. Hope consists in placing our confidence in a certain process of growth and development such that the process is embraced. Marcel (1963) reminds us that the etymological definition of *patience* (which, interestingly, shows some affinity to the root meanings of *dwelling*) is a simple letting things alone or allowing them to take their course: "It is [in] developing an intimacy or connection with the event or circumstances comparable to that which I have with the other person when I am patient with him [that] a certain domesticating of circumstances occurs" (p. 40).

There is the sense that I, as the one who suffers, am no longer in exile and captivity. I have ceased searching for my true home. In finding meaning amid my current circumstances, taking care of the things at hand, and being with others, I am at home. In this sense dwelling resolutely makes of the journey a home. Li Shi Ying, a retired nurse living in the People's Republic of China, tells of her experience of dwelling—one that transformed exile and captivity into home and community:

During the so-called Cultural Revolution, I was considered to be politically undesirable. I was sent far away into the countryside and told to clean and repair toilets. That was my job. There were no jobs lower than that. I was torn away from my husband and two tiny children. I couldn't believe what had happened to me and I thought I would die from loneliness and missing my family and my little children. But then I decided, you can still have a life here. Be the best toilet cleaner and fixer they have ever seen. I learned more about toilets than you could ever believe. I could fix them all. Then I made some friends there [other people who were being "rehabilitated"] and we became wonderful friends. I felt safe and respected and close in their company. We used to laugh and share stories and talk about how it would be when we got back to our families again. When we were sad and lonely and down we would encourage each other. Gradually life went from being barely tolerable to being quite enjoyable at times. I realized I was going to survive my time in the "countryside."

Helen describes how she was able to regain meaning and begin to reconstruct her life following the loss of her dreams, her health, and her husband:

I suffered from pain, and I fell into a really horrible depression. I saw a psychiatrist and numerous types of antidepressants were tried. I also saw a chronic pain specialist. Nothing helped. I had side-effects from the pills and really didn't feel much better. Some days I longed for death. Then one day it came to me that nobody could help me if I didn't want to live and wasn't willing to help myself. But the problem was that even if I wanted to live I didn't seem to be able to help myself. So I said to God "If you are up there and you really care, you had better help me." So there weren't any miracles but I got the idea that I had to maintain a spiritual discipline of meditating and the habit of exercising everyday. So everyday I [lit] a candle and I concentrated on releasing the darkness in myself into the light. . . . Things started to change. I was able to begin to lose weight and to walk short distances and then I met a friend who invited me to swim with her everyday. I lost more weight and became fit and developed a good friend in the process. . . . Five years later I can say that I am happier now.

Norma tells of the time when she was at home, having been diagnosed with multiple myeloma that had broken through in her hip and caused it to fracture:

I just lay on the couch and thought about dying. I was so weak from the chemo and didn't think I had the strength to go on. Two friends refused to give up and they came often and made tea and just sat with me. One day in particular stands out for me. This was when I felt particularly low. One of my friends knew I was a swimmer and she said to me "Norma you have to keep pushing. Swim! Swim! Swim to the surface! You can do it!!" The fact that they were there made all the difference in the world. I felt like I had the strength to go on.

These stories reveal the capacity to weather enormous difficulty in life. One speaks of a certain "domesticating" of that which is alien, another describes coming to a critical decision, and the third describes the resolve to survive. All reveal the hope and sense of safety that come with being able to have one's suffering understood by another. Schweizer (2000) says that "when suffering speaks, it expects an answer from the other-in-language, from the one whom language intrinsically addresses. Suffering that is spoken establishes that the other is no longer in the solitary body but towards another" (p. 234). When suffering is spoken, isolative suffering begins a movement toward another. Celan (1995) expresses the faint but lifesaving signal that accompaniment brings to the one who suffers:

I CAN STILL SEE YOU: an echo
that can be grasped towards with antenna
words, on the edge of parting

Your face quietly shines
when suddenly
there is lamplike brightness
inside me, just at the point
where most painfully one says never.
(p. 299)

Frank (1995), drawing on the work of Levinas and Cassell, says that when the one who suffers is attended to, "a new light . . . begins to shine. . . . Listening and telling are phases of healing; the healer and the storyteller are one. . . . The illusion of being lost is overcome. The sufferer is made whole in hearing the other's story" (pp. 180, 183).

Some stories unfolded profoundly mysterious experiences of Being coming to presence. Some people named this experience God, while in some stories references were made to Providence and "a still small voice," or conscience, that prodded, nudged, counseled, and comforted. Other stories disclosed an experience of presence or God being glimpsed and encountered in the caring and selfless acts of other human beings. Two stories used the word *grace* to describe the propitious arrival of a perfect gift at the right moment, while one story unfolded an experience of "Light" and release.

Katrina shares her experience of sanctuary as a place where God, as benevolent presence, shows up auspiciously in nudgings, synchronous solutions, and the loving, caring actions of a friend:

In thinking back on this time in my life, however, I think that God, or something divine, was watching over me. I wrote to a friend in London, England, and shared with her how I was feeling. It turned out that she was open to coming to Toronto, a city she had visited earlier and liked very much. We were able to work out a deal whereby she became our housekeeper and I paid her. She told me that she couldn't handle my depression, but that she would take care of the practical things, e.g., cooking and other things and keep them running and that maybe by helping to lessen the load, I would be able to begin to heal and she was absolutely right. She had just ended a relationship so the timing for coming to Toronto was right. She stayed with us for 3 years. My sons really loved her and still do. She came into my life at a crucial time.

Melissa, a young woman struggling with rapidly progressing lupus, confronts the loss of her dream to pursue a life of teaching and tells of grief giving way mysteriously to divine light:

I went into my room and crawled into bed. . . . I was devoured by a grief that left me nothing, not even the release of tears. In its wake, my mind became blank, empty and dark, as if a twister had swept across it. I do not know how long I lay like this, but gradually there arose a cry out of my black quiet, a wordless expression of the deepest need. It did not go unheeded. For it was then that the Light came to me, every part of me, filling the emptiness, transforming the darkness. The Light grew ever stronger, until it assumed an unspeakably powerful, beneficent radiance. Not a word had been uttered during these moments, for I did not experience the Light in words, only in images and emotions beyond language. But I knew that I was in the presence of the Source who had created the world and lived in its core. Gradually the Light faded, leaving me, but not alone. Never again alone. For I had been given a revelation and a promise of its presence, in the world, in my life. . . . Despite the disease's continual onslaught, this sense of security stayed with me and sustained me. (Goldstein, 2000, p. 234)

How are we to understand such experiences of absence becoming presence, despair giving way to hope, darkness becoming light, danger becoming sanctuary? Kockelmans (1984) expresses his understanding of danger, turning, and insight as the place where new possibilities, as the illumination of Being as presence, arrive. These experiences are not, and cannot, be produced in a deliberate manner and are not understood with reference to causal models of explanation. Rather, the phenomenon is mysterious, surprising, and paradoxical—"forgottenness" enfolds truth, and danger discloses freedom:

The self-withholding of the truth of Being, which tries to hold it in forgottenness, hides a yet ungranted favor, namely, that a turning will come-to-pass, a turning of Being's forgottenness into Being's truth. Thus, where danger is as danger, there also is the freeing of Being. This turning, however, can happen only abruptly. It is not brought about by anything except Being itself; and it is certainly not brought about in a cause–effect relationship. The abrupt opening up is the flashing of a lightening flash. It brings itself into its own light, which it has brought along. When the truth of Being flashes in the turning of the danger, the coming-to-presence of Being opens up and the truth of Being's issuance come-to-pass. (Kockelmans, 1984, p. 249)

Relating Kockelmans's thoughts to an experience of adversity, it can be understood that life in the everyday and the taken-for-granted manifests a forgottenness of Being. The value, beauty, and gift of life are so easily forgotten in the quest to survive and succeed. Yet it is this very forgottenness that provides the context and necessary conditions in which to experience the turning and jolt of adversity. No awareness or new learning comes without a sense of contrast, negativity, danger, and disjuncture (Gadamer, 1989). Disjuncture is by definition a place of both danger and openness, since it constitutes a gap or dehiscence arising from breakdown, tearing away, and separation. It is into this place of the "wounded gap" of painful awareness, suffering openness, and resolute dwelling that Being arrives as illumination, insight, and truth.

But what is Being, given that it was described in the gathered stories as God, mystery, grace, light, source, guidance, and conscience? Kockelmans (1985) says that Being "is the totality of all meaning" (p. 52). It is not something that humans can grasp and hold still in the sense of being able to ascribe cause and effect and establish a particular and ultimate ground for all that is. Rather,

Being is . . . the holy, the ultimate source of the conserving power that guards beings in the integrity of their Being. . . . Because Being is the holy, it is also the awesome; by its very coming it dislodges and deranges every experience from the patterns of everydayness. It is also the eternal heart of things because it is the innermost source of their presence and because it is the perpetual Being that lets all abiding be. It is the omnipresent and the undefiled. (Kockelmans, 1985, p. 52)

Returning to the stories and conversations gathered for this study, the meaning of dwelling resolutely has been unfolded as an experience of movement and stillness, self-questioning, persevering in the "not yet," and listening patiently and hopefully—movement and stillness described as recollection, repetition, retrieval, refuge, and sanctuary. Everyone, however, does not experience dwelling this way in the "not yet." What I have chosen to name "dwelling resignedly" does not reveal the presence of Being as inexhaustible replenishment. Instead, life is experienced as a humiliating conquest in which one has suffered defeat. In defeat the self closes in on itself, slips its moorings, and drifts languidly without a sense of destination.

Excerpts from the stories of Allison and Gloria, discussed above, are revisited together with the following additional excerpts from conversations. The words of Allison:

There is something that I just don't agree with them about and that is that you are responsible for your own life. I didn't ask to be born and I didn't ask to have all of these horrible things happen to me, so how am I supposed to be responsible for all that?

Gloria describes her view of life following the death of her daughter and, more recently, her son:

When she died I felt that I died too. I haven't been able to enjoy life at all since that time [10 years ago]. Two years ago my son was killed in a car accident. Many people said that I would go to pieces but I didn't. I just felt pretty much the way I have felt for 10 years . . . numb. . . . I can't go back to the way it was [life before the deaths of her children] and I don't like it the way it is . . . so what am I going to do? I just go on.

In the words of Allison and Gloria there is a sense of despair—passive relinquishment to the situation at hand and an acquiescence to life that is experienced not as fulfillment but as intractable, unremitting sorrow. Marcel (1963) explains that

there is in despair the belief that the wound one has suffered is incurable and, moreover, that this wound which is inflicted by separation, is separation itself. It is as if the sufferer says, "I shall never again be anything but the wounded muti-lated creature I am today. Death alone can end my trouble; and it will only do so by ending me myself." . . . The despairing man [*sic*] not only contemplates and sets before himself the dismal repetition, the externalization of a situation in which he is caught like a ship in a sea of ice. By paradox which is difficult to con-ceive, he anticipates this repetition. (p. 40)

Absent from these stories are descriptions of healing solitude, helpful ac-companiment, divine counsel, and reassurance. Instead, the stories un-fold isolation, absence, and meaninglessness.

Adversity as Calling

Calls occur in everyday life for many reasons. As invitations to re-spond to opportunities or summonses to bear witness to important tran-sitions and rites of passage, calls initiate conversations, and they suggest possibilities. Calls may be heard or they may be unheard, disregarded, or refused. I now consider some of the existential and ontological conditions that enable hearing and responding so that positive meanings and new possibilities arrive, and I contrast these ways of being with those that ob-struct and hinder their arrival.

Calling as Discovery and Calling as Concealment

A calling cannot, Marcel reminds us, be heard by a being who is "oc-cupied or cluttered up with himself." Rather, "he [*sic*] reaches out, on the contrary, beyond his narrow self, prepared to consecrate his being to a cause which is greater than he is, but which at the same time he makes his own" (Marcel, 1963, p. 25). One reaches both outward and deeply within to discover the connectedness of all things and to connect with one's self in its very truth. There is, then, an element of emptiness and surrender to this outward and inward reaching, which clears out the clutter and turns down the din in order to hear and connect with others and with oneself.

Marcel has characterized this clearing or emptiness as *disponibilité*. This is an emptiness that is at the same time an availability that fetches back possibilities in the form of a new responsiveness to life, a manner of being in which the doors of one's heart have been left ajar. *Disponibilité*, according to Marcel (1951), means "an aptitude to give oneself . . . and to bind oneself by the gift. Again it means to transform circumstances into opportunities, we might even say favors, thus participating in the shaping of our own destiny and marking it with our seal" (p. 69). Heidegger (1953/1996) illuminates calling as

a mode of discourse. The call of conscience has the character of summoning Dasein to its ownmost potentiality-of-being-a-self, by summoning it to its ownmost quality of being a lack. . . . In the tendency toward disclosure of the call lies the factor of a jolt, which in stopping us has also the character of an abrupt arousal. The call calls from afar to afar. It reaches him who wants to be brought back. . . . What is summoned? Evidently Dasein itself. (pp. 249–253)

As we have seen according to the insights of Marcel, the call is a clearing, an opening, and an availability. But it is also more than that; it is a clearing opened for discourse and covenant. The call and the response to the call constitute a dialogue that takes place within the self. In the stories of Allison and Gloria the call comes as the imperative to make meaning of an apparently meaningless situation. But meaning cannot be made by continuing in the usual manner of being and doing. Great losses require deep, prolonged, and expansive searches to heal. Losses must be moved out beyond the confines of the personal psychological realm to embrace the ontological as well. Nouwen (1996) grasps the significance of this insight when he says that healing the wounds inflicted by adversity is an invitation to move from consideration of one's own pain to be in solidarity with the pain of a common humanity. It is an invitation to find in life a reason to care, some sense of connectedness to others—a way of bearing witness to others' suffering, a manner of participating, a cause that beckons, something larger than oneself.

Unable to respond to the call as an invitation to care and to be in solidarity with others, Gloria and Allison show in their stories, as we have seen, a sense of stagnation, of little or no movement. Rather, they continue to experience themselves as bereft, betrayed, bewildered, ill-equipped, insubstantial, and even unrecognizable. Understanding themselves to be determined by the ravages of fate, they cannot assume ownership of their own lives. Their experience is of being robbed of their possibilities and becoming victims of circumstance. The worlds of Allison and Gloria have become small, narrow, dismal places—places where little is expected of life except more of the same. Significantly, and in contrast to the stories of other participants, Allison and Gloria do not relate experiences in which they reached new insights and were accompanied through treacherous territory by helpful and loving guides. One wonders how life might have been different for them if "asymmetrical gifts" in the form of extravagant loving and caring acts—acts that did not seek recompense—had arrived at the right time. Would new insights have presented themselves, insights that allowed for "recollection" rather than the capitulation of the self?

The stories of others, however, reveal the capacity to notice subtle signs and to be aware of inner resonances that reveal landmarks along the way. Gradually, meaning and direction arrive, but they do not arrive attractively packaged and fully assembled. They turn up fraught with frustration amid the temptation to despair. Yet, as the stories below reveal, attuned listening and a sense of what really counts or matters in life can propel the open, hearing dweller into territory that may be distinctive, challenging, risky, evocative, tender, selfless, poignant, and healing.

As has already been discussed, the call to make meaning amid one's situation cannot be heard by escaping the circumstances at hand but rather by maintaining amid the circumstances a patient enduring and an expectant alertness. This open, willing, attentive enduring weaves new threads into a life-tapestry that has been ravaged by loss. Younger (1995) says that to suffer is to endure, hold out, resist, or sustain. A threat to self or personal identity often brings about the conditions that are necessary, although not sufficient, for an experience of meaning. Suffering brings one close to one's own existence; it makes the self present to the self as a self. Adversity damages the tapestry of the self such that new patterns and figures may need to be woven. Even the background landscape may need to be altered, yet with the reweaving the tapestry achieves a new unity, power, and poignant beauty not in spite of its damage but because it has transcended damage. In hearing and responding to the call there is a sense of deliberately and consciously choosing a new path, but there is also a sense of being chosen or "called" to a different, clearer, deeper, and larger purpose in life. This is experienced as becoming more fully present to one's life and is accompanied by a deepened sense of belonging and caring for others.

Harold tells of finding a gift in the midst of grieving the loss of his son, who committed suicide. The gift comes in the form of a plea from his daughter-in-law that he become her father.

When we brought his body back for the funeral, his wife Susan decided to come too. She had come from a pretty rough background—drinking, fighting, poverty. . . . She was amazed at what she saw when she came up here. For days our friends and family poured into the house, food arrived, people came to sit with us and comfort us. She'd never seen anything like that before and said she wanted us to adopt her into our family. At first I thought she was kidding, but she was serious. So I said "Sure you can be part of our family." Now she comes up here (from the States) for her vacation. We go down there to visit her. . . . [S]he is getting through it, and so are we. I will never get over missing my son, but I can say now that not everything was lost. She has a family and we have a new daughter.

Fiona tells of her discovery that self-healing and meaning in life come from helping others:

Some people ask me how I can do this kind of volunteer work (visit the elderly in nursing homes and the sick in hospital). They think that it must be very depressing and that I must be some kind of saint to do it but I tell them "Don't think too much about it. I really do it for myself." They are kind of surprised when I say that but it's the truth. I found when my marriage ended and my daughter died that I could be overcome with bitterness or I could find a way to help other people who were as scared and sad as I was.

Abraham, in a wonderful example of "resolute dwelling" that transforms bad into good, tells of losing his only son, who was also his best friend. His son was blown up in a bus by a suicide bomber in the Israeli–Palestinian conflict.

I felt that my life had stopped completely, that everything was over for me. I am a religious person, so I had really big questions about where God was in all of this. God seemed cruel and far, far away. I became terribly depressed; I couldn't do anything. I couldn't eat. I couldn't sleep. I couldn't make any sense of it at all. I wanted to die just to be with my son again. Then one day I was reading the book of Job [Hebrew scripture]. . . . [Job] loses his possessions, his family, everything. But he says to God, "Even though you seem to want to kill me, I am going to trust you." I thought that this is what I have to do. . . . So I say to myself, every day I am trusting you. I am not giving up. I am trusting you. I am not giving up and then one day, it starts to make sense to me. I am watching TV. I see Palestinian people weeping and wailing because their sons have been killed by Israeli soldiers. Their coffins are being carried through the streets and suddenly it just hits me. They feel just as bad as I do. Their hearts are breaking just like mine, and I feel so close to them. They are not my enemies; they are my brothers and sisters! And then I know what I have to do. I go to a Palestinian family and I say to them that I am so, so sorry and I tell them that I lost my son too, and then we just all sit down and we weep together. . . . It is like we share one broken heart together. Then we embrace and . . . then the idea takes root. . . . We have to ask more Israeli and Palestinian families to get together and try to find a way to stop the war. Now we have formed an organization for Palestinian and Israeli families who have lost children and want the war to stop.

Sarah and her husband, who struggled with how to "be" in the face of their daughter's choices, describe seeing things in a different light:

We have more insight with regards [to] our own decisions—what makes us happy, more compassion for others, and less need for control (which is an illusion). . . . We see how much of our lives [was] lived for the approval and admiration of others, and try to recognize these traits when they appear in our decisions now. Now, when we meet with adversity, unwanted changes or hardships, we can sometimes remember that there may be an opportunity here to learn or some unexpected gains.

Solomon (2001), who has experienced three life-threatening encounters with clinical depression, relates how this adversity changed him and showed him how precious life is:

A thinner and finer thing has happened to my self; it won't take the kind of punching that it used to take, and little windows go right through it, but there are also passages that are fine and delicate and luminous as [an] egg. To regret my depression now would be to regret the most fundamental part of myself. . . . I impose my vulnerabilities on others far too readily, but I think I am also more generous to other people than I used to be. . . . Since I have been to the Gulag and survived it, I know that if I have to go to the Gulag again, I could survive that also. I'm more confident, in some odd way, than I've ever imagined being. This almost (but not quite) makes the depression seem worth it. I do not think that I will never again try to kill myself; nor do I think that I would give up my life readily if I found myself in war, or if my plane crashed into a desert. I would struggle tooth and nail to survive. It's as though my life and I, having sat in opposition to each other, hating each other, wanting to escape each other, have now bonded forever and at the hip. (p. 440)

Following Marcel, it has been shown that adversity as calling constitutes a covenant that is both a giving and a binding. Adversity as calling is also a discourse in which the self connects with and is called to from its utmost potentiality of being. The call is a call neither to distance oneself from suffering nor to seek to camouflage it nor to assert control over it. The call is to yield to, abide with, and come into an intimate relationship with life's inevitable losses and suffering. This intimate yielding is a patient, hopeful, relaxed dwelling with such that the alienation characteristic of adversity is transformed into connection and belonging. Pain and suffering come to be seen not as things that separate one from life and cause one to feel depleted, lost, and abandoned but as those that establish significance, convey direction, and unite one with a common humanity. Seen from this vantage point, captivity and exile become teacher, and the self becomes learner. Admittedly, change does bring danger and loss, but danger and loss also bring possibilities for deeper meaning, clearer direction, and nobler purposes in life. Living life fully is learning to dwell resolutely in the turning of disruption and disjuncture and listening attentively for the call to one's utmost potentiality and unique purpose in life.

Implications for Healthcare Practice

In this concluding section I bring the parts of this study together and, in keeping with the hermeneutical interpretive tradition, generate a unified text in order to ask how the new understandings generated by this study speak to practitioners of care.

Adversity almost invariably brings individuals into contact with healthcare systems, either because the health problem itself constitutes the adversity or because disease and illness are commonly associated with experiences of hardship, breakdown, and loss. Of the 20 stories and conversations gathered for this study, 12 involve personal experiences of physiological symptoms, disease processes, or loss of function as a result of accident. Such health problems include traumatic injury and diagnoses of cancer, lupus, and liver cirrhosis. Significantly, all the stories in which the adversity is seen as a loss of physical health show diminishment of spiritual and psychological well-being, manifested in such emotional experiences as severe depression, suicidal ideation, wishing for death, fear, anger, anxiety, shame, and marked restlessness and dissatisfaction with life. In the remaining 8 stories and conversations that do not disclose an experience of adversity as a personal health problem per se but rather as an experience in which a spouse, child, or close friend either dies or encounters serious setbacks or health problems, suffering is revealed. The intense experiences in relation to the loss of—and losses experienced by—important others include death of a spouse or child and depression or serious illness of (or separation from) a spouse, child, parent, or sibling. Whether the stories are of personal encounters with disease or loss of well-being associated with deaths and serious setbacks experienced by family members and close friends, it is clear that adversity dislodges the structures of life. The disruption constitutes a severe assault on health and well-being. Restoring health and well-being necessitates coming to an acceptable understanding of the event(s) in relation to the overall direction and purpose of one's life (Eifried, 1998; Frank, 1995; Younger, 1995). Healing involves the restoration of meaning.

It is significant that in the stories healthcare professionals were frequently but not always helpfully encountered. Participants described how some healthcare professionals seemed to intuitively grasp the possibilities in the situation, while others seemed caught up in their habitual ways of being and doing. Some were seen as potentially intrusive or as unwittingly concealing the possibilities at hand. Still other stories revealed the limitations of professional help in the face of human agency when, for example, a decision was taken to refuse professional help or when the lack of desire to live thwarted all professional attempts to intervene.

Sarah tells how health professionals helped her and her family to gain perspective on how to preserve what was important in the face of her daughter's apparently destructive behavior: "They certainly helped us in understanding ourselves and learning to protect what was left of our family from her. For that we will be eternally grateful."

Katrina describes her encounters with health professionals who aggressively treated her husband, who was dying, and who were either completely oblivious or unable to respond to the profound human needs in the situation:

When asked bluntly, "Is he dying?" the doctor always answered with hope, talking of new treatments, and how Daniel had improved from the day before. I didn't see the improvement and I wondered if his children from a previous marriage should be called to his bedside. But the medical staff knew best, didn't they? My husband died . . . alone. We were not prepared.

Her story causes us to ponder how the lack of acceptance of dying by health professionals and their preoccupation with delivering ever more "treatments" protect them from experiencing powerlessness in the face of death. We also see how the emotional unavailability of healthcare professionals isolates the sufferer, driving the suffering ever deeper (Eifried, 1998; Eriksson, 1997).

Helen, on the other hand, helps us to understand that there are times when patients are not ready to accept help, even when it does seem appropriate:

I saw a psychiatrist, and numerous types of antidepressants were tried. I also saw a chronic pain specialist. Nothing helped. . . . Some days I longed for death. Then one day it came to me that nobody could help me if I didn't want to live and wasn't willing to help myself.

By returning to the stories we see that, while health professionals may have been important catalysts in the quest for meaning, participants did not usually place them in the role of main protagonist. Family members, friends, colleagues, neighbors, and fellow parishioners were given a central and constituting role. Harold says, "When we brought his [son's] body back for the funeral . . . [f]or days our friends and family poured into the house, food arrived, people came to sit with us and comfort us." If these stories disclose that family and friends, rather than health professionals, play a central role in helping people get through adversity, then what supporting role can health professionals play in the restoration of meaning? In considering these questions five insights arrive.

The first insight is that we as health professionals can aid the work of suffering by understanding how to be skillfully present. While we need to acknowledge that we can never replace family members, close friends, and neighbors, we can "stand in" temporarily and compassionately until ongoing help arrives. By being present to hear the laments of our patients and their families and by bearing witness to their suffering, we cannot take their suffering away, but we can help to address a source of profound human anguish—the sense of being lost, uncared for, and alone (Younger, 1995). When we are available to our patients in a way that invites them to express their suffering, when we do not hide behind our technical expertise, and when we find opportunities to have healing conversations with patients and their families, we help them to understand each other better and to sustain each other's existence (Frank, 1995; Tapp, 2001). Making suffering endurable, we bring the anguish to expression, thereby offering passage from the bleak isolation of mute suffering to a place where there is hope of connection and belonging. Benso (2000) helps us to understand that such connections can never be imposed; they can be reached only by way of receptive, humble attentiveness:

[Attending] can be successful and can avoid falling into invasiveness only if it lets itself be directed by that toward [which] it tends; if it folds itself upon itself, hollows its activity out, and makes itself passive. . . . Attention waits for the other to make the first move, the first offer to which it will respond. . . . Humility is an act of love of the one who lets herself or himself be taken by the hand and be led by things. (pp. 164–165)

Thus we see that the helpfulness of health professionals resides in their capacity to call forth the conditions in which meaning can be restored. Such conditions involve inviting expressions of suffering while maintaining a tender, receptive openness to the possibilities for human connection in the situation at hand.

As we recognize that when we accompany another we must, following Benso, allow ourselves to be led, and as we consider that such attentiveness inaugurates relationship and connection, a second insight arrives. This is that generous accompaniment and befriending of others who are suffering can be an important part of the healing process for some people who are seeking to make sense of their lives following a confrontation with major threat and loss. The stories of Fiona, whose marriage ended and whose daughter died, and Abraham, whose son was killed by a bomb, speak eloquently of the relief that can come from finding a deep connectivity with others who suffer. Hall (2001) comes to similar conclusions in his research about how AIDS volunteerism enabled those affected by HIV/AIDS to find meaning in their suffering. Specifically, it should be acknowledged that one who has never experienced the adverse phenomenon (whatever it might be) can never have as much insight into the nature of the suffering as one who has. Release from suffering seems to be found in this place of deep connectivity, mutual recognition, and solidarity in suffering. Befriending another and thereby becoming a conveyor of connection and meaning not only seem to offer personal healing but may also offer powerful protection against meaninglessness.

The third insight relates to the understanding that people who are reconstructing their lives following a major loss may be changing in fundamental ways as priorities undergo radical reordering. Recall that Sarah, in learning to dwell with the loss of her hopes and dreams for her daughter, goes from being an exemplar of middle-class respectability and achievement to being an ordinary and worried parent who first wants to hide from sight but then learns to share her burden with friends who care. Abraham risks social ostracism by finding a deep common bond with his supposed enemies. As health professionals we need to understand that people who go through overwhelming adversity are people who may be changing in very profound ways. Helpful accompaniment by practitioners of care is not about patching people up and returning them to life the way it was before the crisis. It is about helping people to dwell toward meaning—to reach beyond themselves—and it is about helping them to understand who they are becoming.

A fourth insight comes from reflecting on the presence of the mysterious and sacred in the stories of those who were able to dwell resolutely. In considering how powerful these experiences were in enabling people to dwell hopefully, patiently, and expectantly, I wonder how healthcare would be different if, amid all of our diagnoses and prognostications, we truly left room for the miraculous and surprising. This is not to suggest abandonment of the empirical and rational but to argue for a respectful, even appreciative, coexistence between that which can be predicted and controlled and that which is undeniably uncertain, indefinite, and intangible. Could there be a place for healing rituals, grace, and prayer in what is considered "best practice"? What if we were able to see in the wounding of the body and mind not only a danger to be covered over as quickly as possible with all the technical know-how available but also, like adversity itself, an opening to new possibilities? Despite our massive knowledge, sophisticated systems, best-practice guidelines, and good intentions, there is much that we don't know, can't control, and need to let be so that possibilities arrive and are not instead closed down.

A fifth insight comes from recognizing the important role of suffering in the process of reaching meaning, freedom, and liberation. By this statement I mean neither to valorize suffering nor to advocate for the cessation of valid and necessary medical treatments. In achieving a balance between looking to and beyond human technology, I am reminded of Solomon's (2001) insights. He strongly urges people to learn as much as possible about psychopharmacological approaches to treating depression so that they can insist on the most up-to-date and appropriate treatments. He inserts, however, an important caveat. Obtaining good psychopharmacological treatment is not to be pursued with the intent of replacing or relinquishing the search for meaning. Rather, it is done with a view to augmenting, energizing, and sustaining the search for meaning in life. Technological advances, including psychopharmacological strategies, may conceal what it means to be human if health professionals approach the loss of meaning in life simply as evidence of chemical imbalance to be rectified. Coming to a new and acceptable meaning necessitates dwelling with suffering rather than denying, distancing, or controlling it. Tillich (1955/2005) helps us to understand that healing does not involve suppression of suffering or diminishing the awareness of conflict and dissonance. Rather, healing strengthens the whole so that within the unity of the body the struggling elements can be reconciled. He offers that healing encounters, whether they be with health professionals or with friends,

aid the healing powers of our soul. They accept us as we are and make it possible to look at ourselves honestly and with clarity, to realize the strange mechanisms under which we are suffering and to dissolve them, reconciling the genuine forces of our soul with each other and making us free for thought and action. (Tillich, 1955/2005, pp. 39–40)

As has been discussed at length, finding meaning in adversity is an experience that ultimately must be brought home, befriended, engaged with intimately, dwelt with resolutely, listened to attentively, and acted upon assertively. Only in this way can the existential possibilities be revealed in terms of who one is and who one can be.

Contributions and Future Directions

Hermeneutical phenomenology is best suited to answering questions about the meaning of human issues and concerns. Because people were invited to "self-select" for participation in this study and the stories gathered were self-authored, it is possible that the stories obtained were skewed in favor of those who found deeper meanings in adversity. Accordingly, it could be argued, those who experienced ongoing loss of meaning or meaninglessness were underrepresented in this study. In addition, the approach used for this study was for the most part retrospective in nature, that is, it gathered reflections more on past experiences than in vivo experiences of ongoing adversity. While this retrospective methodological approach was sufficient to clearly illuminate overall patterns of meaning, it is inadequate for the purposes of tracing minutely the oscillations of everyday dwelling that a prospective study would have revealed. A prospective study stretching over a three-year span that explored people's thoughts and feelings as they lived through adversity might, for example, reveal time- or phase-related dimensions of dwelling as alternating patterns of resigned and resolute dwelling.

Despite these constraints and acknowledging fundamental differences in how knowledge of the human experience can be grasped, this study does resonate with the findings of some empirical studies. In keeping with the work of Brown (1996, 1997), this study affirms that the challenges posed by adversity and the "outcomes" that ensue in relation to it cannot be fully explained with reference to the event itself or in relation to the preexisting personality characteristics of the person undergoing the event. Rather, the challenges posed by adversity reside in the meaning given to the event. This study takes this concept a step farther and illuminates an understanding that it is not merely the meaning given to the event that can be understood in relation to how life unfolds but also the manner of dwelling amid the circumstances that transforms the meaning and alters the life course. Sandler (2001) argues that in order for health professionals to understand how to assist people undergoing adversity, a better understanding of the nature of adversity itself and of the resources that people call upon to become resilient in the face of adversity is required. It is in addressing this particular gap in knowledge that this study makes its contribution.

What is naturally occurring resilience? I offer one definition: the human capacity to dwell resolutely in the face of that which cannot be changed. Accepting such a definition of resilience and using a phenomenological approach to understanding its experience overcomes myriad problems that have assailed the body of work now referred to as resilience research. It does this by skirting the doomed attempts to separate process from outcome and by sidestepping decisions about how much adversity "counts" in relation to quantifiable measures of coping well or coping poorly. Consider that Solomon, despite three bouts with clinical depression, is resilient not because he has conquered mental illness once and for all but because he has come into a patient, intimate, and ongoing abiding with depression. He has made a home of his journey, and he continuously and perseveringly brings his pain home.

Considering that "resolute dwellers" in this study have in many cases described the importance of sustaining friendships that provide a sense of acceptance and a reason to persevere, future study related to naturally occurring resilience could focus in depth on the naturally occurring phenomena of persevering friendships and restorative relationships. Bringing to voice the stories of people who open themselves up to others who suffer and describing how they find the strength to remain present in the face of overwhelming devastation and discouragement could be a particularly compelling avenue of inquiry. Along similar lines, future study could include the phenomenon of volunteerism (Hall, 2001). Asking whether and how the voluntary act of befriending offers a bulwark against meaninglessness and provides a way of recovering meaning in an otherwise meaningless terrain, the experience of not only the befriended but also the befriender could be studied. Finally, and considering the concerns raised by Mahoney (2005) that professional programs are not preparing their graduates to engage skillfully and compassionately with their clients, fruitful avenues of inquiry could take shape.

These studies, ultimately directed at the overhaul of curricula, might begin with trying to understand how to assist students in the "helping professions" to learn to dwell patiently, humbly, and attentively with the suffering person. As knowledge accrued, pedagogies related to suffering could emerge. It is doubtful that such pedagogies could be developed successfully without first revamping curricula to integrate substantive philosophical content. Engaging with the profound questions raised by philosophy about what it means to be human and to suffer would offer academicians and students alike an opportunity for deep reflection, intense dialogue, and meaningful research. In this way our discourses could be refreshed and our professions revitalized.

Conclusion

As I draw this study to a close I realize that I have merely skimmed the surface of how meaning may be found in adversity. What is clear is that I have learned a great deal from the experiences of people who so generously shared their stories. To them I owe a great debt. Not only did they help me to understand how meaning can be found in adversity, but they also stimulated further thought about how to approach life, dwelling resolutely and yielding gracefully in the face of its inevitable upswings and downturns. To find meaning in one's circumstances is, according to Rupp (2005),

> To be grateful for what is,
> Instead of underscoring what is not.
> To find good amid the unwanted aspects of life,
> Without denying the presence of the unwanted.
> To focus on beauty in the little things of life,
> As well as being deliberate about the great beauties of art, literature,
>   music, and nature.
> To be present to one's own small space of life,
> While stretching to the wide world beyond it.
> To find something to laugh about every day,
> Even when there seems nothing to laugh about.
> To search for and see the good in others,
> Rather than remembering their faults and weaknesses.
> To be thankful for each loving deed done by another,
> No matter how insignificant it might appear.
> To taste life to the fullest, and not to take any part of it for granted.
> To seek to forgive others for their wrongdoings,
> Even immense ones, and to put the past behind.
> To find ways to reach out and help the disenfranchised,
> While also preserving their dignity and self-worth.
> To be as loving and caring as possible,
> In a culture that consistently challenges these virtues.
> To remember to say "thank you"
> For whatever comes as a gift from another.
> To be at peace
> With what cannot be changed.

Notes

This paper is based on the following doctoral dissertation: Johnston, N. (2003). *Finding meaning in adversity. Dissertation Abstracts International, 65* (01). (UMI No. AAT NQ86530)

1. Mahoney (2005, p. 338) asserts that psychology has perpetuated five mistakes that have been inherited from philosophical thought. These include the reification of mind–body dualism, the assertion that reason (rationality) is primary and more powerful than emotions and bodily experience, the glorification of the search for certainty and justification, the corruption of the scientific spirit, and the erosion of excellence in education and the academy.

2. Heidegger (1953/1996) suggests that, in questioning and interpreting, our task is "never to allow our fore-having, fore-sight and fore-conception to be presented to us by fancies and popular conceptions but to make the scientific theme secure by working out these fore-structures in terms of the things themselves" (p. 153).

3. Richardson (2002, p. 310) offers a useful synthesis of this genre of literature that describes resilient qualities. Qualities include happiness, subjective well-being, optimism, faith, self-determination, wisdom, excellence, and creativity. In the same article he quotes a special issue of the *Journal of Social and Clinical Psychology* (2000) devoted to research on the strengths, virtues, and positive characteristics associated with resilience. Research is described in relation to the following qualities: morality, self-control, gratitude, forgiveness, dreams, hope, and humility.

4. Among the notions guiding this genre of thought are the ideas that personal growth is a choice in the wake of disruption, that the strengthening of one's access to spiritual sources may accompany reintegration, that adversity may provide the solution to stagnation in life, that searching for a silver lining offers a way to reinterpret the meaning of adversity, and that adversity may come to be seen as a valuable experience.

5. I use the term *story* advisedly here. While the word *story* was used to invite conversations and encourage people to write about an experience of adversity, it soon became clear that those who chose to write stories rather than to engage in a series of conversations were really writing narratives. When I questioned the seven people who wrote stories about what their experiences of writing were like, they remarked that, although the writing was difficult and caused them to relive a difficult time in their lives, it helped them to clarify some things. Wiltshire (1995) offers useful distinctions regarding the increasing levels of reflection and meaning making involved in conversation, telling a story, producing a narrative, and writing a life history. As I thought about the level of reflection involved in moving from a conversation to a narrative, it became clear to me that the people who engaged in a series of conversations with me were using the conversations as a way to put their experiences into perspective, that is, to transform their stories into coherent narratives. For ways in which healing spaces can be constructed so that conversations can become healing narratives see Baker and Diekelmann (1994); Canales (1997); and Tapp (2001).

6. Madison's (1988, pp. 29–30) nine criteria are
    1. coherence—the interpretation presents a unified picture and does not contradict itself; if contradictions exist in the text itself, the interpretation makes sense of these contradictions;

2. comprehensiveness—the interpretation presents a unified picture of the thoughts of the author as a whole;

3. penetration—the interpretation brings out the underlying intention of the author as an attempt to resolve a central *problematique;*

4. thoroughness—the interpretation answers or deals with all the questions that it poses to the interpreted text or that the text poses to the interpreter's understanding of it;

5. appropriateness—the questions the interpretation deals with are ones raised by the text itself; that is, the interpreter avoids using the text to deal with his or her own questions rather than the questions the author was concerned with;

6. contextuality—the author's thoughts must not be taken out of context, that is, without due regard for the circumstances and the historical, social context in which the author was situated;

7. agreement—the interpretation agrees or fits with what the author is saying; this means that the interpreter does not attempt a "hermeneutic of suspicion" whereby the author's words are disregarded as not disclosing what was really intended;

8. suggestiveness—the interpretation is fertile in that it suggests questions that stimulate further research and interpretation; and

9. potential—the interpretation is capable of being extended in that it reveals implications that relate in a harmonious way to each other.

7. By using the word *lending* I mean to convey the notion of allowing the self to be borrowed temporarily by a coercive experience. There is thus the sense that loss of meaning accompanying coercive experience is temporary, and the expectation or hope still remains that at some later point meaning will arrive and will be experienced as the return or retrieval of the self from such a lending.

8. Polkinghorne (1988) writes:

> The plot functions to transform a chronicle or listing of events into a schematic whole by highlighting and recognizing the contribution that certain events make to the development and outcome of the story. Without the recognition of significance given by the plot, each event would appear as discontinuous and separate, and its meaning would be limited. (p. 19)

I suggest that in an experience of adversity the plotline breaks down and events are experienced as discontinuous and separate—chaotic. Thus the challenge in an experience of adversity is to reinvent one's personal plotline so that events that are experienced as random, discontinuous, and meaningless can be woven together to constitute a unifying narrative. For an understanding of the use of narrative in helping people reconstruct their "plotlines" see Fredriksson & Eriksson (2001).

References

Baker, C., & Diekelmann, N. (1994). Connecting conversations of caring: Recalling the narrative to clinical practice. *Nursing Outlook, 42,* 65–70.

Benso, S. (2000). The face of things: A different side of ethics. Albany, NY: State University of New York Press.

Bentley Mays, J. (1995). *In the jaws of the black dogs: A memoir of depression.* Toronto: Penguin.

Brown, G. W. (1996). Social factors and co-morbidity of depressive and anxiety disorders. *British Journal of Psychiatry, 168*(30), 50–57.

Brown, G. W. (1997). Loss and depressive disorders. In B. P. Dohrenwend (Ed.), *Adversity, stress and psychopathology* (pp. 42–68). Washington, DC: American Psychiatric Press.

Canales, M. (1997). Narrative interaction: Creating a space for therapeutic conversation. *Issues in Mental Health Nursing, 18,* 477–494.

Cassell, E. J. (1982). The nature of suffering and the goals of medicine. *New England Journal of Medicine, 306,* 639–645.

Celan, P. (1995). *Poems of Paul Celan* (M. L. Hamburger, Trans.). New York: Persea Books.

Copp, L. A. (1990a). The nature and prevention of suffering. *Journal of Professional Nursing, 6,* 247–249.

Copp, L. A. (1990b). The spectrum of suffering. *American Journal of Nursing, 90,* 35–39.

Copp, L. A. (1990c). Treatment, torture, suffering and compassion. *Journal of Professional Nursing, 6,* 1–2.

Dane, D. (2002, April 6). Dark past, bright future: An abuse survivor rebuilds his life and strives to change a system that fails to protect children. *Toronto Star,* p. L4.

Devito, J. (2001). The faces of hope. *Guideposts: True stories of hope and inspiration, 4*(10), 17–23.

Eifried, S. (1998). Helping patients find meaning: A caring response to suffering. *International Journal for Human Caring, 2*(1), 33–39.

Eriksson, K. (1997). Caring, spirituality and suffering. In M. S. Roach (Ed.), *Caring from the heart: The convergence of caring and spirituality* (pp. 68–84). Mahwah, NJ: Paulist Press.

Frank, A. W. (1995). *The wounded storyteller: Body, illness and ethics.* Chicago: University of Chicago Press.

Fredriksson, L., & Eriksson, K. (2001). The patient's narrative of suffering—a path to health: An interpretive research synthesis on narrative understanding. *Scandinavian Journal of Caring Science, 15,* 3–11.

Gadamer, H.-G. (1989). *Truth and method* (2nd ed.). New York: Continuum. (Original work published 1960)

Gadow, G. (1991). Suffering and interpersonal meaning. *Journal of Clinical Ethics, 2,* 103–107.

Gallagher, K. T. (1975). *The philosophy of Gabriel Marcel.* New York: Fordham University Press.

Garmezy, N., & Masten, A. S. (1994). Chronic adversities. In M. Rutter, L. Herzov, & E. Taylor (Eds.), *Child and adolescent psychiatry* (3rd ed., pp. 191–208). Oxford: Blackwell.

Goldstein, M. A. (2000). *Travels with the wolf: A story of chronic illness.* Columbus: Ohio State University Press.

Grondin, J. (1990). Hermeneutics and relativism. In K. Wright (Ed.), *Festivals of interpretation: Essays on Hans-Georg Gadamer's work* (pp. 42–62). New York: State University of New York Press.

Hall, V. P. (2001). Bearing witness to suffering in AIDS: Constructing meaning from loss. *Journal of the Association of Nurses in AIDS Care, 12*(2), 44–55.

Heidegger, M. (1996). *Being and time* (J. Stambaugh, Trans.). Albany: State University of New York Press. (Original work published 1953)

Kahn, D. L. & Steeves, R. H. (1986). The experience of suffering: Conceptual clarification and theoretical definition. *Journal of Advanced Nursing, 11,* 623–631.

Kahn, D. L., & Steeves, R. H. (1995). The significance of suffering in cancer care. *Seminars in Oncology Nursing, 11,* 9–16.

Kierkegaard, S. (1989). *Fear and trembling/repetition* (H. Hong & E. Hong, Trans.). Princeton, NJ: Princeton University Press. (Original work published 1849)

Koch, T. (1995). Interpretive approaches in nursing research: The influence of Husserl and Heidegger. *Journal of Advanced Nursing, 21,* 827–836.

Kockelmans, J. J. (1984). *On the truth of being: Reflections on Heidegger's later philosophy.* Bloomington: Indiana University Press.

Kockelmans, J. J. (1985). The self and Kant's conception of the ego. In F. Elliston (Ed.), *Heidegger's existential analytic.* New York: Mouton.

Kohut, H. (1977). *The restoration of the self.* New York: International Universities.

Kohut, H. (1984). *How does analysis cure?* Chicago: University of Chicago Press.

Lazarus, R. S. (1999). *Stress and emotion: A new synthesis.* New York: Springer.

Madison, G. B. (1988). *The hermeneutics of postmodernity: Figures and themes.* Indianapolis: Indiana University Press.

Madison, G. B. (1994). Hermeneutics: Gadamer and Ricoeur. In R. Kearney (Ed.), *Routledge history of philosophy: Vol. 8. Continental philosophy in the 20th century* (pp. 290–349). London: Routledge.

Mahoney, M. J. (2005). Suffering, philosophy and psychotherapy. *Journal of Psychotherapy Integration, 15,* 337–352.

Marcel, G. (1951). *Being and having* (K. Farrer, Trans.). Boston: Beacon Press.

Marcel, G. (1960). *The mystery of being: Reflection and mystery.* Chicago: Henry Regnery.

Marcel, G. (1963). *Homo viator: Introduction to a metaphysic of hope.* New York: Harper.

Marcel, G. (1967). *Searching.* Toronto: Newman Press.

Masten, A. W., & Coatsworth, J. D. (1998). The development of competence in favorable and unfavorable environments. *American Psychologist, 53,* 205–221.

Nouwen, H. J. M. (1996). *The inner voice of love: A journey through anguish to freedom.* New York: Doubleday.

Nouwen, H. J. M. (2001). *Turn my mourning into dancing: Finding hope in hard times.* Nashville: Word Publishing.

Orange, D. M. (2000). *Emotional understanding: Studies in psychoanalytic epistemology.* New York: Guilford Press.

Oxford English Dictionary Online. (2005). Oxford University Press. Retrieved August 7, 2005, from http://www.dictionary.oed.com

Picard, C. (1991). Caring and the story: The compelling nature of what must be told and understood in the human dimension of suffering. In D. A. Gaut & M. M. Leininger (Eds.), *Caring: The compassionate healer* (pp. 89–98). New York: National League for Nursing.

Polkinghorne, D. E. (1988). *Narrative knowing and the human sciences.* Albany: State University of New York Press.

Richardson, G. E. (2002). The metatheory of resilience and resiliency theory. *Journal of Clinical Psychology, 58,* 307–321.

Richardson, G. E., Neiger, B., Jensen, S., & Kampfer, K. (1990). The resiliency model. *Health Education, 21,* 38–39.

Rilke, R. M. (1934). Letters to a young poet (3rd ed.; M. D. Herter, Trans.). London: Norton.

Risser, J. (1997). *Hermeneutics and the voice of the other: Re-reading Gadamer's philosophical hermeneutics.* Albany: State University of New York Press.

Rogers, B. L., & Cowles, K. V. (1997). A conceptual foundation of human suffering in nursing care and research. *Journal of Advanced Nursing, 25,* 1048–1053.

Rupp, J. (2005). *The circle of life.* Unpublished manuscript.

Rutter, M. (1985). Resilience in the face of adversity: Protective factors and resistance to psychiatric disorders. *British Journal of Psychiatry, 147,* 598–611.

Sandler, I. (2001). Quality and ecology of adversity as common mechanisms of risk and resilience. *American Journal of Community Psychology, 29,* 1–43.

Schafer, R. (1981). Narration in the psychoanalytic dialogue. In W. J. Mitchell (Ed.), *On narrative.* Chicago: University of Chicago Press.

Schafer, R. (2004). Narrating, attending and empathizing. *Literature and Medicine, 23,* 241–251.

Schweizer, H. (2000). Against suffering: A meditation on literature. *Literature and Medicine 19*(2), 229–240.

Selder, F., Kachoyeanos, M., Baisch, M. J., & Gissler, M. (Eds.). (1997). *Enduring grief: True stories of personal loss.* Philadelphia: Charles Press.

Skinner, E., & Wellborn, J. G. (1994). Coping during childhood and adolescence: A motivational perspective. In P. Featherman, R. Lerner, & M. Perlmutter (Eds.), *Lifespan development* (pp. 91–133). Hillsdale, NJ: Erlbaum.

Solomon, A. (2001). *The noonday demon: An atlas of depression.* Toronto: Schriber.

Steeves, R. H., & Kahn, D. L. (1987). Finding meaning in suffering. *Image: Journal of Nursing Scholarship, 19,* 114–116.

Stern, D. (1991). A philosophy for the embedded analyst: Gadamer's hermeneutics and the social paradigm of psychoanalysis. *Contemporary Psychoanalysis, 27,* 51–58.

Stolorow, R. (1994). The nature and therapeutic action of psychoanalytic interpretation. In R. Stolorow, G. Atwood, & B. Brandshaft (Eds.), *The intersubjective perspective* (pp. 42–55). Northvale, NJ: Jason Aronson.

Stolorow, R., & Atwood, G. (1992). *Contexts of being: The intersubjective foundations of psychological life.* Hillsdale, NJ: Analytic Press.

Stolorow, R. D., Atwood, G. E., & Orange, D. M. (2002). *Worlds of experience: Interweaving philosophical and clinical dimensions in psychoanalysis.* New York: Basic Books.

Tapp, D. M. (2001). Conserving the vitality of suffering: Addressing family constraints in illness conversations. *Nursing Inquiry, 2,* 75–82.

Tillich, P. (2005). *The new being.* Lincoln: University of Nebraska Press. (Original work published 1955)

Werner E. E., & Smith, R. S. (1992). *Overcoming the odds: High risk children from birth to adulthood.* Ithaca, NY: Cornell University Press.

Wiltshire, J. (1995). Telling a story, writing a narrative: Terminology in health care. *Nursing Inquiry, 2,* 75–82.

Wyman, P. A., Sandler, I., Wolchik, S., & Nelson, K. (2000). Resilience as cumulative competence promotion and stress protection: Theory and intervention. In D. Cichetti, J. Rappaport, I. Sandler, & R. Weisburg (Eds.), *Promotion of psychological wellness.* New York: Plenum.

Younger, J. B. (1995). The alienation of the sufferer. *Advances in Nursing Science, 17*(4), 53–72.

4

Narrative Phenomenology

Exploring Stories of Grief and Dying

CRAIG M. KLUGMAN

As a way of putting the death of a loved family member or friend into perspective, people tell stories. They discuss who the deceased person was in life, how the person died, and what their own life has been like since the death. During the conduct of a needs assessment study that inquired about the resources people needed to assist them with grieving and to able to die "well," I became intrigued with the stories people told me. Wondering why people were telling me such stories and what function the stories served, I concluded that telling one's story seemed to be a way of bringing order out of the chaos that ensues from a loss (Becker, 1997). Reflecting on the stories that emerged from clinical practice, I noted that narratives enabled a patient to share an experience with another who did not have direct access to the experience. Through stories clinicians learn not only about symptoms and perceived causes but also about the meaning that these things hold for the patient (Good, 1994). Since stories enable healthcare professionals to gain an understanding of their patients' lived experiences and enable empathy and diverse human engagement, stories offer clinicians a way of enriching their practice.

Narrative Theory

The telling of narratives—whether through oral storytelling or through published books—is a fundamental human activity that allows conversations and experiences to be shared among people and, often, across cultures (White, 1981). Humans use narrative to structure experience, order memory, connect to other people, and build a life history (Bruner, 1987). Narrative humanizes time and action so that people can comprehend events and deal with their emotions (Richardson, 1990). Anthropologist Byron Good (1994) calls this process of constructing a story *narrativizing,* "a process of locating suffering in history, of placing events in a meaningful order in time" (p. 128). In healthcare practice it is evident that patients use narrative to make sense of their illness and to integrate its experience into their life (Good, 1994; Kleinman, 1988). Healthcare providers employ narrative to learn about a patient's illness through empathy, to recognize their own personal medical stories, to connect with other healthcare professionals, and to talk with patients about healthcare (Charon, 2001).

Broadly conceived, narrative is a series of interpreted events connected through time, within which one or more characters change or react to change (Ricoeur, 1981a). A narrative is a text that attempts to make sense of the lived reality of certain characters as they progress temporally from one event to another. Narratives are "kinds of discourse organized around the passage of time in some 'world'" (Polanyi, 1985, p. 10). Norman Denzin (1989) defines narrative as "a story, having a plot and existence separate from [the] life of [the] teller" (p. 48). Philosopher Paul Ricoeur (1981a) explains that a narrative should be "self sufficient," complete without additional explanation or comment. Donald Polkinghorne (1996) defines narrative as "a storied linguistic production of a person's emplotted configuration of life events into episodes or a whole life" (p. 78). According to the *Oxford English Dictionary Online* (2001), *narrative* derives from the Latin *narrare,* which means "to relate, recount, give an account of."

Although some narratives may be told in order to entertain, others are presented for a specific purpose, such as to comment on the world or an experience (White, 1981). "*Stories* are told to make a point, to transmit a message—often some sort of moral evaluation or implied critical judgment—about the world the teller shares with other people" (Polanyi, 1985, p. 12). For example, a narrative may be told to educate, to complain, to motivate, to inform, to sway, or to elicit sympathy and hope. Humans use narrative to transmit ideas, thoughts, knowledge, culture, opinion, and experience, both personal and social.

Ricoeur has had a strong influence on the development of anthropo-
logical narrative theory. His writing attempted to create a philosophical
anthropology that combined phenomenological description with hermeneutic interpretation. From his foundations social scientists have further
developed his work to create the richness of narrative theory. Narrative
has been widely used in qualitative research as a method for knowing
the experience of another. Anthropologists such as Byron Good, Clifford
Geertz, Arthur Kleinman, Sharon Kaufman, and Barbara Myerhoff have
interviewed their participants to learn their life narratives. Narrative is a
method that allows an outsider an inside glimpse into the meaning of
another's world. "Narrative has been viewed as a useful, expansive tool
by those scholars wishing to articulate, from details of the native's point
of view, how individuals construct meanings and negotiate their worlds"
(Kaufman, 2000, p. 341). These tales allow a researcher to see not only
what events have transpired in a community or in the life of an individual
but also the meanings and interpretations that the group or person places
on the events.

My goal in this project was to analyze and interpret narratives of
dying told by witnesses. Heidegger (1977) asserts that we can only describe the dying process, as the person who dies cannot describe the experience of death. I was interested in applying a narrative framework
to examine oral storytelling to discern why people tell these stories. Telling these stories can assist people in their grief work, a process that enables them to reconnect to the community, to reestablish self-identity, and
to facilitate the construction of new experiences. The healthcare practitioner can encourage these stories to be told, thereby gaining an understanding of their importance to the grieving process. This understanding
can enable the healthcare practitioner to engage more meaningfully with
patients and can help grieving persons move forward to create a new life.

In the course of this narrative inquiry into the experiences of dying
as related by family members or friends, I conducted 15 interviews with
participants of various ages. Such narratives can be read on their own for
style, voice, and some lessons about living and dying. However, such a
reading would simply be a "thin description," a superficial approach that
assumes that the surface meaning is the only meaning of the words or actions (Geertz, 1973). Instead, I propose a "deep description" that considers from their own perspectives the culture, history, mythology, psychology, literature, and beliefs of individuals rooted within a culture. As

Heidegger (1927/1964) would say, the participants were "always already" in a culture, and their narratives reflect their own lived experiences.

Much has been written about ways to interpret a transcript. Peacock and Holland (1993) advocate interpretation of text through a process approach. Their method considers how narratives both construct and reflect reality by looking at a text from four different perspectives: cultural, psychocultural, hermeneutic, and psychosocial. "The *cultural approach* also views the narrative as outcome, but focuses on more purely cultural or collective dynamics and on narrative as a gripping formulation of beliefs, values, and ideas basic to a cultural tradition" (Peacock & Holland, 1993, p. 373). Thus, to engage narrative on the cultural level is to understand the framework, plots, characters, and themes that run through personal narratives as well as those that are recorded in historical documents or current literature. The *psychocultural* perspective holds that in narrative a person forms the self by drawing on culturally available plots, symbols, and meanings: "The *psychocultural* emphasizes the place of culturally constructed narrative in psychological processes" (Peacock & Holland, 1993, p. 371). The *hermeneutic* approach focuses on the relationship between those who tell their stories and those who listen. Such an approach assumes that the context in which a narrative is told is relevant to understanding the formation and meaning of the account. The interaction between a specific narrator and a particular audience contributes to new understanding of the story that needs to be heard. Tellers are often searching for new hope, new interpretations, and new outcomes (Good, 1994). Heidegger (1927/1964) points out that it is in "breakdown" that people have the opportunity to grasp new meaning about their lives. The *psychosocial* approach sees narrative as a method that creates relationships and defines social identities between individuals. "Studies of self-narrative as events in social as opposed to psychological processes treat narrative as instrumental in the formation and maintenance of social relationships and collective identity" (Peacock & Holland, 1993, p. 372).

Methods

This grief-narrative project emerged from a larger study designed to develop a resource list of grief support services needed for people living in Texas. The larger study was a joint venture of the Institute for Medical

CRAIG M. KLUGMAN

Humanities and the Texas Partnership for End of Life Care. The instrument developed for this study—"Your Opinion Matters"—was used as a random survey in Galveston and Houston in the spring and fall of 2000. Focus groups and town hall meetings were held during which participants were encouraged to speak about their experiences in caregiving for a dying person. In addition, the participants were asked to describe their experiences with grief. After a dozen of these meetings I realized that we were not receiving information about their perceived needs; rather, participants were sharing narratives about their grief experiences. In order to explore this phenomenon I developed a study that included assembling grief narratives from published memoirs and conducting life history interviews with 15 people from the same geographical area. Life history–based oral history is a discipline whose purpose is to gain understanding through interpretation. Oral history includes rigorous approaches to the conduct of the interview as well as to the preparation and conclusion of the interview that I used throughout this study (Ritchie, 2003).

The project received approval from the institutional review board of the degree-granting university. All participants were provided information about the study and signed informed-consent forms. All names and locations were changed twice during transcription in order to preserve confidentiality. Eligible participants were over 18 years of age and had experienced the death of a close family member or friend.

Participants were recruited through several sources. First, I recruited individuals by recontacting interested "Your Opinion Matters" participants. Second, I approached people at a senior center and in religious communities in the area. The groups were asked if there were individuals who would be interested in participating in this study. The participant pool was constructed by self-selection by those who were willing to talk about death and dying to a person with whom they were not familiar.

The demographics of the participants are presented in Table 4.1. Eight participants were female, while seven were male. They ranged in age from 23 to 76, with a median age of 45. The participants came from a variety of religious backgrounds; however, all of the participants were college educated. Twelve of the 15 participants were European American, 1 was Jewish American, 1 was African American, and 1 was Mexican American. Table 4.1 also lists their relationship to the deceased.

I interviewed each participant once in a place of his or her choosing. The interviews averaged one to two hours in length. Each participant was

Table 4.1: Participants' Demographics

PARTICIPANT	AGE	GENDER	RELATIONSHIP OF DECEASED	AGE WHEN DECEASED DIED	YEARS BETWEEN DEATH AND INTERVIEW
Anne	25	female	friend	19	6
Betty	36	female	mother	18	18
Carol	42	female	grandmother	11	31
Dena	45	female	husband (Bill)	43	2
Eve	46	female	friend (Jennifer)	45	1
Fran	51	female	mother	44	7
Golda	50	female	mother	51	2 months
Helen	76	female	father	35	41
Isaac	23	male	sister	6	17
James	25	male	husband (Joe)	24	4 months
Kurt	26	male	father	22	4
Larry	38	male	father	24	14
Max	50	male	father	50	8 months
Ned	61	male	granddaughter	59	1.4
Oscar	66	male	mother	45	21
Range:	23–76	8 male 7 female		6–59	2 months–41 years
Median:	45			35	7

Source: Klugman, 2001, pp. 209, 211.

asked to speak about the death of one person, and each interview began with an open-ended statement such as "Please tell me about this person, about who he or she was and memories you have of him or her" and "Starting from when you first learned this person was ill or was going to die, please tell me about your experience of their dying and death." This interview process was based on what Becker (1997) describes as "reflexive interviewing." This technique allowed the participant to guide the topics raised and the structure of the narrative. I interjected probing questions that encouraged the respondent to go into greater depth. Thus I acted as a mirror, reflecting back to the participant his or her ideas.

After the interview was completed the tape recorder was turned off, and I thanked the participant for allowing me to share in his or her story. About half of the participants cried during their narrative. I always debriefed the participants, sometimes offering my own experiences in an attempt to help them "come down" from the telling of a painful story. Often we talked about seemingly unrelated topics, such as pets, as a way of returning attention to the present. All the participants reported that the interview experience was positive, healing, and cathartic. Most of them thanked me for taking them on this journey to reconnect with a loved one.

I entered the interview transcripts into a computer using Ethnograph 5.1 software, and the lines of text were numbered. In a first reading of each printed numbered transcript I noted topics and ideas from the interview that became the basis for a thematic codebook. *Thematic code* is a label applied to a section of text that the researcher wants to recall later. The label can refer to ideas, events, metaphors, relationships, actions, emotions, institutions, cultural elements, fears, or any other element of interest. In coding a transcript I marked all sections of text in which a certain theme appeared. For example, all text sections that answered the question of whether the participant spoke with the deceased were coded as "talking." Once the codebook was finalized I used it to test-code several of the interviews. After adjustments to the codes, all the transcripts were freshly coded. Interpretation consisted of looking at all the sections of text across all the interviews that dealt with a particular code and engaging hermeneutically with those texts on cultural, psychocultural, and psychosocial levels.

A second aspect of the study included coding and interpreting published grief narratives. These historical and contemporary works were chosen, in consultation with bioethicist Harold Vanderpool, as being culturally significant to the modern United States. Some of the texts related the deaths of historical or religious figures, including Jacob (Greenspahn, 1987; Hicks, 1962), Jesus (Fuller, 1993; Grant, 1962), Gilgamesh's friend Enkidu (Cushman, 1987; Gordon, 1993; Moran, 1987; Sandars, 1988), Socrates (Plato, 1981), Hector (Homer, 1999), George Washington (Ramsay, 1806; Smith, 1994), Civil War soldiers (Rosenblatt & Rosenblatt, 1992; Wilson, 1996), Ulysses S. Grant ("Hero Finds Rest," 1885; "Closing Scenes," 1885; "His Last Resting Place," 1885; "While Awaiting the End," 1885), Babe Ruth (Beim & Stevens, 1998), Babe Zaharias (Cayless, 1996; Zaharias, 1956), and John F. Kennedy (Parsons & Lidz, 1967; Reston, 1963). Other texts were chosen because they included grief narratives written by professional authors and journalists: Simone de Beauvoir (1985), Jessamyn West (1986), Mark Twain (1990), Rodger Kamenetz (1985), Marilyn Webb (1997), John Gunther (1949/1965), and Mitch Albom (1997). The last set of texts was chosen because they were written by researchers who collect grief stories: Barnard, Towers, Boston, and Lambrimnidou (2000); Byock (1997); Kübler-Ross (1969/1997); and Miller (1992a, 1992b). These works were treated similarly to the collected narratives. All works were coded for theme and plot.

Cultural Approaches to the Grief Narrative

The cultural level of interpretation draws on an investigation into the shared and learned aspects of the text, including frameworks, plots, themes, and purpose. This level asks why one creates a narrative and what cultural elements are borrowed in its creation.

Plots

First, I examined the narratives for plot continuities and similarities. Anthropologist Gay Becker (1997) suggests that all narratives of illness, of which grief narratives are a subset, have a common plot that follows the pattern of "a disruption of life . . . followed by efforts to restore life to normal" (p. 27). Sedney, Baker, and Gross (1994) suggest that these stories include elements such as how the person died, the context surrounding the death, the events leading to and following the death event, and the experiences of family members when they learned of the death.

In the depiction of grief narratives provided by Sedney et al. (1994) and in those I collected and examined, I found many concepts in common with Joseph Campbell's (1949/1973) description of the prototypical hero epic. Campbell discerned that the hero journey myth has three parts: departure, initiation, and return. In the beginning there is the call to adventure, which the hero may immediately accept or try to refuse. Eventually, the hero crosses the threshold into another world. After being initiated into this realm the hero must overcome several obstacles and find the ultimate boon. Finally, the hero returns to the ordinary world and shares the boon with others. Often he or she spends some time living in a dual world of both the other realm and the ordinary (i.e., everyday or prosaic) world.

In the grief narrative the quest cycle takes on specific components. First is the call into the world of medicine, dying, and death. The narrator may struggle through the medical world and overcome obstacles such as being a caregiver, maintaining a deathbed vigil, simultaneously fulfilling ordinary-world obligations, and dealing with the immediate shock of the death. With a sudden or remote death the narrator may not spend any time in the healthcare world but instead enters the realm of grief through a phone call. The narrator then crosses a second threshold into the world of burial and mourning. He or she may need to work with a funeral home to arrange burial or cremation. Most cultures also have other death rituals such as a wake, viewing, or shiva that must be prepared for and observed. Through all these thresholds and realms the narrator must deal with obstacles of organization, finances, and ritual. He or she may need to go through the deceased person's possessions, dispose of an estate, and care for other mourners. In addition to all these duties, the narrator must also face his or her own feelings of grief and reactions to the death of a friend or loved one.

The eventual goal is to return to the world of the living having redefined the self, repaired the disruption in the world of lived experience, made meaning of the event, and reconnected with others. Ann Hunsaker Hawkins (1999), who is a scholar of narratives of illness, holds that the dying person imparts some special knowledge (a boon) to those who witness death. However, the dying person is unable to share his or her boon with the ordinary world. In fact, the focal character of a grief narrative—the deceased—has no voice. He or she cannot describe the death experience because the narrative is not constructed until after that character's death, when he or she can no longer speak. Thus the narrator must complete the myth cycle by bringing the lessons of the deceased's life and dying to the ordinary realm and sharing that knowledge.

Goals of the Grief Narrative

The second step of the cultural examination of grief narratives is to look at the cultural purposes that explain why these stories are told. I identified that the three goals of telling a grief narrative are to reconnect a person to his or her community, to reconstruct the self, and to facilitate the creation of experience.

For a grieving person, one of the causes of suffering is that he or she becomes separated from the community and the outside world. This is reflected in the hermeneutic aspects of narrative, which look at the relationships between tellers and listeners. Entering the world of death and dying isolates a person from other people and from the places he or she frequents in normal life. The act of creating a story and of possibly later telling it is an attempt to reconnect a person to others. The telling of an account requires both a narrator and an audience (Booth, 1988). Whether acting as teller or listener, a person participating in the transmission of a narrative is linked to other individuals (Ricoeur, 1981b). The act of creating a narrative requires the teller to dip into a pool of shared cultural symbols, language and familiar metaphors, and myths to describe experiences that he or she wishes to share with others (Good, 1994). Through these common elements the narrator translates personal experience into a common cultural language that allows the audience to share in the experience (Polkinghorne, 1996). Through constructing and telling these accounts the narrator translates knowing—experience and knowledge—into telling (White, 1981).

Second, narratives serve to help the process of self formation. One's self is one's sense of being, history, and identity; it is who one is and the way one relates to the outer world. This function falls within the psychocultural and psychosocial aspects of narrative. A self is the sum of one's experiences, values, beliefs, self-worth, and attitudes (Ricoeur, 1984). One's personal identity changes through time as a result of experience and relationships. Narrating the self serves to construct a sense of history, linking the self (A) that one remembers being in the past to the self (B) one perceives being in the present and to the self (C) one wants to be in the future. Although these different selves—A, B, and C—may be distinct individuals all contained in the same body, one creates through narrative a sense of the evolutionary history of a person who has changed.

In this way the past appears to lead inexorably to the present, and the future self seems a natural projection from one's current place: "Our sense of personal identity depends upon the continuity of experience through time, a continuity bridging even the cleft between remembered past and projected future" (Bruner, 1986, p. 13). Such a narrative sense of self becomes important because the self one was before the death of a friend or loved one is not the same person as the self after the death. According to philosopher Alasdair MacIntyre (1984), self-identity is based on people's relationships to those around them. One's identity is created as a result of one's role as spouse, sibling, parent, child, cousin, aunt, uncle, colleague, boss, employee, friend, or any other connection one finds meaningful. With the loss of the individual who gave a person that specific relational aspect of identity, the person must rewrite the story of the self. The self that was a parent before the death of a child is no longer a parent in the same way after the child's death. Thus the person must write a story of a new self as the parent of a deceased child or as a person who has no child.

The third reason that one tells a grief narrative is a purely psychocultural phenomenon. The narrator tries to define the death and the ensuing grieving experience. Experience has two meanings in relation to narrative. The first pertains to what a person undergoes as he or she passes through a series of events in real time, a specific instance of personally encountering or undergoing some series of events. As these events transpire in real time they appear to be disjointed, chaotic, and emotional. The person is unable to organize the sequence of events into a coherent order or to interpret them (Ricoeur, 1981a). The function of narrative, then, is to facilitate formulation of the experience to assist ourselves and others to access it (Clandinin & Connelly, 2000).

The second notion of experience is the meaning-laden narrative description a person constructs after the sequence of events has occurred. Thus a person literally reconstructs the experience of his or her past (Polkinghorne, 1996; Richardson, 1990). The teller recalls and recollects fragments of event memories and links them together in a new and ever-changing story (Young, 1987). Such a review can take place only after being separated in time and place from the actual events. From his or her current position in space-time the teller creates meanings and

interpretations of past events. Facts and interpretations cannot be separated; they inform one another (Stivers, 1993). The order of events and
the attachment of meaning are constructed so that the experience appears as a necessary condition for the present to have been reached (Good,
1994). Such thinking requires an individual to accept the notion that there
is no external reality independent from human thought. Even though several people may observe the same sequence of events, each may interpret
them differently, therefore construing different lived experiences. Thus
no single true interpretation—defined as corresponding to an independent external reality—may exist (Clandinin & Connelly, 2000).

Themes

The themes in the stories, like plots, are drawn from the pool of
images and ideas that are present within a culture. A narrator takes the
cultural elements that provide meaning to the story and adds a personal
interpretation. Several themes commonly appear in many of the published as well as the collected narratives. Among the themes are associations such as smells, sound, and light; the role of healthcare providers;
the good death; choosing when to die; isolation; facing one's own death;
the afterlife; and changes in one's own physical body.

SMELLS AND SOUNDS

According to psychologist Trudy Weathersby (2001), certain smells
or sights can stir a memory, bringing a person back to a death or a funeral, especially if that person witnessed the death as a child. An example
of this phenomenon is found in Carol's story. Carol was 11 years old
when her 65-year-old grandmother died from a stroke. She recalls going
to her grandmother's funeral and being shocked by the smell in the
room. There was a large number of fragrant flowers, and Carol found the
smell overpowering. As a result she has always associated flowers with
death:

And I remember her funeral being very fragrant. For a very, very long time, I did
not enjoy the smell of flowers after that. And I don't remember ever smelling
flowers in that concentration ever before that, either. But I started associating
the smell of flowers with death and funerals and my grandmother. So I wasn't the
kind of person that could go and smell a rose and really appreciate it being a rose.
It just smelled like death to me. There were just huge amounts of flowers at this
funeral, just huge.

Flowers are fairly common associations with death. Two other participants who were young when they experienced a death mentioned taking flowers to the grave of the deceased in celebration of a birthday or wedding anniversary.

While smell is often the strongest trigger of memories, some grief associations deal with sounds. Larry was 24 years old when his 75-year-old father died from cancer. He recalls that in the last moments of his father's life the dying man began singing a Louis Armstrong song. Hearing that music today reminds Larry of his father's death and puts him back in the room with his dying father:

So I feel like that was a curse, watching him, those last few minutes. I mean, he s[a]ng. God, it's an old Louis Armstrong song; I had never heard the lyrics to it. But he s[a]ng the lyrics. (Starts to hum.) I can't even remember the name of the song. But he knew the lyrics to it; he knew each and every word to it. And he would sing that song to himself as he went to sleep (pause) and I—I actually didn't care much for old-time rag-style blues, jazz—that's what we call it: old ragtime jazz—before that particular night. That song just kept ringing through my head. It still does. Some nights when I get on stage and I'm scared to perform, that song rings in my head, him singing it. I can't even remember the lyrics. I swear I can't remember the lyrics, but I know the music. Every time I think of that song, I think of the last few minutes with him.

LIGHT

Light is a common feature of historical and collected narratives. In descriptions of the death of President Ulysses S. Grant, he lay dying in bed when a light came through the window and fell upon a picture of Abraham Lincoln. An adjoining portrait of Grant remained dark. When the light disappeared, Grant was found to be dead ("Closing Scenes," 1885). Such imagery of light seems to be associated with the notion of a soul being removed from the physical body.

Betty was 18 years old when her 48-year-old mother died from cancer. In Betty's narrative she describes how the light took her mother's spirit. Her memory was that the light literally had an effect on her mother's body, first causing it to rise and then to fall back once the soul had left:

She had been bedridden for like . . . well, unconscious really, for about a week or something like that. And all of a sudden there was a light in the room and she lifted up from the bed. She went up like halfway. She like sat up in bed. And it's like the light that was shining there took her spirit away or whatever. . . . And then she just lay down. Then she passed away, then. And then the light went away. That's all.

Betty believes in the power of the light, since it appeared to cause her mother to move, which she had not done for about a week. Later in the interview Betty said that the light might have been sunlight that temporarily appeared when a tree branch or curtain moved. However, she still imbues that light with the meaning that a divine force took her mother's spirit.

In both these narratives the light is natural and comes through a window. A window is often seen as a threshold, a way into the interior. For example, Dena was 43 years old when her 47-year-old husband, Bill, died from renal cancer. She interprets the window as a portal for the divine to come into the everyday world to take her husband to heaven.

And the next morning, when I was making the bed, I was remembering—he looked at Jon, he looked at me, he looked out that window—I looked up and it's the eastern sky—and it says he'll come and get us in the east. So even [the sky] had a spiritual significance to me.

At first Bill looks at his son and his wife, possibly saying good-bye. In a later conversation Dena said that when her husband looked out the window she believes he saw a divine presence that took his soul and allowed him to die.

HEALTHCARE

Not surprisingly, healthcare plays a major role in people's stories of death and dying. When participants talk about bad, lingering deaths, they often use medical terminology to describe the illness and treatments. When individuals address healthcare directly, they frequently do so with anger and frustration. Bioethicist Harold Vanderpool (1997) points out that such angry commentary on healthcare dates at least as far back as 1957. A narrator's frustration with healthcare can actually be a lashing out about the lack of control that the dying person has over his or her body and condition. In the following excerpts healthcare providers are viewed as not doing enough, as deceitful in keeping vital information from the patient, as "rude and hostile," and as criminal for not following the patient's desires.

Dena describes how, when her husband was first diagnosed with cancer, the doctors removed a mass and three lymph nodes. Although the doctors assured Dena and her husband that they had removed all the cancer, a few weeks later the lymph nodes were determined to be malignant. Dena blamed the physicians for not being thorough.

They thought they did the arteriogram, though, and the blood mass supply you could see was great. And they thought it was probably about lemon-sized and they took out a football-sized mass. That was the first week of December in '93. And then basically that surgeon told us, "Come back in six months." I—I couldn't get a peace about that. I thought, you know, "Oh well." One of the reasons was they'd taken this inch margin and they only took three lymph node tests and they thought they got everything. That's why they said come back in six months. Well, two weeks later we get a call—it's right before Christmas—and they said it [had] spread to the lymph nodes. How many? 'Cause three was all they took, so that's all they knew.

In some ways Dena faults the physicians for her husband's death because she felt that they were not thorough enough. Similar distrust of healthcare is found in Eve's story. Eve was 45 years old when her 47-year-old friend Jennifer died from breast cancer. Jennifer blamed the doctors for not being honest and forthright about the physical changes she might experience as a result of chemotherapy. As Eve tells the story, Jennifer was angry because she felt as if the doctors had purposely not given her all the information she felt she needed to make an informed choice regarding her treatment:

And then our next conversations as she'd be going through treatment is how horrible it is and how angry she is about not having, not being given appropriate information—that they said, "You may have a little discomfort in swallowing or indigestion." But she was very, very angry in that she had ulcers from her lips all the way through her digestive tract; her feet had very poor circulation as a result of the chemotherapy—she lost all of her toenails; her toes were black and ulcerated. And it was just a really horrible experience.

Anger toward healthcare providers is also a topic in Fran's and Max's narratives. Fran was 44 years old when her 63-year-old mother died from cancer. Fran was angry with her doctor, who was "rude and hostile" and would not talk with Fran or tell her mother the truth about her condition. The physician finally did speak with her, but only after she threatened to fire him.

Max also felt the need to take action against a physician. Max was 50 years old when his 73-year-old father died of cancer. He explains that even though his father had completed the paperwork and made his end-of-life-care desires known, the physicians ignored the patient's and family's wishes. Max believes that the doctors removed the "do not resuscitate" order from his father's chart because they wanted to continue treating him as long as possible:

> He had made very specific positions on his end-of-life treatment and had them drafted by a lawyer in accordance with the state bar association and state medical association, etc., etc., and when we brought them up to a lawyer—I mean to the doctor, he dismissed them as not being a legal document, which is not true. They are—I mean it was. You can imagine the—the—the pain and the drama of sitting outside your father's hospital room arguing with these doctors and having you know—having these things signed with my dad's signature and having 'em dismissed. There were several times when we finally convinced them we had a "do not resuscitate" order in his chart and that was misplaced two or three times. And [he] had a "do not resuscitate" bracelet on him and that was taken off a couple of times too. It was . . . unprofessional and unethical. I'll never forgive them for it.

At first Max hired a lawyer to sue the doctors and seek some sort of vengeance. As time passed, however, his anger waned, and now he just wants the lawyer to send a strongly worded letter to the physicians to teach them about the importance of advance directives. Max wanted his father, not the physicians, to have control over his dying.

THE GOOD DEATH

Not surprisingly, published and collected narratives that center on issues of dying and grief are often concerned with how someone can have a "good death." After experiencing the deaths of her sister from a kidney infection and of her 96-year-old father-in-law from cancer, journalist Marilyn Webb (1997) wrote *The Good Death,* in which she looks at models of dying through the lenses of medicine, law, politics, hospice care, and religion.

The idea of the good death is not limited to published accounts. This theme appeared in five of the collected interviews. According to the participants, a good death provides the patient with the right to decide how and where dying will occur, is painless, is sudden at the end, and allows time for a person to take care of unfinished business and say good-bye.

One aspect of the good death is that the dying person has some choice or control over when he or she dies. Six of the participants said that they believed their dying person chose when to die. Dena believes her husband, Bill, wanted to stay alive long enough to be eligible for full disability and to see his daughter graduate from high school. When Bill realized he would not be able to see his daughter graduate, he asked if they could hold the graduation party early. He died after the party.

Eve feels that a similar motivation kept her friend Jennifer alive. Jennifer's goal was to complete her dissertation proposal defense:

You know, what we concluded (pause) was that she wanted to finish that dissertation so bad[ly] that—I mean, that was like a landmark kind of thing, and she postponed her dying until she got that defense done. She ignored her pain; she ignored how bad she felt and somehow (pause) just tolerated that and just—she would be—dead sooner—that's what we honestly think. She would have died sooner except that she felt like she had to finish that.

The theme of controlling the timing of death is also echoed in Golda's narrative. Golda was 50 years old when her 78-year-old mother died from a stroke and heart failure. Golda's mother had been forced to sell her home in order to liquidate her assets to be eligible for public assistance so that there would be money to pay for nursing home care. Her mother was distraught that the money would go to the government instead of being part of her legacy. She died while the closing papers, including the check, were in the mail. Since the money was not needed for her care, it was, after all, available for her children. Golda believes that her mother chose when to die to preserve the money:

She died as the closing papers for her house were in the mail. She died so that the money didn't go to Medicaid. It was truly amazing. I mean, I—I truly believe she made the choice. I really, really do.

Such descriptions often echo the theme of the good death, which emphasizes a desire to have a death that others would want for themselves.

The notion of control over body, mind, business affairs, and death was important in about a third of the interviews. In the good death, control of pain is essential. For example, Betty gave her mother regular morphine injections to control pain. Dena mentions that control of physical pain and mental suffering was important for her husband, Bill. In addition,

Bill wanted to control the circumstances of his death: he would die only at home, in his own bed, without wearing a diaper.

Fran agrees that a good death should be painless. Her mother was moving and walking around, which should have been quite painful, given her cancer. But because of a stroke that limited control of one side of her body, Fran's mother could not feel the pain, "so in many ways it was quite a blessing that her mind was usually not in reality (pause), because she probably wouldn't have been able to walk—but she just did." Fran's mother's desire for control over her life and death extended even to her finances. Although she was incompetent to control her money, Fran's mother desired to do so until her death.

In some narratives the speaker relates events that were less than optimal or went wrong. In other stories the narrator extols the death as an example of a good death. Betty suggests that her mother's death was "perfect" because she was in control of her treatment and how she died: "She decided which way she wanted to die and stuff. She didn't want to die in the hospital—she wanted to die at home. And she was comfortable. I did everything I could to make her happy." Betty recognizes that she played a major role in helping this "perfect" death occur. By being the vigilant caregiver, Betty made sure her mother's demands were met and that the dying woman was kept comfortable and happy.

In some narratives a sudden death is seen as being a good death for the dying but not for those left behind. Anne was 19 years old when a close friend of the same age died from an undiagnosed congenital heart problem:

But it happened so—I mean, it was much better than if it had been—she found out she had cancer that summer and it had been a year and a half later that she died slowly—but it was—was so abrupt and there were no good-byes and there was nothing.

Carol emphasizes this notion of dying suddenly but not too quickly in briefly describing her great-grandmother's death. She believes that one should die without sickness or lingering illness:

So I'd like to die like my great-grandmother died. My great-grandmother on my mother's side didn't learn English, by the way—figured she didn't have to. She died at 93. I was 2 years old so I don't remember any of this. I was told that she had never been sick a day of her life . . . and that she was sick for about a week and then she died. And that's what I want to do. I want to decide, "Okay, it's time to go." A little bit of decline (snaps fingers)—*pow!*—take myself out. Something like that.

Carol also holds that her great-grandmother decided that it was time to die. In describing her wishes for her own death, not only does she wish to have the health of her grandmother and the suddenness of her death, but Carol also wants to be able to decide when she can die.

ISOLATION

The themes of isolation and loneliness appeared in many of the collected interviews. This separation from others takes several forms, from self-imposed hibernation to being afraid of loneliness to being socially alienated from others. According to death studies scholar Philippe Ariès (1975, 1991), most people die alone. Eve relates how her friend Jennifer isolated herself from friends and from most of her family. Such separation made the dying harder on her friends, who suddenly found themselves cut off and without any way to say good-bye: "So she just cuts herself off from everyone except her immediate family and wouldn't—didn't want to see anybody—didn't want to talk to anybody—didn't want anybody to see her sick." Eve interprets Jennifer's actions as selfish and unfair to her friends. In later passages Eve resents that she never got to say good-bye or have a final conversation.

While Jennifer chose to be alone, Max's father wanted company. In fact, he requested that a family member should always be by his bedside. He had expressed only one thing before they intubated him and that was that he not be left alone: "So there were plenty of children there, so we did stay with him around the clock for about 10 [days]—or maybe even 2 weeks." In some grief narratives the sense of isolation does not come from the dying or from disenfranchised friends but rather from the caregivers who give up their social lives to take care of the dying person. When spending nearly 24 hours a day, 7 days a week with a dying person, a caregiver can find holding down a job difficult and may find it impossible to maintain social relationships with friends. Instead of spending time with friends and coworkers the caregiver is overwhelmed by the needs of the dying person. She or he is often responsible for feeding, administering medications, cleaning soiled sheets, bathing the dying person, changing diapers, and changing wound dressings. The realm of the dying becomes the only world in which the caregiver participates:

It's the experience that so many people [as caregivers] will have or have had, and it's good, I think, for people in general to know that they are not alone. They've never been alone. But when you are going through it you are alone. And that's what makes it so very hard.

As Fran explains, although the caregiver feels completely alone, he or she has a social network of family and friends who can lend support and help, even from a distance. Social service organizations may also provide assistance through respite care and support groups. Often it is left to the caregiver to locate social service organizations that might provide assistance. Unfortunately, many people do not have the necessary knowledge about locating community programs and so do not benefit from these programs. When the caregiver is surrounded only by the dying person and his or her needs, the feeling of being alone can be overwhelming.

MORTALITY

Another common theme in grief narratives is mortality. When experiencing the death of another, one is forced to admit that death exists and that someday it will be the narrator's turn to die. Few people easily face this reality, and for most it is a battle against nonexistence. Simone de Beauvoir (1985) writes: "All men [sic] must die: but for every man his death is an accident and, even if he knows it and consents to it, an unjustifiable violation" (p. 106). This excerpt suggests that even though one knows that every person dies, one rarely thinks of one's own death, since it is viewed as robbing one of life. In four of the collected interviews participants said that the death experience forced them to examine their own mortality. Fear of one's own death includes uncertainty about how it will happen, fear of pain, and fear of dying alone.

Carol claims that watching her grandparents die caused her to worry about the manner of her own death. She fears how she will die more than the concept of death itself:

What scares me about death is the way I'm going to go. It's not the moment of passing—I think that that's going to be wonderful—but it's having cancer—it's getting hit by a truck—it's, you know, it's suffering first. That bothers me. That bothers me.

With Golda's age comes the recognition that most of her life has already been lived and, with it, the certainty of death. Having witnessed her parents' deaths and knowing that she has no control over death, she feels fear and is not sure how to deal with it:

No, I know that this has nothing to do with death stories and it has nothing to do with my mother. I can tell you—and I wouldn't normally do this, so I don't know why I'm saying this now—that I'm pretty terrified of the whole concept. That there's something about being 50 and realizing that more than half my life is over—that is terrifying to me. And partly it's terrifying to think about what happens between now and then. Having watched my father and my mother suffer so greatly, both of them, and not wanting to wind up like either one of them. And partly—just—just, you know, through all those question marks is an acute fear which—because I spent so much time in the intellectual realm, my head keeps saying, "You are being ridiculous." But I can't, and it's sort of this fear that lives in me all the time, which I think is absurd. But I don't know how to get rid of it and I don't know how to keep it in perspective. So that's weird—I don't know. And that's not just triggered by my mother's death, but it certainly was exacerbated by it. Maybe it's just being 50, you know. Like, I ought to be 50.

For other participants the concern is not so much how they will die but rather the fact that they too will ultimately die. When people experience the death of someone who is of the same age and social circumstances, they are forced to acknowledge the possibility of their own death. Eve describes this unsettling reality: "It's just unbelievable the number of people that I'm—have known since—in the last couple of years—that are my age that are dying. And pretty much all of them are dying of cancer, for whatever reason."

If being middle-aged—like Carol, Golda, and Eve—begins a process of confronting the reality of one's own death, then reaching a greater age may exacerbate these continuing thoughts of death. When talking about her father's death at 80, Helen, who is now 76, finds herself thinking often about death and dying. She said to me in the first 5 minutes of the interview, "I'm 76—ha. I myself am going to realize that I am older than—perhaps pushing—when my father died. I mean, that comes into my head. I am very conscious of death now—very."

AFTERLIFE

With concerns about one's own mortality come questions about an afterlife. Such concerns have long been part of human experience. Klenow and Bolin (1989–1990) report that nearly 70% of 1,069 survey respondents expressed a belief in some sort of an afterlife. Similarly, a 1985 Gallup study indicated that 71% of the population of the United States believed in the existence of an afterlife. Thirteen of the 15 people interviewed for this current study affirmed a belief in some sort of existence after death. They described the afterlife as a reincarnation, a reunion, a paradise, or a dark place. These data seem to be at variance with what Melvin Krant (1974), Elisabeth Kübler-Ross (1969/1997), and Gardner Murphy (1959) wrote in the 1950s through 1970s, that the notion of an afterlife is no longer an important part of American death thought. Thus it may be reasonable to question whether current thought may be moving from scientific perspectives to more spiritual and religious understandings.

Golda said that her religion, Judaism, provides no definitive answers as to what happens after death. However, she has visions of her father being in heaven. When asked whether religion influenced her ideas of death and dying, she laughingly said,

Only the frustration in the sense that it doesn't give us any answers. . . . When my father died I could visualize him up there with his brothers who were dead and my grandparents. I mean I could just—sitting on a cloud somewhere, you know.

Golda's response is not surprising. Klenow and Bolin (1989–1990) report that only 17.2% of their Jewish respondents expressed belief in an afterlife—the lowest response of any religion. They attribute this to the religion's unclear position on the matter.

Three of the participants saw the afterlife as reincarnation. Carol believes that after death a person spends some time in heaven and then returns to earth in some form. She traces her beliefs to an unusual Christian church to which her grandparents belonged. Its services last 3–4 hours and consist of a medium channeling messages from the deceased to the living:

And [Bill] believes in reincarnation; my grandmother did too. They were a very interesting brand of Christianity that believed in medium séances, levels of heaven, guardian angels that guide you through your life and meet you after your life and help you review your life. And reincarnation, that we—we'd get a chance to come back and do things differently as a different person.

Others expressed different ideas about the afterlife. Those with more traditional Christian religious upbringings expressed a belief in heaven. Anne said that as part of her Catholic upbringing she was taught to believe that after death one goes to heaven, where families are reunited and the deceased keep watch over those they left behind on earth. She has not yet decided whether to adopt this teaching as her own personal belief. Describing the influence of her beliefs on her view of death, Anne said:

Well, I've always—from my father—known that when you pass away—and I still believe this—that you are going to a much better place. And this (pause) I guess I can say—I was talking about my father and how he used to tell us that—in his words, that whenever you die you're going to go to a place where you're never hungry, you're never cold or you're never too hot, you're never uncomfortable and never experience pain (laughs). I don't know if he was giving us some sort of paradise, but maybe . . . that was a paradise that you go to when you pass away. And that you're going to be in this—that was a place called heaven, you know, and—but all of us will have an opportunity to go to heaven. And I never experienced—I never had the experience of him having talked about Satan or hell or any of that. And after just, you know, talking to other friends, they're, like, "Well, there's heaven and there's hell." And—but my (pause)—I mean, I still feel that. When I pass away or, you know, I'm going to go to a better place, like he described.

Isaac, who has adopted his Catholic father's lessons about heaven, depicts an idealistic Christian afterlife where one is rewarded for good works and relieved from suffering that occurred on earth. He is sure that he will go to a better place after death. Others' religious beliefs may not, however, be a source of comfort. In situations like these help may be required to put one's beliefs about the afterlife into an acceptable perspective. James was concerned about his partner Joe's place in the afterlife. Given that Joe was gay and had committed suicide, which are two major sins in the Catholic Church, James was uncertain what would happen to his partner after death. He had visions of Joe being tortured in a dark and painful place. He was assured by a priest that, because of the mental illness and suffering he had experienced on earth, Joe would spend very little time in purgatory and would then go to heaven:

When the priest said that, you know, because of the belief in purgatory and that suicide is (pause), you know (pause), I guess is a sin (pause). That—that he said that he—he truly believed that Joe would spend very little time in purgatory before going to heaven because Joe suffered so much in life and . . . had such a heavy cross to bear—which he did (pause). So I believe he's in heaven, and after those first few weeks, you know, when I told you I was having visions of him in a dark place, I'm thinking maybe that was him being in purgatory. But after those first few weeks, then I started feeling his presence real strongly in church. And I said that's where I knew . . . now [he's] in heaven. I don't feel him as much in church anymore, so I am sure he is in heaven.

PHYSICAL BODY

A major theme in both published and collected narratives is the movement and appearance of the physical body. From previous excerpts it can be recalled how Larry and Betty describe how their loved one's body rose up and then lay back down after the soul had left. Writers Simone de Beauvoir (1985) and Philip Roth (1991) poignantly describe how, while bathing their parents, they were struck by how frail and insignificant they looked at the end of a vigorous life.

Max, however, relates to his father's body through its strength. He mentions that, when dying, his father was restrained and slept most of the time. Despite having tubes running in and out of his body, Max's father displayed strong movements that resembled walking. Max interprets these movements as his father's wanting to be away from the world of healthcare and death:

You know, we'd sedate him and he'd wake up and he didn't know where he was and he wanted—he wanted to get out. And they had to restrain him after a while. I mean, he had all these tubes in him and everything. He was such a strong person that he—I had to do all I could to hold him down in the bed, that's how strong he was, even at that point. He—he kept moving even when he was sleeping—he kept moving his feet like he was trying to get out of the bed and out of the room and out of the hospital. You know, he would always be edging himself over that way.

Max takes comfort in the notion that his father was a physically strong person, one who had the fortitude to fight the imposition of interventions intended to delay his death. As discussed earlier, Max struggled to have his father's wishes honored and the life support removed. However, the hospital was adamant that such care be continued. Carol, on the other hand, does not view the body as resisting unsought intrusions but rather as an enemy that, after a long life of service, betrays and forces a person to relinquish health: "It just—it just makes me despair of how the body can betray you." Death, then, for Carol represents being betrayed by one's own body.

Golda's mother experienced a sense of being disconnected from a portion of her body. After a stroke she lost the ability to relate to one half of her body.

And they did the CAT scan and the doctors came back and said it was a massive stroke. And she'd lost all the feeling—she lost all her—she lost one side of her body. And apparently she'd lost knowledge of the existence of that side of her body, which is apparently a fairly normal response, but it's hard to comprehend it. But you'd say to her, "Raise your right hand," and she'd raise her right hand. When you'd say, "Raise your left hand" . . . she'd raise her right hand. And [she was] fully [alert and] thinking completely. So she didn't—so it was difficult for her to comprehend that she had lost the use of her body.

Eve's friend Jennifer, who had breast cancer, was, on the other hand, extremely aware of her body and her appearance. As Eve tells the story, Jennifer's breast was integral to her sense of being attractive:

The first time she'd ever talked about anything like this before was that she was—really didn't want to have a mastectomy because that was one part of her body that she liked. And even though she was very attractive, she didn't see herself as being attractive, and so she was really, really uncomfortable with what she was going to look like afterwards. And she was really—in her word, she was very attached to her breast. She loved her breast and that was kind of like the worst part of her body that—if something had to be removed or she had to lose a part of her body—that was the worst for her.

For others, the body is not something that betrays and disfigures a person but rather something sacred and holy to be honored. Dena describes how she and her son cared for the body of her husband, Bill, and she links this care to a religious parable, thereby imbuing the ritual of washing the body with meaning and spiritual significance:

We called hospice and we also called the willed body program and they had someone come over. And now I'm going to sound like I'm advertising, because it was such a wonderful way to be handled. We called our pastor and close church friends. People immediately came over. I laugh a little bit because, you know, we picked out what Bill was going to wear. And he had Eternity cologne; the first year we found out that he had cancer I started buying Bill Eternity cologne because I said I [would] love him for eternity. And he had never used the bath bottle; that was not part of the man that he was, you know—that was a girly thing. And Jon [her son] and I—boy, we prepared the warm water and we put that stuff—he smelled good from head to toe. They offered to prepare the body, but I just thought that was another privilege, you know, just like Mary and Mark [sic] and them preparing Jesus' body. And how would I like it [if I could choose between] a stranger, who may or may not look at the spiritual aspects of what's happened, or family to do this. And so it really was—I think Jon and I were linked in a way—in an incredible way—as we did that.

For Dena, the act of washing and perfuming her husband's body was a reverential activity that linked her to her religious beliefs, connected her to her son, and provided an expression of her undying love for her husband.

The excerpts and interpretations offered above serve to illustrate how elements drawn from images and beliefs held in common by cultural groups are woven into grief narratives. Plots, goals, and themes used in the telling and construction of a story come from a common cultural lexicon and form a basis for sharing experiences with others. The act of sharing the story, using elements common to the narrator and the community, enables a sense of connection and helps individuals to deal with their grief.

Psychosocial Approaches to Grief Narratives

Psychosocial approaches ask how the narratives affect social relationships and an individual's social identity. Grief narratives have two psychosocial functions (Peacock & Holland, 1993). The first preserves memories of a life (Miller, 1992a) by keeping the deceased person alive socially and culturally through the narration of his or her life and death. The narrator thus enables the deceased to continue performing a social function and playing an important role in society. The second role played by the grief narrative is to educate others and gain insight oneself about life, death, dying, grief, and caregiving. Through stories about a deceased person the narrator not only teaches others but also, through telling and retelling these stories, gains insights and learns from the life and death of his or her friend or family member.

Published Literature

Jessamyn West, a Quaker, dedicates her 1986 book, *The Woman Said Yes: Encounters with Life and Death,* to her mother and sister as a celebration of their lives: "With love for Grace and Carmen and to celebrate their courage." West's book consists of two distinct accounts. In the first she describes her battle with tuberculosis and how her mother nursed her to recovery over several years. Her mother's death at the end of a long life receives very brief mention. The second part of the book deals with the death of West's sister Carmen. Years after both their parents have died Carmen is diagnosed with bowel cancer, and West nurses her sister through the dying process. Carmen decides against aggressive treatment. Instead, she spends her time reliving memories and preparing for her death. Knowing the pain and indignity associated with a long-drawn-out death, West serves as a midwife, helping her sister to leave this world in accordance with Carmen's wishes. Unlike many grief narratives, which tend to be rather removed and distant as the author goes through his or her own reactions and needs, West's work is fraught with emotion as she concentrates on her sister's experience. Her description of her sister's death serves as a tribute in that it describes how Carmen died as she lived—on her own terms. The book also performs an educational purpose, offering the viewpoint that refusing medical treatment is not giving up but rather is a choice.

In his beautifully written 1985 book about his mother's life and death the poet Rodger Kamenetz (1985) explains that his mother visited him in three dreams. In those visions she prompted him to write her narrative as a way to complete her life by giving it structure. His book serves as a memorial and a testimony to a lived life: "Now in the wake of that dream, word after word has risen and fallen, broken and receded. This book is one wave, her legacy and her will" (Kamenetz, 1985, p. 116).

Mitch Albom, a sports journalist, is the author of *Tuesdays with Morrie*, a *New York Times* best seller and Oprah Winfrey Book Club selection. This 1997 work describes Albom's 14 visits to his former college professor Morrie Schwartz, who is dying of amyotrophic lateral sclerosis (ALS). Most of the sessions were tape-recorded, though some are offered from Albom's memory. Schwartz and Albom took on the publication of this book as a joint project. This project was a way for Schwartz to offer his life's lessons to a wide audience and to achieve a type of immortality by leaving his mark: "'Mitch, . . . I want to tell you about my life. I want to tell you before I can't tell you anymore.' His voice dropped to a whisper. 'I want someone to hear my story. Will you?'" (Albom, 1997, p. 63). Albom is the conduit through which Schwartz can continue to teach others. Thus the book is a memorial to Schwartz's life as well as a lesson for others on the meaning of living and dying.

Other writers have viewed stories of dying as an opportunity to educate and to build community through bringing death into the living room for discussion and personal growth. Surgeon Sherwin B. Nuland wrote *How We Die* (1993), in which he discusses the many ways in which people die, such as from heart disease, old age, Alzheimer's, accidents, suicide, euthanasia, AIDS, and cancer. Through his *New York Times* best-selling book Nuland wanted to make dying less mysterious:

I have written this book to demythologize the process of dying. My intention is not to depict it as a horror-filled sequence of painful and disgusting degradations, but to present it in its biological and clinical reality, as seen by those who are witnesses to it and felt by those who experience it. Only by a frank discussion of the very details of dying can we best deal with those aspects that frighten us the most. (Nuland, 1993, p. xvii)

Nuland's project is to make death public rather than something that happens behind closed hospital doors. In the final chapter, "Lessons Learned," he suggests that the physician, family, and patient need to learn to accept the inevitability of death. He also suggests that witnesses to death should use that experience to create a richer life.

Physician Ira Byock's 1997 book, *Dying Well,* begins with a short narrative of his father's death, an event that inspired him to write. As a hospice director Byock had seen death before, but for the first time he experienced death as a person, not as a medical practitioner. Byock's project explores the possibility for growth in dying. He presents inspirational stories of dying patients and offers moral lessons from each. Among Byock's suggestions for creating a meaningful death are writing one's own death narrative, learning to be dependent, letting go, and finding dignity in terminal illness.

Stories Gathered from Interviews

Grief narratives enable the teller to share the story of a life. Five of the eight participants interviewed for this study explained that talking about memories of the deceased helped keep those memories fresh and renewed the deceased's presence in their life. In a narrative invited as part of this study, Betty describes how telling her mother's grief narrative serves to maintain the memory of her mother by expanding the number of people who are aware of her life and death:

I guess it's okay—I mean, it's good. I guess that, you know, it gives—extends the memory that, you know, somebody else, even though you have never seen her or anything like that, but, you know, it extends the memory. . . . Keeps her alive or something.

Laurel Richardson (1990) writes that through narrative "the past can be retrieved and relived in the present" (p. 23). When we tell about our memories, we bring relationships from the past to life in the present, and memory turns into lived experience. Larry tells how he keeps the memory of his father alive:

Talking about him, remembering him, illustrating him, whenever I do stand-up [comedy] illustrating some of the weird, wacky moments that he was associated with that was part of . . . helps me remember him, helps me keep his spirit alive just like any other member of my family, you know. One thing about him I'll never forget about him, you know—I'll never forget any of them—I'll never forget any of the things that—I'll never forget. I may forget a lot of things but I'll never forget everything. The important stuff will always be there, you know.

Larry explains that talking about and remembering his father is an expression of his love for his dad. Larry does not converse about his father with other people so much but rather uses accounts of him as part of a stand-up comedy act. Keeping the memory of a deceased person in the now of lived reality maintains the deceased as part of social reality.

Telling helps Dena hold on to memories, especially when the material objects collected over a lifetime have disappeared. She had to sell most of her marital assets to pay off the debts that had accumulated during her husband's illness. Dena explains how talking about her husband is the only monument she has to him, since there is little physical evidence left that he ever existed:

The—oh goodness—like the lady in the financial institution that broke down and cried. It's those kinds of people that still come up to me and tell me what they remember about Bill that . . . it just makes me so proud. Because even though we've had to sell vehicles and, you know, the insurance money's gone—you know, all those kind of practical things that you would have left to remind you of someone. Bill doesn't have a grave; he donated his body. . . . I've tried real[ly] hard to get him a marker in the veterans' memorial and, do you know, they can't find his service records. But it's amazing how fast you can wipe out signs of an age or a life.

As mentioned previously, Bill donated his body to science, so there is no grave where he is buried or a place that can be visited. But Dena desires to maintain Bill's social identity through some means. Since a physical reminder is not possible, she tells his story.

The grief narrative is often told not just to memorialize individuals but also to make their life or experience a lesson in living and dying. Fran says that she tells her grief narrative as a way to inform people of what may occur when caring for an ailing parent. Her goal is to enlighten others so that they know they are not alone, even though they may feel alone when they are going through this experience. Fran wants to help people who may find the process psychologically difficult and have thoughts of suicide:

The fact that someone even wants to hear it, I think is—it's a good thing that someone would be interested in—in that. That's a good thing because it's the experience that so many people will have or have had and it's good, I think, for people in general to know that they are not alone. They've never been alone. But when you are going through it, you are alone. And that's what makes it so very hard. So. But now I just—I think in my own way—I think it's—it's my form of teaching and offering experience to help in any way that might count. 'Cause I think it can—which is why I want to make a book out of it because I—there's a lot of people out there that are getting into that suicidal state and all because they are so alone. And they're not alone and it doesn't—you hate your mother and it doesn't, you know—it's just a reality, you know, how things can be then.

Much of Fran's account describes her own mental state and how she avoided succumbing to suicidal thoughts caused by her depression, frustration, and isolation as a caregiver. By sharing her story she helps other caregivers establish social relationships.

Similarly, James took his partner's death as an opportunity to educate others about the mental illness from which Joe suffered. James remembers Joe's death as a time when he received a call to work in psychiatry to help others as well as to start a foundation to help inform and educate others about mental illness. He also hopes to advocate for legislative reform to improve the care and treatment of those suffering with mental illnesses. James recognizes that in such work he may have to deal with the deaths of patients, but he thinks that, after the loss of Joe, he can handle it:

I think it brings more awareness (pause) to them about maybe mental illness and (pause) its implications, which is something that I am trying to do right now, or eventually—that I want to raise an awareness when I get into medical school and all. . . . And so I'm refocusing that energy into—I want to go to med school and study psychiatry and help really severe people like Joe. Maybe if I help them it will be like helping Joe. But, as in all that—working with a high-risk group I am going to lose somebody the same way I lost Joe. . . . It won't be the same. It will be more of a professional thing but it'll still sort of hurt. And so I want to do that. I want to build, I want a foundation in his name to subsidize (pause) those who can't afford mental health care. I want to raise public awareness, especially [about] how the legal system [treats those with mental illness].

James is still working toward fulfilling his goal. When I met him five years later he was a fourth-year medical student applying for a residency in psychiatry.

Hermeneutic Approaches to Grief Narratives

In the hermeneutic approach one examines the act of sharing the narrative. The focus is on the relationship between a specific teller and a specific listener (Peacock & Holland, 1993). Thus analysis looks at the intersubjectivity of the narrative experience. In this section I examine how the act of sharing the narrative changes the narrator, enabling him or her to change and grow. The dialogic exchange is an essential part of this process. The listener is expected to contribute to the story, to suggest new avenues of interpretation and meaning. According to Russian literary theorist Mikhail Bakhtin, narratives are unfinalizable (Morson & Emerson, 1991). That is, through the telling the narrator receives oral and body language feedback that opens new possibilities and interpretations, which in turn leads to a reframing of the experience itself (Iser, 1978; Polkinghorne, 1996). The narrator finds unexpected and surprising directions for the story.

Such surprises can lead to rethinking the experience, but they primarily serve to assist the narrator to reconstruct the self. Becker (1997) calls this "healing biographical discontinuities through narrative" (p. 224). In the grief following a death an individual searches for a new narrative of the self, since the meaning of the old self has changed (Riches & Dawson, 1996). As discussed under the goals of grief narrative, the death of a relational anchor forces a person to reassess his or her self-identity. With the loss of a child a person may no longer be a parent, sibling, grandparent, aunt, or uncle. The hermeneutic aspects of the grief narrative assist a person in re-creating the relationship upon which a portion of his or her identity is founded. Since this process is by nature dialogic, it also serves to reconnect the person with others in the community. According to Sedney et al. (1994), telling a grief narrative can "(a) provide emotional relief (b) help make an experience meaningful, and (c) bring people together" (p. 289).

Published Narratives

In *A Very Easy Death* feminist writer Simone de Beauvoir (1985) writes about her mother's death. The reader finds within this text an estranged mother and daughter. Beauvoir comes to her mother only because the woman is dying. Beauvoir writes that simply by holding her mother's hand on her deathbed she is lying to her mother, for that act suggests reconciliation and love (Beauvoir, 1985). This book reads as if Beauvoir is attempting to work out her own conflicted feelings toward her mother, and in that way it serves as a catharsis, a releasing of emotion. In a sense, Beauvoir is trying to create a good death, a good narrative for her mother, but she finds that no such thing exists. The title of the book comes from a comment a nurse made to Beauvoir after her mother died, that the woman had a very easy death. Her mother had forgone much aggressive and painful treatment, so in some ways her death was easy, but the irony that Beauvoir builds into the account shows that in fact no death is easy.

Philip Roth's (1991) *Patrimony* is the story of his father's dying and death. Throughout the text Roth seems to come to terms with his grief and what it means to be an orphaned adult. This book reads as an attempt to achieve meaning in and a new understanding of the loss of his relationship with his father. Roth has tried to build a self that does not include having his father near him. In the act of translating his private experience into public language he seeks a cathartic release to the pain of grief.

Collected Narratives

Bakhtin believed that there is little difference between written and spoken communication (Morson & Emerson, 1991). Thus the same approach that one takes to a published work can be applied to oral narratives. Although telling a grief narrative to a researcher is not a recognized form of therapy, Robert Neimeyer (1999) encouraged his patients to write their grief narratives to assist them in reconstructing their worldview and sense of self. Several participants in this study described the experience of telling the story as therapeutic. Although Eve was asked the same open-ended questions as all the other participants in the study, she felt challenged to consider issues about which she would not ordinarily think:

I feel really good that you asked me questions that made me go places that I didn't really want to go, and [that] the other people that I've talked to are really just listening and don't want to push me. It's their purpose. They didn't see their purpose as being therapeutic in any way, so they didn't push me to go places that, you know, might bring up some emotion.

Telling a grief narrative often helps the narrator come to a new understanding of himself or herself and arranges the pieces of the puzzle in such a way that life can be reconstructed. For example, during our conversation Eve discussed how she had prayed for a sign or some contact from her deceased friend Jennifer. Eve mentions that previous discussions of Jennifer's death have caused her to value her relationship with her own parents, enabling them to be more affectionate with one another. This breakthrough, she decides, was a divine gift from Jennifer:

It really changed our relationship a lot. And it would be neat not to have to talk about that particular event [Jennifer's death], but that I was, for the first time in a long time, going and hugging them and embracing them and (pause) got immediate "Hey, we like this" and hugging back and asking for more and (starts crying) (pause). I hadn't ever talked about that out loud, and I guess it just dawned on me that (pause) in looking for, like, a visitation or something from Jennifer (pause), it is. You know, that's like it. That was a gift that she gave to me and my family. That grieving over her and what she'd been through, you know, managed to be a breakthrough for me to be openly physically affectionate with my parents, but I hadn't been in 20 years. So, I mean, could I ask for a better gift for someone? Thanks, Jennifer. And I had never put those (pause) two things together like that, you know (pause). Like, that—was like a gift that there was, like, maybe some kind of divine intervention for that to happen, you know?

Through telling her narrative Eve realizes that her relationship with her parents has changed. The hermeneutic exchange between Eve and me led her to a new interpretation of previous events.

Sometimes in the course of telling the narrator may reinterpret thoughts and feelings about the deceased person. Helen was 35 years old when her 80-year-old father died from a stroke. She held strong feelings of bitterness toward her father, whom she recalled as being aloof and rarely offering her the affection she craved. However, during our talk she recalls a forgotten memory:

Oh God, I'm just remembering—boy, that popped into my head—I'm just remembering that he was the one who met me at the train when I fled from my only attempt at really getting married (laughs). Good ol' Pop. . . . You know, that's a nice memory. Thank you, Craig. Because he certainly didn't shirk my emotionality then, did he? I've got it in my head somehow that he failed me a little on emotion and not feeling. And I'm really glad—thank you, I'm really glad to remember that he's the one they sent to the station to get me off the train. And he and I went and had a soda and he went and got something—something they had in those days—tranquilizers. And I read Marcus Aurelius—my God, what a memory. Boy, that was a—but I'm drifting off, I know, but I'm very grateful to you. I'm really grateful for that "aha." See, I have a little resentment, yeah. I have a little resentment, but I keep—I'm always trying to rationalize it a little by saying "What the hell do you want for a parent, sweetie?" Who is a perfect parent? That's insane, there is no perfect parent. And it clearly makes me feel a little dizzy to criticize my father. So this is—thank you.

As a result of our discussion Helen recalled a hidden memory that led her to reinterpret her relationship with her father.

Golda also gained new insight into her relationship with her deceased mother. She decided that perhaps her combative relationship with her mother was due to the fact that the narratives of her mother's independent life stop at the time when Golda was born:

I, you know—this is a weird exercise, 'cause I don't—I'm not sure that I ever thought about this till this very, very second, but I wonder if—I've always had sort of a combative relationship with my mother and was always sort of embarrassed by her when I was young because she didn't do anything. And I wonder if I didn't just feel guilty about that . . . that all the stories stopped when I was born.

Through narrating her story Golda begins to examine her feelings toward her mother. She begins to sense that what bothered her about her mother—that she "didn't do anything"—may have been a result of her mother having to nurture and care for Golda. Thus Golda begins to reinterpret her understanding of her mother.

The act of telling a narrative leads some narrators to realize they still need to work on their pain from the loss. Ned was 59 years old when his 17-month-old granddaughter drowned. When I ask him what it is like to relate his story to me, Ned explains that it reminds him that he still has much to think about concerning this death:

Well, it was obvious there were times that tears were close to the surface (pause), which suggests to me that (pause) maybe I need to (pause)—suggests to me (pause) that I have not paid enough attention to that recently. That I have allowed—that I have allowed the busyness of my life (pause) to prevent me from (pause) giving much thought or reflecting intentionally, focusing on her and our loss.

Through sharing the story the narrative changes in order to help the narrator reconstruct a life. Re-creating the identity, though, can be done only through reconnecting with others. Sometimes the reinterpretation comes about simply from making the time to tell the story.

Even though all people construct these narratives, they are not often shared. Some of the participants said that in the year after a death people close to them would listen to their story. After that it was as if a fence had been erected, and the stories were no longer allowed to be brought out in public. However, some, such as Golda, had never shared their story with anyone. This project allowed participants to revisit the experience surrounding the dying and to once again talk about this topic. All of the participants expressed gratitude for or a level of comfort in being able to tell their grief narrative. The result for many of the participants was a sense of catharsis, a feeling of relief that they could step beyond ritualized cultural expectations. Given that individuals change over time, periodically revisiting these key events in a person's life allows a transformation in the self and in his or her relationship to the world.

Of particular interest was the fact that not one of the interviewed participants made eye contact when telling his or her narrative. In the United States maintaining eye contact is considered polite, as it demonstrates that the listener and the teller are both interested in what is being said: "A person who does not maintain eye contact may be perceived as not listening or not caring" (Purnell & Paulanka, 1998, p. 18). However, I found that all the participants avoided looking at me when telling their stories. Helen closed her eyes, and when I asked her about this she said,

Well, I'm reliving it. When I go—I can see him. What's fun about this is that for years I've lived here—I don't think of my father in the backyard anymore. . . . But the reason that I'm doing this, and I'm so glad, 'cause this has been much—I think it's—I happen to think it's a much better idea not to look at you. Oh God, you might have had people that couldn't have done this without looking at you. I didn't want to be looking at what you were—you know, making a contact. I have found this very comfortable to sit, and when I close my eyes I go back, love. Very particularly you have evoked my father in those old baggy trousers. And I'm very pleased. . . . You've let me evoke my father.

Being offered the opportunity to tell a narrative in a way that minimizes intrusion seems to offer people an opportunity to both preserve important memories and come to new and sometimes more acceptable understandings of themselves and of their loved ones.

Psychocultural Approaches to Grief Narratives

The psychocultural approach asks how an individual draws on culturally available plots and symbols to form the self and to formulate the experience (Peacock & Holland, 1993). The narrator is trying to make sense of a set of seemingly chaotic events that he or she underwent. The events by themselves have no meaning and lack symbolism, themes, and interpretation. The act of telling the narrative is the act of defining the self and of constructing the experience through emplotment and subjunctivizing. The narrator takes the events and gives them a plot, time line, meaning, interpretation, theme, and character to create the experience.

Viewed from this approach, narratives that are offered verbally appear to be uncontrolled and unstructured (Frank, 1995). Since published texts are by their nature ordered, structured, and polished, they have already been emplotted. Five of the 15 interviews conducted for this study reveal strong psychocultural elements. Often narrators of these tales have trouble relating what happened immediately after the death because they have been unable to create a coherent story. All of the narratives in which young people died lend themselves to this approach. Anne's friend died from an undetected congenital heart problem. Isaac lost a sister to an unknown sudden cause. James's partner committed suicide. Ned's grandchild drowned. Sudden death leaves no time for the witness to prepare for the loss. The grieving person feels the shock of abrupt loss and is later forced to make sense of what he or she may view as a meaningless, senseless, or preventable death.

James explains what he was thinking and feeling immediately after learning of his partner's suicide:

It was numb (pause)—nothing's running through it. Just absolute shock (pause). I still go into mental shock (long pause). I—I don't know what ran through my mind those first few weeks, I think (pause). In fact, I don't remember what happened at all those first few weeks afterwards. Wow.

James's sense of chaos is associated with a lack of memory: he does not recall what happened in the first few weeks. Telling his narrative is an attempt to recall and make sense of the events.

Ned relates how raw and fragmented everything felt in the weeks following his granddaughter's death and how he needed time to make sense of it all:

No, I (pause) would've needed some time (pause). A couple of things I tried to remind myself of in going through the experience (pause). The first was simply to allow myself to go through it and not to (pause), you know, not to be (pause) the instructor, not to be (pause) the macho male, not to (pause) be the disconnected person in charge while everybody else, you know, around me was not in charge. [I] intentionally attempted not to do that but to allow myself to experience (pause) the pain, allowed myself to cry when I needed to cry, allow myself to (pause) yell or shout if I needed to, and obviously in appropriate places (pause). And at least for the first month or month and a half I think it would have been impossible to (pause)—for me to have made much of a story out of it (pause), you know. And it certainly (pause)—I would say at least the four to five weeks after her death (pause) are kind of—are vague recollections. They were very powerful (pause). I mean, it was a very powerfully emotional time and so I was severely depressed and (pause) minimally functional. And I was aware of that and tried to allow myself to be that way and not to (pause)—and not to change it.

The most sense that Ned could make of his experience was simply to acknowledge that overwhelming events had occurred and to give himself permission to feel and experience them.

Narrative Phenomenology

Phenomenology is about the study of the structure of experience. It raises questions about how people choose their words, how ideas come to them, and how they tie their experiences together through images, symbols, themes, and plots. As a branch of philosophy, phenomenology concerns itself with our place in time and space, our actions, our intentionality, and our embodiment. In engaging with the text—that is, published narratives and verbal stories—questions can be asked that allow the interpreter to see the context in which the narrative was developed, the meanings it holds, and the functions it performs. In the end, narrative is about living and about making sense of a series of events that occur in a life.

Enabling people to tell their accounts and teaching people to listen can help individuals deal with their grief and encourage others to accept death and dying as a part of life. The value lies not so much in determining how people construct and reconstruct experience and the self in an abstract sense but rather in how people can assist others to make meaning of the loss and continue living. Healthcare providers not only have but can also make opportunities to assist people to make meaning and to continue living fully. The power of narrative phenomenology lies therefore in the process of engaging people in remaking their own world by making sense of their life experiences and their grief.

Narrative phenomenology is also useful for other purposes. Rita Charon (2001) suggests that inviting narratives offers a way for healthcare providers to connect with patients, to empathize with them, and to share common experiences with other providers. While Charon emphasizes the importance of the healthcare provider's absorbing and processing of the narrative, I am in favor of a much more active stance being taken by health professionals. Considering the benefits that accrued to individuals in this study from telling their stories, I believe that health professionals could and should be educated to become expert listeners and story facilitators. More than mere witnesses to grief and suffering, practitioners should actively invite narratives, both verbal and written, paying attention to the symbols invoked, the themes that emerge, and the function that telling the story seems to serve. In this way important memories can be preserved, new and acceptable interpretations of problematic experiences can be found, life and death can be put into perspective, and important lessons that have been learned can be shared with others. By overcoming isolation and restoring community, stories of chaos and loss can be transformed into narratives of deep meaning and personal enrichment. People of all ages, experiencing grief at various levels of intensity, should be actively encouraged to share their grief narratives verbally and in writing. After all, telling stories is what we as humans do to make sense of our lives and, indeed, to make sense of existence itself.

References

Albom, M. (1997). *Tuesdays with Morrie.* New York: Doubleday.

Ariès, P. (1975). *Western attitudes toward death: From the Middle Ages to the present* (P. M. Ranum, Trans.). Baltimore, MD: Johns Hopkins University Press.

Ariès, P. (1991). *The hour of our death* (H. Weaver, Trans.). Oxford: Oxford University Press.

Barnard, D., Towers, A., Boston, P., & Lambrimnidou, Y. (2000). *Crossing over: Narratives of palliative care.* New York: Oxford University Press.

Beauvoir, S. de (1985). *A very easy death* (P. O'Brian, Trans.). New York: Pantheon.

Becker, G. (1997). *Disrupted lives: How people create meaning in a chaotic world.* Berkeley: University of California Press.

Beim, G., & Stevens, J. R. (1998). *Babe Ruth: A daughter's portrait.* Dallas: Taylor Publishing.

Booth, W. C. (1988). *The company we keep: An ethics of fiction.* Berkeley: University of California Press.

Bruner, J. (1986). *Actual minds, possible worlds.* Cambridge, MA: Harvard University Press.

Bruner, J. (1987). Life as narrative. *Social Research, 54*(1), 11–32.

Byock, I. (1997). *Dying well: The prospect for growth at the end of life.* New York: Riverhead Books.

Campbell, J. (1973). *The hero with a thousand faces.* Princeton, NJ: Princeton University Press. (Original work published 1949)

Cayless, S. E. (1996). *Babe: The life and times of Babe Didrikson Zaharias.* Urbana: University of Illinois Press.

Charon, R. (2001). The patient–physician relationship—narrative medicine: A model for empathy, reflection, profession, and trust. *Journal of the American Medical Association, 268,* 1897–1902.

Clandinin, D. J., & Connelly, F. M. (2000). *Narrative inquiry: Experience and story in qualitative research.* San Francisco: Jossey-Bass.

Closing scenes. (1885, April 16). *New York Times,* p. 1.

Cushman, R. E. (1987). Gilgamesh (J. Haight & A. S. Mahler, Trans.). In M. Eliade (Ed.), *The encyclopedia of religion* (Vol. 13, pp. 401–403). New York: Macmillan.

Denzin, N. K. (1989). *Interpretive biography* (Vol. 17). Newbury Park, CA: Sage.

Frank, A. W. (1995). *The wounded storyteller: Body, illness, and ethics.* Chicago: University of Chicago Press.

Fuller, R. (1993). Jesus Christ. In B. M. Metzger & M. D. Coogan (Eds.), *The Oxford companion to the Bible* (pp. 356–366). New York: Oxford University Press.

Gallup, G. (1985). *Religion in America—50 years: 1935–1985; The Gallup report.* Princeton, NJ: Princeton Religion Research Center.

Geertz, C. (1973). *The interpretation of cultures.* New York: Basic Books.

Geertz, C. (1983). *Local knowledge.* New York: Basic Books.

Good, B. J. (1994). *Medicine, rationality, and experience.* Cambridge: Cambridge University Press.

Gordon, C. H. (1993). Gilgamesh epic. In B. M. Metzger & M. D. Coogan (Eds.), *The Oxford companion to the Bible* (p. 254). New York: Oxford University Press.

Grant, F. C. (1962). Jesus Christ. In G. A. Buttrick (Ed.), *The interpreter's dictionary of the Bible* (Vol. 2, pp. 869–896). Nashville: Abingdon Press.

Greenspahn, F. E. (1987). Jacob (J. Haight & A. S. Mahler, Trans.). In M. Eliade (Ed.), *The encyclopedia of religion* (Vol. 7, pp. 503–504). New York: Macmillan.

Gunther, J. (1965). *Death be not proud: A memoir.* New York: Perennial. (Original work published 1949)

Hawkins, A. H. (1999). *Reconstructing illness: Studies in pathography* (2nd ed.). West Lafayette, IN: Purdue University Press.

Heidegger, M. (1962). *Being and time* (J. Macquarrie & E. Robinson, Trans.). New York: Harper & Row. (Original work published 1927)

Heidegger, M. (1977). *Basic writings* (Vol. 1, D. F. Krell, Ed.). New York: Harper & Row.

A hero finds rest. (1885, July 24). *New York Times*, p. 1.

Hicks, L. (1962). Jacob (Israel). In G. A. Buttrick (Ed.), *The interpreter's dictionary of the Bible* (Vol. 2, pp. 782–786). Nashville: Abingdon Press.

His last resting place. (1885, July 24). *New York Times*, p. 1.

Homer. (1999). *The Iliad* (W. H. D. Rouse, Trans.). New York: Signet Classics.

Iser, W. (1978). *The act of reading: A theory of aesthetic response.* Baltimore, MD: Johns Hopkins University Press.

Kamenetz, R. (1985). *Terra infirma.* Fayetteville: University of Arkansas Press

Kaufman, S. R. (2000). Narrative, death, and the uses of anthropology. In T. R. Cole, R. Kastenbaum, & R. E. Ray (Eds.), *Handbook of the humanities and aging* (2nd ed., pp. 342–364). New York: Springer.

Kleinman, A. (1988). *The illness narratives: Suffering, healing, and the human condition.* New York: Basic Books.

Klenow, D. J., & Bolin, R. C. (1989–1990). Belief in an afterlife: A national survey. *Omega: The Journal of Death and Dying, 20*(1), 63–74.

Krant, M. J. (1974). *Dying and dignity: The meaning and control of a personal death.* Springfield, IL: Charles C. Thomas.

Kübler-Ross, E. (1997). *On death and dying.* New York: Touchstone. (Original work published 1969)

MacIntyre, A. (1984). *After virtue* (2nd ed.). Notre Dame, IN: University of Notre Dame Press.

Miller, N. K. (1992a). Autobiographical deaths. *Massachusetts Review, 33,* 19–47.

Miller, N. K. (1992b). Facts, pacts, and acts. *Profession, 92,* 10–14.

Moran, W. L. (1987). Gilgamesh (J. Haight & A. S. Mahler, Trans.). In M. Eliade (Ed.), *The encyclopedia of religion* (Vol. 5, pp. 557–560). New York: Macmillan.

Morson, C. S., & Emerson, C. (1991). Global concepts: Creation of prosaics. In *Mikhail Bakhtin: Creation of a prosaics* (pp. 15–63). Stanford: Stanford University Press.

Murphy, G. (1959). Discussion. In H. Feifel (Ed.), *The meaning of death* (pp. 317–340). New York: McGraw-Hill.

Myerhoff, B. (1994). *Number our days: Culture and community among elderly Jews in an American ghetto.* New York: Meridian.

Neimeyer, R. A. (1999). Narrative strategies in grief therapy. *Journal of Constructivist Psychology, 12,* 65–85.

Nuland, S. B. (1993). *How we die: Reflections on life's final chapter.* New York: Knopf.

Oxford English Dictionary Online. (2001). Oxford University Press. Retrieved September 14, 2005, from http://www.oed.com

Parsons, T., & Lidz, V. (1967). Death in American society. In E. S. Shneidman (Ed.), *Essays in self-destruction* (pp. 133–170). New York: Science House.

Peacock, J. L., & Holland, D. C. (1993). The narrated self: Life stories in process. *Ethos, 21,* 367–383.

Plato. (1981). *Five dialogues* (G. M. A. Grube, Trans.). New York: Hackett.

Polanyi, L. (1985). *Telling the American story: A structural and cultural analysis of conversational storytelling.* Norwood, NJ: Ablex.

Polkinghorne, D. E. (1996). Narrative knowing and the study of lives. In J. E. Birren, G. M. Kenyon, J.-E. Ruth, J. J. F. Schroots, & T. Svensson (Eds.), *Aging and biography: Explorations in adult development* (pp. 77–99). New York: Springer.

Purnell, L. D., & Paulanka, B. J. (1998). *Transcultural health care: A culturally competent approach.* Philadelphia: F.A. Davis.

Ramsay, D. (1806). *The life of George Washington.* Retrieved June 22, 2000, from http://www.earlyamerica.com/lives/gwlife/index.html

Reston, J. (1963, November 23). Why America weeps. *New York Times,* pp. 1, 7.

Richardson, L. (1990). *Writing strategies: Reaching diverse audiences* (Vol. 21). Newbury Park, CA: Sage.

Riches, G., & Dawson, P. (1996). Making stories and taking stories: Methodological reflections on researching grief and marital tension following the death of a child. *British Journal of Guidance and Counseling, 24,* 357–365.

Ricoeur, P. (1981a). *Hermeneutics and the human sciences* (J. B. Thompson, Trans.). Cambridge: Cambridge University Press.

Ricoeur, P. (1981b). Narrative time. In W. J. T. Mitchell (Ed.), *On narrative* (pp. 165–186). Chicago: University of Chicago Press.

Ricoeur, P. (1984). *Time and narrative* (Vol. 1, K. McLaughlin & D. Pellauer, Trans.). Chicago: University of Chicago Press.

Ritchie, D. A. (2003). *Doing oral history: A practical guide* (2nd ed.). New York: Oxford University Press.

Rosenblatt, E., & Rosenblatt, R. (Eds.). (1992). *Hard marching every day: The Civil War letters of Private Wilbur Fisk, 1861–1865.* Topeka: University of Kansas Press.

Roth, P. (1991). *Patrimony: A true story.* New York: Simon and Schuster.

Sandars, N. K. (Ed.). (1988). *The epic of Gilgamesh.* New York: Penguin.

Sedney, M. A., Baker, J. E., & Gross, E. (1994). "The story" of a death: Therapeutic considerations with bereaved families. *Journal of Marital and Family Therapy, 20,* 278–296.

Smith, R. N. (1994). *The surprising George Washington.* Retrieved January 26, 2001, from http://www.nara.gov/publications/prologue/george1.html

Stivers, C. (1993). Reflections on the role of personal narrative in social science. *Signs: Journal of Women in Culture and Society, 18,* 408–425.

Twain, M. (1990). Appendix A: The death of Jean. In M. Kiskis (Ed.), *Mark Twain's own autobiography* (pp. 245–252). Madison: University of Wisconsin Press.

Vanderpool, H. Y. (1997). Doctors and the dying of patients in American history. In R. F. Weir (Ed.), *Physician-assisted suicide* (pp. 33–66). Indianapolis: Indiana University Press.

Weathersby, T. (2001). *Death and dying self-assessment.* Retrieved May 21, 2001, from http://dying.about.com/health/dying/blans1.htm

Webb, M. (1997). *The good death: The new American search to reshape the end of life.* New York: Bantam.

West, J. (1986). *The woman said yes: Encounters with life and death.* New York: Harcourt Brace Jovanovich.

While awaiting the end. (1885, July 24). *New York Times,* p. 1.

White, H. (1981). The value of narrativity in the representation of reality. In W. J. T. Mitchell (Ed.), *On narrative* (pp. 1–23). Chicago: University of Chicago Press.

Wilson, J. M. (1996). *I have looked death in the face: Biography of William Porcher DuBose, soldier, philosopher, theologian.* Kingston, TN: Paint Rock.

Young, K. G. (1987). *Taleworlds and storyrealms: The phenomenology of narrative.* Dordrecht: Martinus Nijhoff.

Zaharias, B. D. (1956). *This life I've led: My autobiography as told to Harry Paxton.* London: Robert Hale.

5

Wish Fulfillment for Children with Life-Threatening Illnesses

BONNIE EWING

Introduction

Children with life-threatening illnesses are subjected to numerous treatments and procedures. They often experience enormous physical and emotional pain and suffering as attempts are made to prolong their life. Desperately dependent on the medical system for their survival, these children and their families often experience hopelessness and helplessness due to the many hospitalizations, painful treatments, and procedures they must endure.

As a life-threatening illness progresses, children come to realize that their body is changing and becoming more fragile. Their self-esteem suffers as they sense that they are not growing and developing in the normal way that they once did (Hynson, Gillis, Collins, Irving, & Trethewie, 2003). Becoming aware that they are different from other children, they feel lonely and isolated. Bluebond-Langner (1978) writes that dying children are unlike other children because they will not "become" (p. 213). Society measures their worth by what they do now, unlike other children, who have time to prove themselves.

Within all of the physical and emotional turmoil in these children's lives is the anxiety brought on by their experience of *being-toward-death*.[1] How is fear of death experienced by children with a life-threatening illness? How do these children face living with uncertainty? Do they dream and think about possibilities for the future?

Wish-granting organizations seek to offer a form of escape or a respite from these difficulties; they invite the children to enter a world of fantasy or dreams by thinking of a special wish, one that they desire above anything else. With this invitation an assumption is made that having a special wish fulfilled creates a sense of hope and joy that may help these children transcend the difficult and sorrowful conditions that they must endure before death. However, when a child is diagnosed with a life-threatening illness, real-life limitations affect the outcome of this special wish experience, regardless of what adults might hope or believe may happen. Children with a life-threatening illness exist within the context of impending death. They experience suffering in the form of physical pain, anxiety, anger, separation and loss, and fear of death. Hope, in the form of wish fulfillment, may make a difference by providing a more meaningful existence for the children—or it may not.

Wish-granting organizations believe that they are providing uplifting experiences for children with a life-threatening illness. Adult volunteers and professionals develop and advocate for approaches that will help to ensure that the fulfilled wish will be beneficial for these children. Parents also share their impressions of their experiences of wish fulfillment with volunteers from the organization and sometimes with the media. All, including volunteers, parents, and professionals, may benefit, however, from further exploration of what special wish fulfillment means to the child.

Significance of the Study

Although adults hold strong beliefs about the importance of wish fulfillment for dying children, there has been no research that explores what the experience of having a special wish fulfilled means to a child with a life-threatening illness. We cannot assume that a child feels the same way as an adult would about the experience of having a special wish become a reality. Also, because their verbal language is unsophisticated, children cannot be relied upon to convey the complexity of meanings of having a special wish fulfilled. Therefore, children are in a prime position to be misunderstood by adults (Garbarino, Stott, & faculty of the Eriksson Institute, 1992). Research specifically designed to give children a voice was needed.

It is of paramount importance to learn what having a special wish fulfilled means to a child with a life-threatening illness, because miscommunication and misunderstanding between adults and children may be detrimental to both children and parents. For example, some adults, including parents and professionals, believe that it is better to protect children from the pain of knowing; they therefore avoid discussing problems related to the child's illness or they may provide vague answers. In some cases they even lie. The expressed desire to protect children by concealing information is often an indication of the adult's discomfort with issues of loss, pain, illness, and death (Bluebond-Langner, 1978).

Furthermore, caregivers need to know how a child experiences having a special wish fulfilled so that they may provide appropriate care to the child and the family. Superimposed upon all of the physical issues that the child is facing are other, complex emotional challenges that may be expressed only with great difficulty. Given the difficulty that children frequently have in communicating their feelings verbally to adults, assumptions are often made about the nature of these challenges that the child is facing. In particular, it is assumed that children with a life-threatening illness are facing extreme anxiety and fear about death and could benefit from a respite from these feelings through the granting of special wishes and retreats into fantasy. Considering that understanding of the child's experience in relation to having a wish granted is lacking, the purpose of this study was to illuminate through interpretation of their drawings the children's experiences of having a wish granted.

The artwork collected for this study lives on as testimony to how these children experienced having their wishes fulfilled. The drawings serve as an enduring portrayal of an experience that was desired and hoped for within the struggle of living and dying.

Background

As cofounder of a chapter of the Make-A-Wish Foundation, I became actively involved in granting wishes for children with a life-threatening illness. As I observed the children as they had their special wish fulfilled, I became increasingly interested in knowing more about what this experience meant to them. Intuitively, I sensed that the children needed a change and that they chose to have a special wish fulfilled as an alternative way of dealing with the unbearable circumstances that surrounded them. Many of the children wanted to go to Walt Disney World. Others wanted to go to another country. Some wanted to meet special celebrities, and others simply wanted toys or computer games.

As I considered the kinds of wishes children chose, I wondered about the significance of the experience for them. Remembering an adolescent with cancer who was admitted to the hospital not long before he died but who refused to remain in the institution, I recalled that he had begged to go to the Super Bowl. His wish was fulfilled, and he had a wonderful time; he died three weeks later. I wondered what it meant to him to choose this alternative intervention in place of the life-prolonging therapy that he would have received in the hospital. Could it be that he wanted to feel "normal" by going to a ball game like his peers, or did going to the game have a significance for him that remained elusive for me?

What could it mean to these children to have a special wish fulfilled during a time of great uncertainty in their life? I thought it might be possible that having a wish fulfilled could create stronger family bonds and that it might engender a sense of hope. Hopefulness is believed to directly influence the health of an individual by helping that person work at regaining or augmenting health or accepting death. Hope is fundamental to the child's survival and is an important element in the will to live (Gaes, 1987; Hinds, 2004; Kübler-Ross, 1983). Hope counters despair and fends off the closing down of a future of possibilities and is also considered by many to be both basic and essential to healing. In the healing relationship hope is not something given or provided to an individual, nor is it a personality trait. Hope is experienced and exchanged by both the healer and the one being healed (Benner, 1984).

Of interest to me was the relationship between hope and the granting of a child's wish. A wish is something that a person desires and hopes to obtain (Freud, 1953/1965). Psychological explanations suggest that once one's basic needs are fulfilled, desires of the intellect begin to unfold. Gratification of one's needs and desires may increase self-esteem and self-worth and may contribute to having a positive outlook on one's life, which may aid in healing (Maslow, 1998). There are other ways to understand and interpret the phenomenon of hope. Hope and wishing are intertwined with the idea of future possibilities, since wishing for something engenders the hope that the wish will come true. When a child is dying, however, future possibilities are limited by illness. When one has the sense that the future has been changed or shortened by serious disease, the present can take on greater immediacy and importance. Children with a life-threatening illness live in the present, and their future possibilities remain uncertain.

When I reflected on the experiences of children with a life-threatening illness who have had their special wish come true, I wondered how their feelings of alienation, uncertainty, isolation, loneliness, and fear of death showed themselves in the context of having their wish fulfilled. It seemed possible that having a special wish fulfilled could change a child's understanding of his or her existence and being-toward-death.

Reflections on these children bring to mind a passage from the poem "On Children," from *The Prophet* (Gibran, 1923):

> You may give them your love but not your thoughts.
> For they have their own thoughts.
> You may house their bodies but not their souls,
> For their souls dwell in the house of tomorrow, which you cannot visit,
>   not even in your dreams.
>
> (17)

Meaning and Artwork

One of the primary ways in which children speak meaningfully to us is through their artwork (Kübler-Ross, 1983). Art is a practical children's activity that reveals hidden meanings through symbols and images. Since children do not have linguistic sophistication, artwork provides an avenue for uninhibited expression of their experiences in order to make meaning manifest (Rollins, 2005). Heidegger (1960/1993b) writes that art brings something into being from its essential source. Art grants a clearing in which artist and artwork can *be*. Art may allow the artist to experience a clearing through artwork. Art is a way to create openness, a region that is free for all things to be expressed. Heidegger (1960/1993b) states: "[T]he clearing, the open region, is not only free for brightness and darkness but also for resonance and echo, for sound and the diminishing of sound. . . . The clearing is the open region for everything that becomes present and absent" (pp. 383–384).

Through metaphorical thinking children use symbols and images in their drawings to represent elements in a situation that they are trying to understand. Embedded meanings are manifested in symbols and images that may then be interpreted to bring to expression what the children are unable to articulate (Fontana, 1993; Piaget, 2001; Rollins, 2005; Welsh & Instone, 2000).

The fact that children are unable to clearly articulate their experiences through verbal language has further implications. Heidegger

(1971) writes: "Where word breaks off no thing may be" (p. 60). Without a means of expressing themselves, it is possible that children cannot even *think* about certain aspects of their experiences. Art provides that means of expression and communication. Art is a form of language that reopens the possibilities of thinking and communicating their experiences of their illness and of having a special wish fulfilled. Thus drawings may both provide the children with a much-needed vehicle for expression and also provide the researcher a way to interpret the meaning of having a special wish fulfilled within the context of having a life-threatening illness.

The Study

In this study I hoped to reveal the shared meanings and common practices embedded in the symbols of the artwork of children who have had their wish fulfilled. Beginning with the question "What is the meaning of having a special wish fulfilled for a child with a life-threatening illness?" I sought to acquire a deeper understanding of how children with a life-threatening illness experienced having a special wish fulfilled. Hoping to add to the body of healthcare practitioners' knowledge of children's experience of dying, I aimed to better understand the needs and problems of the child who has a life-threatening illness. A better understanding was important because miscommunication and misunderstanding between adults and children may be detrimental to the child. Eight drawings were chosen for analysis and interpretation.

Assumptions

This study was based on the following assumptions:

1. The shared practices and common meanings embodied in the experience of a phenomenon occur within a context of common symbols with shared meanings.
2. People who share a common experience (e.g., children with a life-threatening illness who have a special wish fulfilled) use symbols in their drawings to reflect the meaning of that experience.
3. Interpreting the symbols and their relationships as expressed in the drawings provides an understanding of the meaning of that experience.
4. The children in this study share common practices and meanings

because of the commonalities of living with a life-threatening illness,
even though they are different in chronological and developmental
ages.

The assumption that commonalities exist is based on the premise
that children with a life-threatening illness are members of a culture
who share a common background and participate in common meanings.
A culture shares common experiences, thoughts, actions, activities, and
expressions. Common themes and common meanings are therefore expected in a study of human beings who have a common cultural background (Benner & Wrubel, 1989). As Gadamer (1988) states, "[I]t is the
task of hermeneutics to illuminate this miracle of understanding, which is
not a mysterious communication of souls, but rather a participation of
shared meaning" (p. 69). These children, through their experiences, live
in a world of shared meaning.

Key Terms

Dying is the process of ceasing to live. It is a time when a child is
fighting to live and medical professionals are attempting to stave off
death.

Wish granting in the context of this study is the practice followed
by the Make-A-Wish Foundation. A child's wish is fulfilled after the child
explores three different wishes. Children are chosen after referrals from
family, friends, or professionals. The referring individual is told to contact
the family so that they in turn can contact the organization if the child
desires to have a wish fulfilled. This process protects the child from unwanted suggestions by well-meaning individuals. Skilled volunteers then
establish the child's readiness to have the wish granted. The child's condition, even though he or she is ill, is considered to be an important factor
in his or her capacity to experience enjoyment in the fulfillment of the
wish. The preference is that the child be in a state of good health at the
time the wish is granted. However, it is deemed more important to grant
the child's wish even at or near the time of death than to have the child
die without having the wish fulfilled.

Drawings are pictures containing symbols and images that communicate thoughts, understandings, and concerns. Symbols and images comprise a vocabulary in artwork and contain multiple meanings that can be
interpreted by the viewer.

Life-threatening illness, as defined in this study and by the Make-A-Wish Foundation, is a state of illness in which the child will most probably not live past the 18th year of life.

Participants

The children whose artwork was gathered for this study had their wishes fulfilled by the Make-A-Wish Foundation. This organization grants special wishes to children with a life-threatening illness who are from 3 to 18 years of age. At the time of writing this paper some of the children who had submitted artwork were still alive, while others had died. Some of the participants were known to the researcher, but others were not. Twelve pictures were given to the researcher, and eight of these were chosen for the study. As part of a project organized by the Make-A-Wish Foundation, each child drew one picture. The children whose drawings were accepted ranged between the ages of 6 and 14; their parents had given the organization permission for public use of the drawings. Since life-threatening illness and degenerative disease cause children to regress physically and psychosocially, no attempt was made to select participants using criteria based on chronological age when arriving at a decision as to which children's drawings would be accepted for the study.

Method of Inquiry

Hermeneutic inquiry was used to unveil the meaning of having a special wish fulfilled for children with a life-threatening illness. Meaning was uncovered through interpretation of the expression of their experiences in their drawings. Hermeneutics is both a philosophical position and a method of understanding the lived experience of an individual. It is a process of making intelligible that which is not yet understood (Bernstein, 1991). The hermeneutic process seeks to render understanding explicit through interpretation of meanings contained within symbols and images. Gadamer (1960/2003) explains:

[H]ermeneutics must be so determined as a whole that it does justice to the experience of art. Understanding must be conceived as a part of the event in which meaning occurs, the event in which the meaning of all statements—those of art and all other kinds of tradition—is formed and actualized. (p. 164)

By interpreting the drawings in their totality and looking at their parts in relation to the whole, the underlying shared meanings of children with a life-threatening illness who have had their special wish fulfilled were discerned.

Approval to conduct the study was obtained from a Human Subjects and Research Review Committee, and permission to use the artwork of the participants was obtained from the Make-A-Wish Foundation. A meeting was conducted with the president of the foundation chapter, who verified the names of the children, ages, diagnoses, and wishes granted and that public relations permissions had been obtained. In addition, the files of the participants were reviewed to determine that the necessary clearances had been obtained. Eight drawings were selected, and all identifying information was removed.

The drawings were obtained at a holiday gathering where children were given colored markers and asked to draw a picture of the wish that they had had fulfilled. The children were free to express themselves while in a group with other children. Using drawings that had been obtained in this relaxed atmosphere was preferred because children are less inhibited and are able to express themselves more freely in a situation where formal demands are not placed upon them (Garbarino et al., 1992).

The eight drawings selected for the study were rich in symbols, images, colors, configurations, and patterns that revealed the meaning of having a special wish fulfilled for children with a life-threatening illness. Meaning in artwork is contained within the symbols and images that the viewer is able to discern. Symbols and images are expressions of the artist in a metaphorical language and contain multiple meanings in which there is a shared understanding between the viewer and the artist (Edwards, 1986). The viewer has the opportunity to engage in a dialogue with the artwork to uncover the multiple meanings being expressed.

To dialogue with artwork means that an understanding occurs in which the pictures can be brought to language by the viewer. The symbols, forms, images, colors, patterns, and configurations call forth thoughts, ideas, and feelings. The drawings chosen for the study were those that evoked dialogue and best exemplified how the children experienced having a special wish fulfilled. The drawings chosen contained symbols that most clearly revealed the actual wish that the child had had fulfilled, such as a picture of Mickey Mouse, indicating that the child had gone to Walt Disney World. Drawings were selected that included images of the wish that the children and their families had experienced. Considering the symbols embedded in the drawings provided a way to understand emotional expressions, body-image disturbances, and family dynamics. Pictures that appeared devoid of symbols, images, or patterns showing the wish that was fulfilled were not selected for inclusion in this study.

Philosophical Context

This study seeks to disclose meanings embedded within the actions and practices of children with a life-threatening illness who have had their wish fulfilled, as revealed in their drawings. During infancy individuals begin interpreting themselves in light of their cultural background (Leonard, 1989). Hidden skills, practices, and linguistic meanings in the culture are pervasive and make our world intelligible to us. This background understanding creates possibilities and conditions for our actions. According to Heidegger (1927/1962), the understanding of being is embodied in social practices, language, cultural conventions, and historical understanding. He states that through our way of being in our world we come to know. Meanings are shared by individuals who share common cultural practices and a common language. Language provides the means by which human beings can reveal hidden meanings through interpretation of experiences. Yet "meaning is always coming into being through the 'happening' of understanding" (Bernstein, 1991, p. 139). Without understanding, meaning cannot come to be.

Heidegger (1927/1962) suggests that each of us comes to interpret and understand a phenomenon through a prior awareness, or *fore-structure,* of understanding. This a priori understanding about a phenomenon is believed to arise from one's everyday involvement in the world. In the context of this study, fore-structure means that I, the researcher, had a prior awareness of the phenomenon of having a wish fulfilled based on my life's experiences, which include habits, skills, and ways of living that were acquired from my culture. Fore-structure is a threefold structure upon which all interpretation is grounded; it consists of fore-having, fore-sight, and fore-conception. *Fore-having* in this case refers to the fact that I came to the artwork with a familiarity that was based on background practices from my professional world; this familiarity is part of what made the interpretation possible. *Fore-sight* accounts for my point of view, and *fore-conception* means that, because of my background, I had an expectation of what to anticipate in the artwork.

Fore-structure is the link between interpretation and understanding. It is the way one enters the hermeneutical circle of ontological thought.

In this study fore-structure was an entry point into the artwork of these children that accounted for my thoughts about the meaning being expressed in their artwork. It was the way that I developed a beginning understanding of how the children experienced having a special wish fulfilled within the context in which they lived. Through my personal background and professional experiences as a pediatric nurse and as a wish-granter for children with a life-threatening illness, I interpreted pictures and brought them into verbal language as they "spoke" to me through the metaphorical language of the artwork, which embodied meaning within symbols, images, and patterns. This language provided a way for me to interpret the stories that the children were trying to express.

Gadamer (1960/2003) states that there is an ontological sharing in a picture. The symbol in a picture has a representational function. It is a manifestation of something that is present but that is not yet revealed. Art may be the best available language for children wanting to express complex ideas and emotions. Drawing affords children opportunities to communicate ideas meaningfully. Since adults tend to communicate predominantly in a verbal manner, drawings present us with the challenge of deriving our understanding from immersing ourselves in the language of the artist.

Interpretation of the Drawings

Each of the children's drawings was transcribed into a written text by describing it in detail. An explication of the meanings was carried out, taking into account that the understanding of activity is holistic and contains multiple meanings. The drawings were analyzed according to a modification of an analysis process described by Diekelmann and Ironside (1999). Each drawing was examined for the physical qualities of the picture, such as forms, configurations, and structural elements. In addition, symbols and images were studied in relation to the whole picture. A description of each picture was written that related the parts to the whole and the whole in relation to the parts. A dialogue with each picture was allowed to develop in order to assimilate and synthesize the meanings that emerged through reflection upon the symbols, images, configurations, forms, and patterns in the drawings; for example, the symbol of water and how it was drawn in one child's picture suggested water play and the beauty of the ocean as well as the threat from its power. Back-and-forth questioning was then undertaken in an effort to understand these artistic expressions in relation to living with a life-threatening illness and having a special wish fulfilled.

Themes were discovered as they emerged from the initial understanding of the pictures, and an interpretive summary of the themes was written that disclosed both the implicit and explicit meanings. Interpretations were constantly challenged by returning to the drawings and to the written exegeses. These challenges affirmed, extended, or overruled interpretations. In addition, questions were brought forth and answered through a process of reflection during which I was able to call upon my experiences, both personal and professional, to gain a further understanding of the meanings being expressed in the artwork. The drawings were reanalyzed for clarification as the themes were developed and reinterpreted, a process that reflects the hermeneutic circle, in which interpretations are complete but never-ending. Finally, a constitutive pattern that reflected all the recurring themes was identified and written. A constitutive pattern is a thread that runs through the themes, is present in every theme, and is thus found in every text. This procedure allows for a continuous interaction with the text that may reveal contradictions and inconsistencies in the interpretive process (Diekelmann & Ironside, 1999).

Findings of the Study: Themes

The findings of this study are summarized by the constitutive pattern "living in limbo." This constitutive pattern represents a common idea found in all of the selected drawings. In addition, five themes were identified: being a child—playing, wishing, and hoping; "Why can't I be like the rest of the kids?"; "I am trying to balance things"; "I am all alone"; and "I need to find a comfortable place to be."

Theme: Being a Child—Playing, Wishing, and Hoping

The drawings of the children revealed many common practices of being a child—playing, wishing, and hoping—as expressed in the various forms of play embodied in the wishes that they requested to have fulfilled. In play children often try to live out their hopes and dreams. Through fantasy, or mental play, children adapt to the tensions, anxieties, and fears they experience about themselves and their world. Fantasy is a way to negotiate tormenting emotions and deal with conflicts. It is a way to alter the situation to make the child feel safe and better.

Walt Disney World, a place devoted to the concept of play, was most popular among the wishes that were fulfilled. Four out of the eight children whose drawings were included in the study chose Walt Disney World as their favorite wish. What is it about Mickey and Minnie and the Magic Kingdom that so enthralls children? These children were enticed by a place filled with stimulating lights, noise, and action. They were willing to endure the crowds in the heat of the day that make even normal, healthy children exhausted. Our culture sends out messages that Walt Disney World is a wonderful place where children can have fun and play. One need not be afraid in a place filled with magic, music, lights, and laughter. Perhaps these children believed that in the Magic Kingdom all things are possible.

Mickey and Minnie are humanlike mice who are dearly loved by young and old alike. In the cartoons these little mice meet challenges in their day-to-day lives and most of the time overcome their difficulties, sometimes by a twist of fate (Updike, 1995). But one of their most important features is their ability to live forever. Their overall appearance changes little; they never age and they will never die. They exemplify a way to continue, to be immortal, a way that holds the promise of hope for a future in which one can be happy, secure, and safe from harm.

In their drawings some of the children projected body-image disturbances onto Mickey. For example, in some of the pictures Mickey is missing his nose, and in one picture he has no arms. Psychological research (DiLeo, 1973; Rollins, 2005) shows that children with a life-threatening illness will often omit parts of their own body when they draw pictures of themselves. Such omissions of parts are posited to be reflections of their body-image disturbances. In this study, however, children projected their disturbances onto Mickey, making him more like themselves. They seemed to fuse with Mickey. This movement toward fusing with Mickey may in part be related to the fact that a child who is suffering from a life-threatening illness needs a sense of pride and self-respect and that self-esteem becomes diminished because of physical discomforts and alterations in self-image (Hinds, 2004; Rollins, 2005). The child needs to be recognized as a whole person, not only as an ill person. Fusing with Mickey or becoming more like him may help the authors of these artworks achieve the self-image they seek.

Interpretive phenomenology offers other possibilities for interpreting and understanding than are offered by psychology. Heidegger (1927/1962) suggests that we human beings experience each moment as it relates to our past as well as to our sense of future possibilities:

> Only in so far as Dasein *is* as an "I-*am*-as-having-been," can Dasein come towards itself futurally in such a way that it comes *back*. As authentically futural, Dasein *is* authentically as *"having been."* Anticipation of one's uttermost and ownmost possibility is coming back understandingly to one's ownmost "been." Only so far as it is futural can Dasein *be* authentically as having been. (373)

Children who have their wish fulfilled come to their experiences in the context of the lives they have lived thus far but also with the awareness that their future possibilities may be limited. Their life is shortened because of their illness, and while the children are alive they may have limited options. Thus, any experience in the present may hold within it their past experiences and their wishes for future possibilities.

A 9-year-old boy with osteogenic sarcoma chose a computer as his wish (see figure on following page), and an adolescent with Hodgkin's lymphoma chose a pinball machine. It is extremely important to a child's growth and development to master activities in order to move forward on the continuum of life (Freyer, 2004). The opportunity to develop and practice skills in the context of play encourages the child to continue to be involved in life, thereby fostering his or her desire to grow, develop, and become. Waechter (1987) emphasizes the necessity and importance of promoting the feeling that the dying child can continue to develop and grow. If the child senses that others are giving up, he or she will feel abandoned before death, which is a most unconscionable way for a child to experience the process of dying.

The fulfillment of the wish helps the child to be, in terms of his or her ownmost possibilities, not to be merely a "dying child." In play the psyche and the soma can come together as the child creates, imagines, and fantasizes about things that make him or her become something other than what is present. Wishing offers children the possibility of being and becoming different from the being in which they currently find themselves. In play and in wishing the child can be a whole person, active in making choices, creating, and reaching out to the world.

The fulfillment of a special wish that involves play may be a way for the child to become more harmonious in mind, body, and spirit. It gives

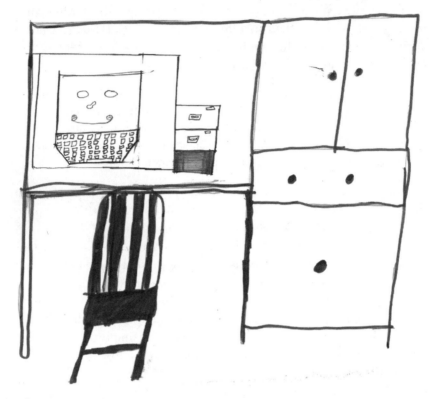

Playing

the child opportunities to reenvision and understand anew his or her difficulties in coping with a life-threatening illness. This reenvisioning introduces something joyful and hopeful. The child may imagine the process
of dying, but he or she can also imagine that there are other ways of living. Because the child with a life-threatening illness must live a life filled
with hospitalizations, technical procedures, and separations from family,
the fulfillment of a wish can help the child to realize that there are alternatives to his or her present existence. The fulfillment of a wish was a
form of play that the children selected as being most special to them. Play
offered these children a hopeful way of seeing and understanding themselves. Did play produce a sense of renewal of life, a feeling of going on,
a continuation of existence?

According to Gadamer (1960/2003), play is a natural process. In play the mode of being is close to the movement of nature. We are a part of nature, and the meaning of play is pure self-presentation. In their play children present to others what exists for them. For example, children enjoy dressing up and want others to recognize what is being presented. Likewise, in their artwork children want others to know what they have presented. They want others to know who they are and what they are trying to express. Through their pictures the children in this study appear to have presented themselves and what existed for them—among other things, the play of their wishes.

The ease of play becomes an absence of strain. It does not mean that "there is any real absence of effort but refers phenomenologically only to the absence of strain. The structure of play absorbs the player into itself and thus frees him [*sic*] from the burden of taking the initiative, which constitutes the actual strain of existence" (Gadamer, 1960/2003, p. 105). Having their wish fulfilled may have helped to ease the strain of the burdens of their illness for these children whose lives were threatened. Children try to alleviate their difficulties through play as they become engrossed in what they are doing. When children do something pleasurable such as playing a game or enjoying the water of the ocean, these activities can induce a state of relaxation. Relaxation generates a state of calmness and peacefulness that is healing to the body, mind, and spirit (Benson, 1975; Dossey, 2004).

These children, who were part of a unique culture of children with a life-threatening illness, shared common experiences—revealed in their drawings—of being emotionally conflicted as they had their dreams fulfilled. They harbored feelings of joy and happiness as well as pleasure, anger, and fright. In their everydayness they lived enmeshed within a context of uncertainty. Living on the brink between life and death, they were struggling to survive, but what kind of life is it when survival is struggle? It is a life of trying to hold on to what exists while being uncertain of what each day might bring. They were living both knowing and not knowing what might happen. Their bodies were changing in a way opposed to what they desired. Their lives were driven by a struggle to live, but they were unable to fulfill their wishes for a normal childhood. They existed with a deep-seated concern about not being able to fully live out their lives, lives that would normally involve plenty of wishing, hoping, and playing. Thus, embedded within the fulfillment of their wishes were complex concerns about living and dying.

Theme: Why Can't I Be Like the Rest of the Kids?

Before his wish was granted, an adolescent drew himself as apathetic and haggard. Reclining on the couch in plain clothing, with his eyes closed and hair disheveled, he looked listless and disengaged. After he received a pinball machine, however, his drawing of himself showed a person who was well groomed, wide-eyed, and energized. Emphasizing his masculinity, he drew himself with a large upper body and large muscles. A comparison of the before and after pictures conveyed further information. This young man did not draw some parts of his body, and in both instances he drew side angles of his body. In the before picture the left half of his body is hidden. In the after picture his right hand and arm are concealed from view. As he grasps the machine with his left hand he reveals only three fingers. Was there something about his bodily changes that he was trying to reveal?

When one does not feel well physically and one's body image is altered, self-esteem becomes diminished (Rollins, 2005). Children who do not feel good about the way they appear often feel uncomfortable and embarrassed. In addition, children with a life-threatening illness worry about the functioning of their body parts. Sometimes they try to deny their illness and pretend that they are like others. They pretend that they are not ill so that their parents will not be upset.

Because they are overwhelmed by the complexities that occur with illness, children with a life-threatening illness often regress physically, socially, and emotionally (Hinds, 2004). As the disease takes over their body they lose performance and function. Changes in body image create shame and feelings of being abnormal, resulting in decreased self-esteem. Sometimes the children become aggressive because they harbor hostility, and they act out their anger. They may become depressed and ridden with anxiety and guilt about being sick (Spinetta, Rigler, & Karon, 1987). They do not know how they will be able to use their body from day to day. They wonder if their body will continue to function, since they are unable to walk and talk as they did when they were not ill. They wonder if they will be able to go on breathing and if their hearts will continue to beat.

Theme: I Am Trying to Balance Things

A child who suffered from a degenerative disease that progressively took away his ability to balance could not run, jump, and play like normal children. His picture of Mickey Mouse suggests that there is another Mickey inside the character, one who is able to walk down a narrow path. This Mickey-within-a-Mickey looks delicately balanced and may even be ready to dance.

Does the fulfillment of a wish give such children a way to experience vicariously what it might be like to be more balanced and in control? In his day-to-day life this child was experiencing a loss of physical control. One can appreciate that his emotions were also out of control. The drawing shows a dark sun in a dark sky that leads one to conclude that things would be out of control on Earth if the sun did not shine. The order of Earth would become chaotic, and life would cease to exist. An object in the picture strongly resembles an overturned dinghy. This boat suggests the idea of things being upside down. It is not difficult to appreciate that children with a life-threatening illness feel that their world is upside down. The lines of the boat in this drawing are scribbled, uncontrolled markings that are seen not only in drawings by children with muscular disease but also in pictures by children who have a great amount of anxiety (DiLeo, 1973; Rollins, 2005). The child who drew the boat with scribbled lines may have been revealing the anxiety that children with a life-threatening illness frequently experience.

According to Heidegger, anxiety makes one feel "unsettled." Anxiety reveals to us the possibility of death. Heidegger (1927/1962) states that "anxiety is essentially being-toward-death" (p. 310). Anxiety discloses *Dasein,* which is open to future possibilities. Death is the possibility of the impossibility of existence. In children with a life-threatening illness anxiety about death may be combined with anxiety brought on by the sense that their life is out of balance.

Furthermore, the child who drew the dark sun and the uncontrolled upside-down boat may have been revealing through symbols a struggle not only with his own feelings of anxiety about confronting death but also with the anxiety imposed by a culture that has difficulty accepting death as a part of life. Our culture does not recognize that to be human is to be toward death. It often views death as a symptom to be treated, prevented, or even overcome. Our culture places a burden upon children with a life-threatening illness by using technology and hospitalization as means to extend life, even at the cost of causing emotional and physical pain. The children are caught in between, trying to survive as the professionals attempt to save their lives. They want to relinquish the pain, sorrow, and sadness that come with dying.

Like other children in this study, the child who drew the overturned boat and the dark sun was trying to maintain a sense of balance, which is revealed in his choice of colors. Half of the picture is drawn in black; the other is drawn in bright colors. The sun is divided in half vertically, showing two different suns, one that seems to be smiling and one that looks angry and sad. One eye of the sun is shut and the other eye is open. These images give one a sense that the child was balancing a dark and unhappy aspect of his life with fun, brightness, and pleasure. His drawing shows how children with a life-threatening illness try to balance feelings of unhappiness with happiness and their anxieties with things that are calming.

While balance is a way of staying in control physically and emotionally, it also has an ontological meaning that is related to healing. Balance is the sense of peacefulness that one can attain through integration of mind, body, and spirit (Dossey, 2004). It does not necessarily follow that balance can bring about a cure, but balance can bring a person a sense of peace within the self in which healing can occur.

Theme: I Am All Alone

Often one of a child's greatest fears is of being alone in the dark. In darkness children often cry uncontrollably. They feel insecure, overwhelmed, and frightened; they seek attention from their mother or other adults. Feeling helpless and anxious, they crave love and cuddling. Within the fear of blackness and darkness is a primitive fear of nothingness.

Heidegger suggests that death forces upon us the question of the meaning of being. Death is the ontic end point of life that reveals nonbeing. With death all beings disappear, and only the nothing seems to be left (Heidegger, 1927/1962). Children with a life-threatening illness are forced to confront fears of not-being, or nothingness. Children who fear dying often think of what it might be like to be without parents, brothers and sisters, home, and friends (Bowlby, 1973; Davies, Collins, Steele, Pipke, & Cooke, 2004). They are afraid of what it would be like without their home and the familiar places that they know. They may wonder if there will be anything after death. Such feelings give rise to anxiety, terror, anger, despair, and depression. Many children are unable to verbalize their feelings about death. They frequently experience anxiety and exhibit behaviors such as crankiness, aggressiveness, and irritability (Lyon, Townsend-Akpan, & Thompson, 2001; Wolfe, 2004).

In one picture of the Magic Kingdom (see figure on page 209) a child shows a preoccupation with dying. A path that at first glance looks like a moat also resembles a box situated between what look like grass and water. The box is shaped like a coffin. With the exception of Mickey Mouse, who is inside the box, not a single person is visible. Mickey is entirely alone. Mickey's eyes, however, are open, which makes him look as though he is alive. He even has a smile on his face. Could he be at peace? In our culture we frequently tell children that when they die they will be at peace. The child's picture shows how children with a life-threatening illness think about dying. They often try to comfort themselves with beliefs that death will be a peaceful and pleasurable experience.

In another picture a young boy drew a picture of himself standing happily with all of his family members, but he is separate from them. While he seems to be smiling and enjoying the experience, he has positioned himself apart from his family. The literature suggests that children with a life-threatening illness often feel separate and different from other family members because, by virtue of their illness, they are not healthy like the rest (Hynson et al., 2003). How, then, did he experience the fulfillment of his wish?

The family was included in the depiction of the fulfillment of his dream but absent in other drawings. Family relationships become strained when a child is seriously ill. Parents have tremendous difficulty coping with the prospect of losing their child. They may overindulge the child at times; they may also distance themselves from friends and other family members as protection from the pain of the final separation that will occur with death. Relationships between the child with a life-threatening illness and his or her siblings are also altered (Rollins, 1990; Giovanola, 2005). The dying child receives more attention from parents, which strains relationships with brothers and sisters, who consequently feel left out. Children with a life-threatening illness are aware of these family dynamics and have difficulty coping with them (Arnold & Gemma, 1994; Davies & Connaughty, 2002).

Theme: I Need to Find a Comfortable Place to Be

The children's pictures revealed symbols of nurturance in the form of food, shelter, and parental caregiving. Children who are dying seek to find a place of comfort. They are threatened by anxiety, by being-toward-death, and by the need to find a comfortable place to be. A place of comfort could be an actual place in which to live, such as a home, or it could be a form of nurturance, such as food or the security of a mother's arms. A comfortable place is one that is safe and sheltered, where children are free to be themselves. The artwork of the children reflected the need to find a place of comfort. All of the children, in their own ways, revealed their common feelings and shared practices of seeking shelter and security while having their dreams come true.

Nurturance is the sum total of food, shelter, protection, and physical and psychological security (Van Eys, 1983). To nurture a child will conceivably help the child grow and develop further into a healthy adult. Children depend on their parents as well as other members of their culture to meet their needs for survival. To be nurtured is to be comforted and cared for by others. According to Heidegger (1927/1962), care is the "formally existential totality of Dasein's ontological structural whole" (p. 237).

Often both children and adults go about their day-to-day activities, such as eating, without giving them much thought. According to Heidegger (1927/1962), daily activities are carried out in the ready-at-hand mode of being, in which meaning is embedded in activities that provide us with an understanding of our way of being in the world. It is frequently when things go wrong, or when there is a break in the normal pattern of activity, that this meaning is revealed to us. For example, our normal patterns, such as eating, will change because of illness, when sometimes we eat less or develop a distaste for certain foods. But for a child with leukemia (a life-threatening illness), embedded within the action of eating are many issues that pose challenges for the child.

Children with a life-threatening illness frequently cannot retain food because of the medications they take. They are caught in a web of trying to maintain their weight and look good while at the same time feeling periodically nauseated and looking anorexic. They wish to find a place where they can be themselves and put aside the concerns of the body. Food suggests nurturance, being cared for, and being protected by love.

Symbolically, food is equated with life, health, and growth. Meeting the need for food as well as for shelter, protection, and love is a way in which families care for their children (Watson, 1985).

In certain ways children are also cared for by their culture. Professionals such as nurses and doctors claim they give care to sick and dying children. When examining the healthcare given by professionals, one must question what kind of care and nurturance these children receive within the curative healthcare system. The children are subjected to painful procedures, hospitalizations, and invasive techniques as well as surgeries and medications that change their body image. The caregivers in their day-to-day life are often part of a hospital staff, and frequently the care that is offered is impersonal, causing the child to feel depersonalized. A disease is treated or a part of the body needs to be fixed—the child is frequently not treated as a whole person (Bluebond-Langner, 1978; Rollins, 2005).

Heidegger (1927/1962) says that care constitutes all of our involvement in the world and that there are two forms of caring. One form "leaps in" and takes over; it can foster dependency and lead to domination. The other kind of care "leaps ahead" and cares for the other so that his or her own potential for being remains open; this kind of caring focuses on the person and his or her possibilities, not on the task at hand. There are times when people require someone else to care for them, such as when they are seriously ill. At such times it is important that caregivers recognize the individuals' potential to be themselves and that they assist them to become involved in their own care as much as possible. To use Heidegger's distinction, the caregivers need to leap ahead as far as possible, even when it may be more tempting to leap in.

In a young boy's picture his mother is present. No one can replace the love a mother provides. The bond that forms is the strongest of all bonds, and separation is difficult for mother as well as child. Young children need their mothers in order to grow and survive. Mothers provide food, love, security, and protection so that children can grow (Bowlby, 1973; Brazelton, 1984).

The boy's mother is there as they walk into the water. His mother is close to him in the sense that she is standing at the same depth. However, her position is also the farthest away. Perhaps the distance between his mother and himself in the picture suggests that the child was struggling with conflicting feelings about the closeness he felt toward his mother and the changes that may have occurred in his relationship because of having a life-threatening illness. Mothers are often torn between wanting to overprotect their seriously ill children and wanting to maintain a distance that serves as a cushion softening the pain of impending death (Bjork, Wiebe, & Hallstrom, 2005). In this child's drawing it looks as though his mother's eyes are blurred or covered. Might it be that the child is concerned that his mother is shielding herself from his suffering? Or perhaps the child is fearful that his mother does not see his pain or worries. Many children with a life-threatening illness are afraid to let their parents know how they feel inside. They want to make things better for their families, who are also suffering, so they sometimes pretend that they are well.

Some of the pictures show castles that are recognizable as the Magic Kingdom. Heidegger (1977) claims that at the root of *building* is "to dwell" or "to stay in place." To dwell is to reside in a place by keeping things safe from harm. Dwelling occurs when we protect, preserve, and care for something or someone (see figure on following page). Were these young children, so vulnerable and sensitive, seeking the castle as a place to dwell? They needed a place to stay where they could be free from harm. They were tormented by illness and traumatic separation from their parents, families, and friends due to hospitalizations. They suffered from the effects of medications and surgeries that altered their bodies and made them feel less than whole. They needed nurturance, protection, comfort, and a sense of belonging.

Constitutive Pattern: Living in Limbo

Interpretation of the pictures revealed one constitutive pattern, which is the highest level of hermeneutic interpretation. The constitutive pattern must be present in all texts (Diekelmann & Ironside, 1999). It runs through the texts as a common thread that links them, thus revealing further meaning. The common thread in the studied drawings of having a special wish fulfilled for the child with a life-threatening illness is "living in limbo." Limbo is a state of being midway between two extremes. To live in limbo is to exist in the in-between. Historically, limbo was thought of as the region between heaven and hell where souls—such as those of unbaptized babies, who through no fault of their own were barred from

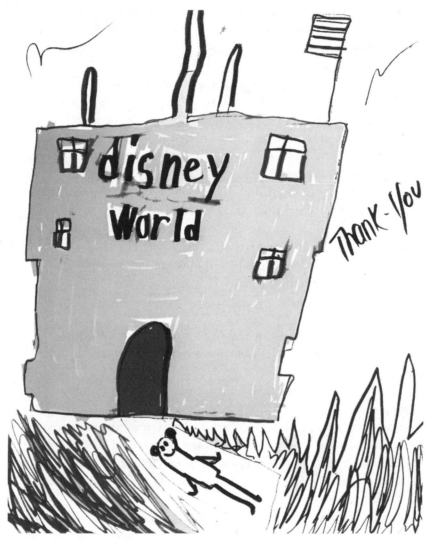

Dwelling

heaven—simply had to wait. Limbo is the in-between of existence, being neither here nor there; it is a staying in place, a state of being held captive or being forgotten. The state of limbo is a struggle for the individual who is in it. One has a desire to achieve something, to get to the desired place, to accomplish the task. However, being unable to reach the desired goal causes a tension, a sense of confinement, an imprisonment in which one cannot move toward the point where one wants to be (Halvorson-Boyd & Hunter, 1995).

In their drawings the children with a life-threatening illness who had their special wish fulfilled reveal a tension that is like a tug-of-war. While they show the pleasure of having a special dream fulfilled, they likewise depict their struggle of living and dying. They are living their lives being abnormal but wanting to be normal. They know that their bodies are changing but do not know what exactly is happening. They experience isolation and loneliness but seek comfort and love. They are unsure about what is happening to them, and they crave certainty. They are afraid of the dark and need brightness and cheerfulness to help ease their fear. They understand that their parents are suffering and so they try to please them. They want to play but sometimes cannot. They live a life of pain and emotional complexity in which things are out of control, and they seek to balance things out with pleasure, joy, and hope.

New Understandings of Having a Special Wish Fulfilled for a Child with a Life-Threatening Illness

Since I began this research 10 years ago I have been continually captivated by the artwork provided by children with a life-threatening illness who have had a special wish fulfilled. I believe their drawings are a gift, and I cherish them. The pictures continue to exist long after the death of the children who drew them. Their art is the children's unspoken words that contain secrets of their experiences waiting to be understood.

The children were not easily able to share their stories verbally. Their language was too unsophisticated to express their deepest feelings. I recall how they would talk about their trips, toys, and other wishes. They would often smile and speak of what they had done, where they went, or what they received. I realize now that I was coming to understand the *what* of their experiences, but the *how* of having their special wishes fulfilled could be understood only through explicating the meanings embodied within their artwork.

I recall a 10-year-old girl with leukemia who shared that she had a very nice time at Walt Disney World. I asked if she had met Mickey, and she responded with a smile and a nod and then became very quiet. Sensing that there was more about the trip that she was unable to express, I asked the little girl if she would draw a picture for me about her experience, and she quietly did exactly that, producing a portrait of Mickey. Later, however, when she was with a group of other children who had had their special wish fulfilled, she enthusiastically drew a different picture of Mickey. It occurred to me that she seemed more comfortable expressing herself in the company of others who had a life-threatening illness.

These children comprised a culture of their own. They shared experiences of how it was to have a special dream fulfilled while living with a life-threatening illness. Their artwork was a way of expressing their shared practices and common ways of living. As a group they had a shared understanding of what was unique to them. Art was a means for them to share with others what they could not express in verbal language. In reference to art Heidegger (1960/1993b) states:

Being a work, it always remains tied to preservers, even and particularly when it is still only waiting for them to enter into its truth. Even the oblivion into which the work can sink is not nothing; it is still a preservation. It feeds on the work. Preserving the work means: standing within the openness of beings that happens in the work. This "standing-within" of preservation, however, is a knowing. Yet knowing does not consist of mere information and notions about something. He [*sic*] who truly knows beings knows what he wills to do in the midst of them. (p. 192)

As a preserver of these children's artwork I wanted to know more about the *how* of their experiences of having their special wish fulfilled by unveiling what had been concealed. Heidegger (1960/1993b) states that art involves caring for things in their context and within their historical significance. Art is a way of both appreciating and understanding other beings. Works of art are not merely a collection of symbols but contain within them the collective shared practices and meanings of people who comprise a culture that is historically situated and part of a broader context. The children with a life-threatening illness who had their wish fulfilled comprised a culture of their own that was situated within the social fabric of which they were a part. Their artwork contained their habits, common experiences, expressions, and ways of relating to others in their world. Art was a way for the children to reveal what mattered to them. It was an entry that opened up the way for others to come to understand what was being expressed.

Heidegger (1960/1993b) argues that art contains ambiguities that both conceal and reveal our way of being. In the essence of the work there is something worthy of questioning. Art is the creative preserving of truth. Truth is the unconcealment of being. Understanding of being creates a clearing in which what matters and is meaningful shows up. The children expressed their experiences in their drawings. Contained within them were experiences of the fulfillment of their wish while they suffered from the pain and anxiety of having a life-threatening illness. Their artwork provided a way for others to understand what they were trying to communicate about their experiences. The artwork in this study contained joy and sorrow, happiness and sadness, dark and light, hope and fear. This art preserved meaning within symbols, constructs, and figures—and by the absence of such forms of expression. It was the children's way of being in the world. Their truth was unconcealed and revealed the meaning of their experience.

To understand what was being revealed in the pictures I was required to dwell with them. Heidegger (1954/1993a) claims that we need to dwell with the things around us to allow them to open themselves up to us. I wanted to preserve and protect not only what the children drew but also what they were trying to say. The drawings offered a way to understand something more about their experiences. The children were speaking through symbols and images to whoever might want to listen to how they experienced the fulfillment of a dream. I became the children's interpreter, attempting to unveil what they were trying to communicate. According to Heidegger (1927/1962), each of us is constantly interpreting our world. We are able to interpret meaning because of cultural history and shared background understanding. Interpretation is our way to understand knowledge that is embedded within our shared practices. By dialoguing with the pictures I have come to understand, through my personal lens, more about the essence of the children's experiences. There was much more to having a special wish fulfilled than simply receiving a toy or going on a trip.

New Questions

What originally was explored as the meaning of having a special wish fulfilled for children with a life-threatening illness has revealed new questions: What is the meaning of living in limbo for children with a life-threatening illness? What does it mean for children with a life-threatening illness to live in the in-between?

The culture influences how children think about themselves and their world and fundamentally shapes the way children grow and develop. Children in return influence how the culture evolves and changes. "Every culture carries within it an image of the ideal self. It is usually flattering and ennobling, a picture of what we are to be and to hope for, not what we still are" (Callahan, 1993, p. 120). In Western culture our image of the ideal self holds that we should live life to the fullest in terms of who we are, what we can become, and what we can do for our society. Society places great value on individuals who are fit, healthy, economically sound, and productive and ascribes little worth to the sick, dying, and indigent.

This concept of the ideal self, as it comes to be projected by Western cultures, assumes that it is our right as autonomous individuals to control our living and our dying. We believe that nature can be brought under human control and made to do whatever we want. We expect and demand a healthy life, and we choose to engage in a battle against death. Our medical subculture upholds these notions of the ideal self by using medical technology as ammunition to fight a war against death (Callahan, 1993). In Western culture adults in general and healthcare practitioners in particular demonstrate their ways of caring for dying children by working strenuously and unceasingly to prolong their lives. By fostering the use of advanced technology, our culture communicates that it is unacceptable for children to die. The mere thought of the death of a child is almost unthinkable. We try to prevent the child's death at all costs because we believe that it is outrageous, unjust, unfair, and intolerable for a young child to die. Thus we justify the use of powerful technology to extend the lives of our dying children.

The dying child symbolizes the failure of Western culture to overcome nature. Even with technology that supposedly gives humans a way to conquer nature, we fail at times to keep our innocent young children alive. The dying child is evidence that our culture has failed to protect its young by staving off disease. The death of a child proves that humankind is unable to overpower nature. Children with a life-threatening illness are often pushed to become brave warriors. They may be forced to muster up courage and strength in an ongoing battle against death. These children must learn to live in limbo, in the in-between of life and death. To live in limbo is to live a life of uncertainty. Living in the in-between is both knowing and not knowing what is happening. A tug-of-war is at play. As a part of the self advances toward death, the other part struggles to stay alive. Children with a life-threatening illness exist in the limbo between these two extremes.

In my experience as a pediatric nurse I have found that children with a life-threatening illness, who are already living with uncertainty, begin to realize there is confusion, hiding, fear, and denial within adult society. They come to realize that their society does not highly value those who are sick. They may feel embarrassed at and ashamed of having a serious illness. Eventually, many come to feel that they are not to speak openly of dying. How must it feel to be fragile, young, and dying and to live daily with physical and emotional pain when they are just budding into life? They are different from other children, and they know they are not always accepted as normal children. They are caught in a web of trying to live while they are dying and trying to die while they are living. They are living, but their life is lived on the brink of death. Their lives become like a seesaw. One day they are up and the next day they are down, never knowing what the next moment will bring.

Anxiety and Being-Toward-Death

I have cared for many children as they died. I have observed how their fear intensifies as the children realize that, at the end of a long, exhausting pathway of medical interventions and hospitalizations, they will still lose the battle to live. I have witnessed many of these children crying for help and reaching out to others in desperation, trying to alleviate the anxiety that comes with sensing that life is taking a downward course and coming to an end. Children who were once vibrant and full of life now experience their lives as being turned upside down and out of control, and they realize how powerless they are to change things.

Craving certainty, children with a life-threatening illness want desperately to control life's events. They wish and hope to be healthy and happy once again. Some children maintain their hope for health by becoming more spiritual. A 9-year-old with a life-threatening condition wrote:

I WISH

I wish there was a bird from God
and got me well

from His wings on me,
and got me well.
(Berger, Lithwick, & seven campers,
1992, p. 195)

I have observed that the children who live with these illnesses often feel alone and confused by the changes that have occurred in their day-to-day lives, not only from their illness but also from other complexities. Their families are often overwrought with sorrow and despair. Their daily activities have changed, and their relationships with their peers may no longer be the same. They suffer from feelings of loneliness and often have difficulty expressing their emotions. Moustakes (1961) states:

Feelings of loneliness must often be hidden in childhood. They are too frightening and disturbing—like any intense, severe, disturbing emotion the feelings must be curbed, controlled, denied, or if expressed, quickly resolved or eliminated through busy activities and goals. (p. 40)

Children are often afraid to let others know how they feel. They come to learn that nice children have nice feelings. Eventually, they show only an expurgated and edited version of their inner life.

Their sense of loneliness becomes intensified as people avoid them, treating them as though they had a contagion. They feel rejected by friends, extended family members, and other people to whom they may once have felt close. Even many health professionals avoid working with dying children. Children with a life-threatening illness and their families thus often feel singled out and rejected by their culture. Why do people find it difficult to be with children who are desperately in need of our care? What is it about dying children that our culture finds difficult to face?

The dying child calls forth an even more deeply embedded problem for our culture than was mentioned above. The dying child is an individual who will not *become*. Life will be unlived, and a life unlived is one that is unfulfilled. The dying child is like a mirror that reflects an image of a time when we will no longer be. But even worse than the reminder that each of us will die is the fear that we too may die before we have reached fulfillment. One of the deepest fears embedded within the fear of death is the fear of living an unfulfilled life. The life that is unfulfilled is a life in which wishes and dreams are put on hold. It is a life that is cut off from the things we wanted to do or be. It is a life in which our desires, choices, and hopes for a future will not be realized.

Much of our time as children is spent thinking about what we want to become, do, or see. From the time we are very young and begin to speak we frequently talk of our future. We speak of who and what we would like to become, such as a policeman, teacher, nurse, doctor, artist, or architect. Phrases such as "When I grow up I want to be . . ." are common among children as they fantasize about a future that contains various possibilities. Our wishes and desires help us to go on with life. Thinking of fulfilling our dreams gives us a sense of hope for the future. But, coming face to face with a dying child, we see in full view a life that will not be lived out, a future that is no longer there. The dying child's life is one that will never be realized to its fullest. The child exists in the in-between, living while dying and dying while living and doing neither to the fullest. While in limbo the child is staying in place and not moving forward; limbo is a region where one can exist but where one cannot fulfill one's dreams.

My interpretation of the pictures suggests that in the face of the torturous struggles of prolongation of life through technological means our culture shows its solicitude for dying children by attempting to offer a means of fulfilling life in some way before death. To show concern for the dying child, society demonstrates that there are ways a child can experience what it might be like to fulfill his or her dreams. The fulfillment of a special wish, a dream come true, is one way in which society attempts to help the child to cope with the enormous difficulties that he or she must face. It is a way to fulfill the child's hopes and dreams for the future.

Being and Becoming

The fulfillment of a special dream gives the child a chance to become. The child can become the person he or she always wanted to be, can meet somebody special, or can obtain something he or she never thought possible. Having a special wish fulfilled is considered precious by members of our culture who believe that they are indeed helping the child to bring life to fulfillment in some way.

The fulfillment of a special wish is like a diamond, a jewel that sparkles in the mind of the child and of our culture. The gem is precious, something to fantasize about, to possess and hold on to. But diamonds are multifaceted and do not sparkle from all angles. Even the most perfect diamond has flaws or microscopic defects that cannot be seen by the naked eye. The jewel holds within it a promise of the play, fun, and enjoyment that are normal parts of a child's life, but it also contains within it the tension, suffering from pain, isolation, and loneliness that occur within a context of living while dying and dying while living. The need for fun and play is inherent to being a child. The fulfillment of a wish is a way of being. Play is a way of coping and gaining control. It is a way for the child to overcome difficulties. Gadamer (1960/2003) claimed that play draws the child into its dominion. It fills the child with its spirit. The experience is a reality that surpasses the child. Play has an "absolute autonomy" (Gadamer, 1960/2003, p. 111) in which a change takes place, a transformation in which the individual as a whole changes to become his or her true being.

The fulfillment of the wish as a form of play gives these children a chance to rise above a life that is fraught with problems and sorrow. It allows children with a life-threatening illness to transcend the reality of their disease, treatments, and processes of dying to come closer to becoming true children again. Contained within the idea of having fun and doing something thrilling is a sense of hope. It is a way for the children to be, at least temporarily, *children,* not dying children. This sense of being a child holds deep meaning because it is the way for children to continue to live and grow. The fulfillment of the wish is a way of recapturing how it is to simply enjoy life while feeling healthier and happier, if only for a brief interlude. I have observed children who have their wish come true rise to the occasion, both looking and feeling better. They will even dress up and seem once more like their peers in order to experience the special dream.

How precious is this jewel of the special wish! It is a way to reenergize, to look forward and feel that something beautiful and magnificent can excite and renew things. The fulfillment of the wish is a way to regain a sense of hope. Even though a child's most fervent wish may be to live— or possibly to die and end the suffering—the fulfillment of a special wish may be a dream come true and may provide a sense of pleasure and joy that helps children to feel more comfortable. Each of the children's joyful smiles in the pictures was different, but each revealed that having one's dream come true is a pleasurable experience.

In my experience with children who have a life-threatening illness I have observed their need for distraction from their pain, sorrow, and loneliness. The fulfillment of the wish is a way to combat negative thoughts and feelings. Loneliness and uncertainty can give rise to the creation of pleasurable fantasies that can become reality (Moustakes, 1961). According to Freud (1953/1965), wish fulfillment is a way to reduce anxiety. In fantasy the child can think of pleasure in order to avoid pain. To be a player on a favorite baseball team, to meet the president and talk to him, or to spend some time with a superstar may be so special that it will help to alleviate anxiety through the pleasurable effects that the child experiences.

Not only does the child experience pleasure, but family members also seem to experience some relief from suffering through their participation. Children who are ill and dying often blame themselves for the devastation that surrounds them. The fulfillment of the wish offers a way to bring them closer to their parents. It is a way to please their parents rather than to hurt them. In addition, brothers and sisters generally become a part of the special event too, which brings the whole family together.

The child's friends are often more accepting if they hear that he or she is going somewhere special or meeting a celebrity. They can join in on discussions about the dream. Some friends even become a part of having the dream come true. A sense of unity comes about as the child enjoys discussing the wish with other people. In some cases the child's entire school becomes involved in the fulfillment of the wish by raising money. Thus the dying child can feel more normal by participating actively in life with family and friends as opposed to being passive, feeling sick, and experiencing loneliness. Through fulfillment of the wish the child can also become actively involved with the community. Many social groups and churches raise and contribute funds. Other voluntary organizations offer goods and services to help make the dream become a reality.

Many people who are involved in granting children's wishes believe that the fulfillment of the wish is a respite. It is a way to "get away from it all." The children can temporarily escape from hospitals, nurses, doctors, and painful procedures. Even healthcare professionals lend their support, affirming that leaving on a trip, for example, will be helpful. They rally around to help make the fulfillment of the wish special, for example, joining in when a special celebrity comes to visit the hospital.

Technification and the Culture of Dying

Might the fulfillment of the wish for a child with a life-threatening illness be a way to satisfy the needs of our culture? Is the fulfillment of the wish a way for the culture to "look good and feel better" so that it can uphold its ideal self as healthy, content, and productive? Does the child in some way sense that he or she must be part of pleasing the culture? These questions bring us back to the deeper issues regarding the dying child in relation to our culture. In their short time on earth dying children discover that life is for the living. The child is part of an order in the culture. The living hold a priority, and the activities of the culture are centered around them (Bluebond-Langner, 1978).

The child exists within a social fabric that cannot comfortably accept death, especially of its young. It is a culture that upholds health and longevity as its image of a life worth living (Callahan, 1993). Death will occur someday, but most members of Western culture tend to think of death as something that happens to other people, and everyone thinks that if it must happen to him or her, it will happen well in the future.

Western society has invested extensively in technology as a way of warding off death and perpetuating the illusion that nature can be conquered. Heidegger (1977) suggests, however, that modern technology covers and obscures the *being* of beings and ultimately itself. Technology both reveals and conceals. Technology is a revelation of truth as a means for the revelation of being but one that hides its own essence. Technology encourages us to hide from our own way of being (Heidegger, 1954/1993a), including being-toward-death. We attempt to stave off death by extending life through extraordinary means, spending enormous sums of money to develop and distribute medical technology.

We avoid facing the fact that we all will die one day by upholding the belief that life should be preserved at any cost. The result is that we cause dying people to suffer emotionally and physically agonizing deaths. We traumatize children with painful procedures and hospitalize them, causing them to feel alone and afraid. We subject them to bodily manipulations and surgical procedures that further create a fear of mutilation and body-image disturbances, and we expect them to accept that what we do is good for them. Although technology has saved lives and can restore health and quality of life, with technology we also wreak havoc on the gentlest of our members and hurt their loved ones because we do not want to face the inevitability of death.

I am reminded of all the times that I spent in the pediatric intensive care unit attending to machinery to keep children alive. I observed numerous children go to their death while attached to machines such as respirators and cardiac monitors. The unit was a center for much thought, debate, and discussion about conditions such as septicemia, cardiac surgery, cancer, and brain trauma. While most of the children lay comatose, their doctors, nurses, and numerous other healthcare providers discussed the course of their disease and performed high-risk procedures. While I feel that we made life-saving decisions, I also believe that we lost touch with the children and how they wished to live their lives. We were practicing in a state of limbo in which we knew what compassionate and humanistic care ought to be but were not achieving the desired end. We were concerned with diagnosing diseases and treating them, but what kind of care were we giving to the children? Perhaps we were leaping in and taking over for them without caring for the individual child, so that our caring, rather than being focused on the person and his or her possibilities, was focused on the tasks at hand.

I wanted desperately to provide comfort for the children and to practice in a more humanistic way. I wanted to create a peaceful, gentle atmosphere by holding the children and reaching out to their parents to provide comfort. In addition, I realized how important it was for me to feel human in this highly technological environment. I wanted to feel more inspirited and connected with my patients, but instead I found myself spending time with machines. The experience of attending to machines rather than communicating with the children left me feeling dissatisfied. In many ways the curative care that we provided was dehumanizing, isolating, and insensitive to the children. It also had a profound effect on me, since I felt that I was not able to give the compassionate and sensitive care I believed the children needed as they were dying (Matzo, Sherman, Penn, & Ferrell, 2003). Heidegger (1977) argues that technology separates individuals from the essence of their existence. He states that our preoccupation with technology causes us to separate "mortals" from their primordial way of existing and being. An overwhelming preoccupation with material things obscures our quest for spiritual understanding. Technology is like dogma, which possesses a worldly power that ignores the subtle affairs of the mind and heart (Mitcham, 1994).

We must in some way transcend technology so that we are not overcome by it (Furman, 2000). Somehow we must come to understand our existence at a deeper level. Healthcare providers need to recognize their own needs, paying attention to what enables them to feel whole and healthy and in touch with their patients. Providers are commonly frustrated by the demands of giving. They experience compassion fatigue as a result of the conflict they feel between performing the numerous tasks and duties they are responsible for and wishing to attend to their patients' emotional needs. The essence of being is recognition of the totality of the individual and the relationship of the person to the world and the universe (Heidegger, 1927/1962). Thus healthcare providers and dying children alike exist in relation to the community, the culture, and the world, finding their place by engaging in the universal processes of life.

Being with One Another

Might there be something in the phenomenon of fulfillment of a dying child's wish that reveals more to us about our relationship to one another? Is there something about having a special wish fulfilled for the child with a life-threatening illness that reveals our way of being? Observing children, watching them grow, and experiencing their joys have a profound effect upon those around them. We often look to children for our own enjoyment, and we glean a sense of the joy of life from them. Seeing smiles on their faces or making them feel better helps us feel better too. Children inspirit us, reconnecting us with the wonder of life that we knew when we were young. Because—in the normal scheme of things—they will live on after we are gone, our children offer a way for us to feel that we are immortal.

But what are we really doing when we work to fulfill their dreams? Some healthcare professionals become deeply involved in the dying child's experience of having a dream come true, while others remain on the fringes of the experience, contributing services in small ways. Yet somehow all want to be part of the experience of knowing that a dying child has been helped and cared for in some way. Heidegger (1927/1962) argues that wishing is rooted in care. Wishing ontologically presupposes care. We show concern and care for children with a life-threatening illness by fulfilling their dreams.

Heidegger (1954/1993a) states that we are dwellers. Dwelling is our way of being interconnected with one another through care. Care is our human way of being. The essence of dwelling means to remain in place and to be brought to peace. The word *peace* means "free from harm and danger," "preserved from something," "safeguarded." "To free" actually means "to spare." "Real sparing is something positive and takes place when we leave something beforehand in its own essence, when we return it to its essential being, when we free it in the proper sense of the word into a preserve of peace" (Heidegger, 1954/1993a, p. 351).

We are coming together, trying to overcome the complexities that surround dying children in a technological society by continuing to try to preserve the way of being of these children. In our coming together to fulfill their wishes we are trying to preserve something important—the joy, laughter, and fun that children experience just by being who they are. We are attempting to help them become closer to their families and find a place of peace and comfort. The drawings of the children who had their special wish fulfilled depicted a need to find a place of comfort and an attempt to balance the complexities in their lives. The balancing of body, mind, and spirit has been linked to healing, whereby a state of peaceful existence is brought to fruition (Siegel, 1986). The person who experiences healing experiences a sense of being interconnected with others, with his or her world, and with the universe. As the healer shows concern and care for the one receiving healing, both become united in the healing process.

The fulfillment of the dreams of these children provides them as well as adults with a way of coming together to find a sense of peace. The "wish child," the family, contributors, concerned members of the community, physicians, nurses, and volunteers unite in this experience. They come from all walks of life to participate in the experience and share in the joy and hope that the fulfillment of the wish brings to the child. Joy and hope have also been linked to healing. Such states can bring about a sense of peaceful integration, a state of calmness and serenity of mind, body, and spirit (Siegel, 1986). By fostering a sense of peace through our interconnectedness we are caring for our dying children and we are dwelling with them. By safeguarding and preserving their essence, their playful way of being children, we are safeguarding our humanity as human beings. As their protectors and through the fulfillment of their wishes we are attempting to transcend technology by counterbalancing its negative effects with other ways of being that help the child to maintain a sense of hope. We are seeking alternative ways of safeguarding the essence of being in a culture that seeks to hide from its own essence.

Our Future, Their Future

Our children are our future, and through fulfillment of their wishes we are trying to give back to dying children the sense of future that the process of dying takes away. We are cultivating hope, which embodies the notion of a future. To hope is to believe that something more is possible. In their wish to visit Walt Disney World the children revealed that they desired to go to a place where anything might be possible, a place where dreams come true. Some of the children also drew symbols of spirituality, such as crosses and circles. A circle, the universal symbol of wholeness, may connote a future life that contains other possibilities.

Heidegger's thoughts on *Dasein* reveal the understanding that each of us is always seeking future possibilities:

As long as Dasein lives there always remains something which it can be, but is not yet. Dasein is like a painting which is never completed; it always has further possibilities not yet realized, aspects, events, accomplishments which are not yet a part of its actuality. In fact, the picture will never be completed until death. This is the final arc of the circle of existence, the missing piece needed to complete the picture. (Demske, 1970, pp. 372–373)

Thus the fulfillment of the wish may provide a way for children to be free to become open to future possibilities both in life and death. The children can have fun, play, and hope and dream about the future, which helps them to understand that something else might be possible. Through fulfillment of their wishes the children can feel the experience of being cared for and safeguarded by others, thereby becoming more at peace. Children who experience peace within themselves may then come to realize a life with other possibilities.

The fulfillment of their dreams seemed to provide a sense of future possibilities for them in both living and dying. It seemed to give them the idea that this world is filled with joy, happiness, and excitement and that they could experience this joy in a way that was new to them. The fulfillment of their wishes may also have given them an idea of joy, hope, and peace in terms of what the next world might bring, possibly even more of the joys of childhood, introducing the possibility and sense of something more to be achieved in the next world, something that they might not ever be able to find in the world in which they now lived.

Children with a life-threatening illness are walking the line between this world and the next, never knowing which world the next day will bring. They live with the uncertainty of not knowing which world is better. They exist with the tension between living as dying (living in a world while dying) and the possibility of dying as living (dying and going to a better place where everything will be wonderful). Within the context of uncertainty the fulfillment of a child's wish may be a way of both holding on and letting go. The fulfilled wish may give the dying child a glimpse of what could be or should be the hope of relief in the next world. Thus the child may gain the courage to let go of this world and die soon after the wish is granted. On the other hand, fulfillment of the dream may suggest that there are more possibilities to be pursued in this life, thus fostering the desire to hold on to this life for longer.

Implications for Future Research, Education, and Practice

The implications arising from this study for further research and practice include the need to understand how the experience of having a wish fulfilled could be integrated into the care of children with a life-limiting illness as an alternative and complementary therapy. Specifically, the manner in which the inclusion of wish fulfillment makes a difference to children, their families, health professionals, and the volunteers involved in granting wishes bears further study. National and international initiatives are currently under way to develop new approaches to the practice of palliative care in pediatric settings (Matzo et al., 2003). Since the prognosis of children with a serious illness is often unclear, approaches that integrate curative and palliative care are often necessary. Given the importance of sustaining hope and keeping in mind wish fulfillment as a complementary therapy directed to this end, future research to explicate the relationship of hope and healing (of both a physical and spiritual nature) is warranted.

In considering how wish fulfillment could make a difference for children who are seriously ill as well as for their families, wish fulfillment might be studied as a way of engendering a sense of empowerment in children, thereby enabling them more easily to express desires, make choices, and influence the decisions often made by adults on their behalf. With a heightened sense of agency, children might be in a position to express choices pertaining to treatment options, and dying children might even be able to express the desire to cease treatment and let go.

As a therapy that counterbalances the heavy burden of suffering imposed by conventional technologically based approaches, wish fulfillment could also be studied ethnographically as an interweaving of relationships that ameliorate the isolation imposed by a child's suffering by bringing community members together to offer a gift to the child and his or her family in a way that eases suffering and offers hope. Moreover, an ethnographic study of this nature might reveal what it means to community members to be involved in bringing a child's hopes and dreams to fruition. The question of whether their involvement in granting wishes enhances a sense of meaning and purpose in their own lives might be studied.

Such a study might also illuminate what it means to a family to have an opportunity to spend time together, outside of hospital walls, engaged in play and in the creation of special memories. The fulfillment of a special wish as a way of bringing the entire family together to play and enjoy the pleasures of life might be studied in light of whether it strengthens family relationships and coping and builds a storehouse of memories that ease grief and bereavement after the child is gone.

This study also suggests that conventional treatments intended to perpetuate life should be evaluated carefully against the benefits thought to be secured, in particular by focusing more intentionally upon the preservation of quality of life for children who are dying. By preserving quality of life through activities that emphasize fun and by helping children to continue to create, dream, and achieve important goals at a time when they might otherwise feel only defeat, despair, and sorrow, wish fulfillment offers one among several ways that could be studied in relation to how quality of life might be preserved for children with a life-threatening illness.

Future study could also inquire further into the experiences of providers who are caring for dying children. In particular, the conflict that healthcare professionals experience in relation to perpetuating the lives of their patients through extraordinary technological interventions, compared to preserving quality of life through palliative, complementary, and alternative therapies, could also be studied (Ferrell & Coyle, 2002).

While it is possible for many children with a life-threatening illness to have their wish fulfilled through the efforts and funds of wish-granting organizations such as the Make-A-Wish Foundation, it may be impossible for some children who have a life-threatening condition to have their dreams fulfilled in this way. The practical and financial limitations of organization chapters, the scarcity of volunteers in certain locations, and the inability to raise funds for travel may constitute insurmountable challenges to granting some wishes. In such cases the benefits of having a special wish fulfilled might possibly be approached through alternative means. Healthcare professionals could consider taking imaginary trips with children, through fantasy, to "magic kingdoms." By actively engaging in play with these children and encouraging them to dream about other possibilities, practitioners of care can engender hope and alleviate suffering. Less costly activities, such as a visit from a clown, may also offer respite and secure similar benefits for the child. Such approaches remain to be researched, written about, and integrated into the educational curricula of health professionals.

Taking into account the role that art played in this study in providing insight into the experiences of dying children, I suggest that healthcare providers such as nurses, counselors, and art therapists might work together to bring children's suffering to expression through encouraging them to draw their experiences, concerns, and hopes for the future within the context of having a serious illness. In this way children would be able to communicate feelings that might be too complex to express in words, and they might also be encouraged to continue dreaming and drawing, thereby giving expression to their hopes and fears. Such drawings could give health professionals a way of gaining a deeper understanding of the needs and wishes of children who have a limited future as well as a way of engaging more intimately with the children themselves.

The significance for health professionals of being able to engage more intimately with dying children and their families has far-reaching implications. By considering that all relationships involve mutual exchanges it could be understood that when health professionals are able to engage with their patients in a way that promotes healing (e.g., by helping the child and family move toward acceptance of a peaceful death for the child), the health professionals are affected positively. By studying how health professionals help children and their families find meaning in their circumstances and how they find caring for the dying child meaningful, we might develop a better understanding of how preserving the personhood of the child and comforting the family enable health professionals to find satisfaction and a sense of calling in their work. Studying such phenomena in depth might reveal, for example, that by providing comfort to our patients we not only humanize the process of living and dying but also receive something special ourselves. Since Kübler-Ross (1983) has argued that dying children, being wise beyond their years, are our teachers, it seems reasonable to assume that if we as healthcare professionals opened ourselves to the wisdom of dying children they could teach us to care for them in newer and better ways. And perhaps in opening ourselves up to what the children can teach us about caring in life, we healthcare professionals might even come to develop a different set of priorities and a more meaningful way of living.

Allowing for the importance of integrating measures to promote quality of life for dying children into practice, educational strategies related to palliative care could also be studied. Moving beyond conventional knowledge intended to provide guidance on physical care of the dying child, such educational approaches could be developed to enhance practitioners' comfort in staying engaged with their patients in the face of impending death. These educational objectives could also emphasize how to bring joy and humor into the lives of children who need holistic care (Hayden-Miles, 1995).

Having a special wish fulfilled could be studied as a hopeful phenomenon in Western culture—a culture that often seems impoverished in relation to replenishment of humanity and sources of deep meaning. Signifying that there is more that can be done for dying children than prolonging their lives with every technological means available, wish fulfillment offers a way for society to perhaps begin to understand itself differently through the preservation of play and the safeguarding of humanity.

Conclusion

Reflecting on my experiences as cofounder of a chapter of a wish-granting organization, on my understanding of what having a wish granted means to children within the context of living and dying, and on what I have learned through my many years working in pediatric nursing, I realize that I have received significant benefits. Being a part of a movement devoted to ameliorating suffering and bringing joy not only provided a wonderful sense of community but also gave me a deeper appreciation of life. This deepened appreciation and my dissatisfaction with conventional approaches to caring for children led in turn to a strong desire to cherish and safeguard all that is poignantly precious about life, especially the lives of children who are dying. Given the difficulty of bringing the experiences of dying children to voice, I sought to offer them a different medium of expression—their artwork.

In concluding this study I offer health professionals several challenges. The first is to continue to find the causes within and beyond our work that connect us to our patients and to each other in ways that provide a deep sense of meaning and purpose in our lives. The second is to find new approaches (such as artwork) to bring that which cannot be said—or is extremely difficult to say—to expression so that the isolation of suffering is overcome. The third is to open ourselves up to a whole range of innovative and complementary therapies that provide comfort, enable dreaming, invite new possibilities, and keep hope alive.

Note

1. Heidegger (1927/1962) identifies being-toward-death as a common phenomenon in human experience. Human beings of all ages, healthy or ill, are aware that they will one day die, and this awareness is an essential part of their understanding of their day-to-day existence.

References

Arnold, J. H., & Gemma, P. B. (1994). *A child dies: A portrait of family grief* (2nd ed.). Rockville, MD: Aspen.

Benner, P. (1984). *From novice to expert: Excellence and power in clinical nursing practice.* Menlo Park, CA: Addison-Wesley.

Benner, P. (1994). The tradition and skill of interpretive phenomenology in studying health and illness, and caring practices. In P. Benner (Ed.), *Interpretive phenomenology: Embodiment, caring, and ethics in health and illness* (pp. 99–108). Thousand Oaks, CA: Sage.

Benner, P., & Wrubel, J. (1989). *The primacy of caring: Stress and coping in health and illness.* Menlo Park, CA: Addison-Wesley.

Benson, H. (1975). *The relaxation response.* New York: Avon.

Berger, L., Lithwick, D., & seven campers (1992). *I will sing life: Voices from the Hole in the Wall Gang Camp.* Boston: Little, Brown.

Bernstein, R. J. (1991). *Beyond objectivism and relativism: Science, hermeneutics, and praxis.* Philadelphia: University of Pennsylvania Press.

Bjork, M., Wiebe, T., & Hallstrom, I. (2005). Striving to survive: Families' lived experiences when a child is diagnosed with cancer. *Journal of Pediatric Oncology Nursing, 22,* 265–275.

Bluebond-Langner, M. (1978). *The private worlds of dying children.* Princeton, NJ: Princeton University Press.

Bowlby, J. (1973). *Attachment and loss, Vol. 2: Anxiety and anger.* New York: Basic Books.

Brazelton, T. B. (1984). *To listen to a child.* New York: John Wiley.

Callahan, D. (1990). *What kind of life: The limits of medical progress.* New York: Simon & Schuster.

Callahan, D. (1993). *The troubled dream of life: Living with mortality.* New York: Simon & Schuster.

Coles, R. (1992). *Their eyes meeting the world: The drawings and paintings of children.* Boston: Houghton Mifflin.

Davies, B., Collins, J. B., Steele, R., Pipke, I., & Cook, K. (2004). The impact on families of a children's hospice program. *Journal of Palliative Care, 19*(1), 15–26.

Davies, B., & Connaughty, S. (2002). Pediatric end-of-life care: Lessons learned from parents. *Journal of Nursing Administration, 32,* 5–6.

Demske, J. M. (1970). *Being, man, and death: A key to Heidegger.* Lexington: University Press of Kentucky.

Diekelmann, N. L., & Ironside, P. M. (1999). Hermeneutics. In J. Fitzpatrick (Ed.), *Nursing research digest* (pp. 33–35). New York: Springer.

DiLeo, J. H. (1973). *Children's drawings as diagnostic aids.* New York: Brunner/Mazel.

Dossey, B. M. (2004). Nurse as healer: Toward the inward journey. In B. M. Dossey, L. Keegan, C. E. Guzzetta, & L. G. Kolkmeier, *Holistic nursing: A handbook for nursing practice* (4th ed., pp. 39–53). Rockville, MD: Aspen.

Edwards, B. (1986). *Drawing on the artist within.* New York: Simon & Schuster.

Ewing, B. (1996). *The meaning of having a special wish fulfilled for a child with a life-threatening illness: A hermeneutic inquiry.* Unpublished doctoral dissertation, Adelphi University, Garden City, NY.

Ferrell, B., & Coyle, N. (2002). An overview of palliative nursing care. *American Journal of Nursing, 102,* 26–30.

Field, M. J., & Berman, R. (Eds.). (2003). *When children die: Improving palliative and end-of-life care for children and their families.* Committee on Palliative Care and End of Life for Children and Their Families. Washington, DC: National Academies Press.

Fontana, D. (1993). *The secret language of symbols: A visual key to symbols and their meanings.* San Francisco: Chronicle Books.

Freud, S. (1965). *The interpretation of dreams* (J. Strachey, Trans.). New York: Avon. (Original work published 1953)

Freyer, D. R. (2004). Care of the dying adolescent: Special considerations. *Pediatrics, 113,* 381–388.

Furman, J. (2000). Taking a holistic approach to the dying time. *Nursing, 30,* 46–49.

Gadamer, H.-G. (1988). On the circle of understanding. In J. M. Connolly & T. Keutner (Eds.), *Hermeneutics versus sciences?: Essays by H.-G. Gadamer, E. K. Specht, W. Stegmuller* (pp. 68–78). Notre Dame, IN: University of Notre Dame Press.

Gadamer, H.-G. (2003). *Truth and method* (2nd ed.; J. Weinsheimer & D. G. Marshall, Trans.). New York: Continuum. (Original work published 1960)

Gaes, J. (1987). *My book for kids with cansur: A child's autobiography of hope.* Aberdeen, SD: Melius & Peterson.

Garbarino, F., Stott, M., & faculty of the Eriksson Institute. (1992). *What children can tell us.* San Francisco: Jossey-Bass.

Gibran, K. (1923). *The prophet.* New York: Knopf.

Giovanola, J. (2005). Sibling involvement at the end of life. *Journal of Pediatric Oncology Nursing, 22,* 222–226.

Halvorson-Boyd, G., & Hunter, L. K. (1995). *Dancing in limbo: Making sense of life after cancer.* San Francisco: Jossey-Bass.

Hayden-Miles, M. (1995). The meaning of humor for nursing students within the student–clinical instructor relationship: A hermeneutic inquiry (Doctoral dissertation, Adelphi University, Garden City, NY, 1995). *Dissertation Abstracts International, 56,* 06B. (UMI No. AAT9531710)

Heidegger, M. (1962). *Being and time* (J. Macquarrie & E. Robinson, Trans.). New York: Harper & Row. (Original work published 1927)

Heidegger, M. (1971). *On the way to language* (P. D. Hertz & J. Stambaugh, Trans.). New York: Harper & Row.

Heidegger, M. (1977). The question concerning technology. In *The question concerning technology and other essays* (W. Lovitt, Trans., pp. 3–35). New York: Harper & Row.

Heidegger, M. (1993a). Building dwelling thinking. In D. F. Krell (Ed.), *Basic writings* (A. Hofstadter, Trans., pp. 347–363). San Francisco: HarperSanFrancisco. (Original work published 1954)

Heidegger, M. (1993b). The origin of the work of art. In D. F. Krell (Ed.), *Basic writings* (A. Hofstadter, Trans.; pp. 143–203). San Francisco: HarperSanFrancisco. (Original work published 1960)

Hinds, P. (2004). The hopes and wishes of adolescents with cancer and the nursing care that helps. *Oncology Nursing Forum, 31*, 927–934.

Hynson, J. L., Gillis, J., Collins, J. J., Irving, H., & Trethewie, S. J. (2003). The dying child: How is care different? *Medical Journal of Australia, 179,* S20–S22.

Kübler-Ross, E. (1983). *On children and death.* New York: Macmillan.

Leonard, V. W. (1989). A Heideggerian phenomenologic perspective on the concept of the person. *Advances in Nursing Science, 11*(4), 40–55.

Lyon, M. E., Townsend-Akpan, C., & Thompson, A. (2001). Spirituality and end-of-life care for an adolescent with AIDS. *AIDS Patient Care & STDs, 15,* 555–560.

Maslow, A. H. (1998). *Toward a psychology of being* (3rd ed.). Princeton, NJ: Van Nostrand.

Matzo, M. L., Sherman, D. W, Penn, B., & Ferrell, B. R. (2003). The end of life nursing education consortium (ELNEC) experience. *Nurse Educator, 28,* 266–270.

Mitcham, C. (1994). *Thinking through technology: The path between engineering and philosophy.* Chicago: University of Chicago Press.

Moustakas, C. E. (1961). *Loneliness.* Englewood Cliffs, NJ: Prentice-Hall.

Piaget, J. (2001). *The language and thought of the child* (3rd ed.). Boston: Kegan Paul.

Rollins, J. A. (1990). Childhood cancer: Siblings draw and tell. *Pediatric Nursing, 16,* 21–27.

Rollins, J. A. (2003). New initiatives in end-of-life care. *Pediatric Nursing, 22,* 292–293.

Rollins, J. A. (2005). Tell me about it: Drawing as a communication tool for children with cancer. *Journal of Pediatric Oncology Nursing, 22,* 203–221.

Sahler, O. J. Z., Frager, G., Levetown, M., Cohn, F. G., & Lipson, M. A. (2000). Medical education about end-of-life care in the pediatric setting: Principles, challenges, and opportunities. *Pediatrics, 105,* 575–584.

Siegel, B. H. (1986). *Love, medicine, & miracles: Lessons learned about self-healing from a surgeon's experience with exceptional patients.* New York: HarperCollins.

Spinetta, J. J., Rigler, D., & Karon, M. (1987). Anxiety in the dying child. In T. Krulik, B. Holaday, & I. M. Martinson (Eds.), *The child and family facing life-threatening illness* (pp. 50–60). Philadelphia: Lippincott.

Updike, J. (1995). Introduction. In C. Yoe & M. Yoe (Eds.), *The art of Mickey Mouse.* New York: Hyperion.

Van Eys, J. (1983). Feeding the dying child: Ethical decision-making in a new guise. In J. E. Schowalter, P. R. Patterson, M. Tallmer, A. H. Kutscher, S. V. Gullo, & D. Peretz (Eds.), *The child and death* (pp. 315–327). New York: Columbia University Press.

Waechter, E. H. (1987). Death, dying, and bereavement: A review of the literature. In T. Krulik, B. Holaday, & I. M. Martinson (Eds.), *The child and family facing life-threatening illness* (pp. 3–31). Philadelphia: Lippincott.

Watson, J. (1985). *Nursing: The philosophy and science of caring.* Boulder: Colorado Associated University Press.

Welsh, J., & Instone, S. (2000). Use of drawings by children in the pediatric office. In S. Dixon & M. Stein (Eds.), *Encounters with children: Pediatric behavior and development* (pp. 571–589). St. Louis, MO: Mosby.

Wolfe, L. (2004). Should parents speak with a dying child about impending death? *New England Journal of Medicine, 35,* 1251–1253.

6

Moral Meanings of Caring for the Dying

SHELLEY RAFFIN BOUCHAL

What is it like for nurses to care for dying individuals who are suffering? I have experienced and reflected upon this experience in countless ways. As an educator I found that this particular journey heightened as I pursued and completed doctoral studies. I began this inquiry at the side of nine palliative care nurses who willingly, openly, and quite profoundly participated in my journey to understand nurses' experience of caring for dying individuals who are suffering. Their willingness to open up their experience to me exemplified their commitment and obligation to palliative care nursing.

Nursing has made many important contributions to palliative care. Historically, nurses have cared for dying individuals who are suffering, and the alleviation of suffering has been a cornerstone of caring, compassionate nurses (Lindholm & Eriksson, 1993). "Nurses are, or should be[,] . . . people who have professed an allegiance to those who suffer lives of enormous and sometimes unbearable pain" (Caputo, 1993, p. 243). Nurses who are committed to caring for the very ill accept full responsibility for their actions; they are willing to risk suffering with others and willing to be a witness to suffering. Those who refuse commitment by becoming detached, callous, or cynical in the face of suffering are "spectators" to life rather than "witnesses" (Taylor, 1991). Nurses create embodied relationships by making a conscious choice to be fully aware of their own bodies and to remain present to the patient, thereby creating a moral space for suffering. Their actions stem from a moral obligation to suffer with others. Nurses are called to consider their moral obligations in all situations, in all encounters, and with all patients.

Nurses do not have the luxury of simply looking in on or overseeing the dying journey; they must engage with illness and pain, becoming fully present to the suffering person. "Nursing practice situates us in the midst of the lives of people where suffering takes place" (Moules, 2000a, p. 5). The obligation or intention to understand suffering is a deeply ethical one. "Obligation is what is important about ethics" (Caputo, 1993, p. 18). Beyond obligation, nurses also have a passion to understand, and this passion moves us beyond assumption. In the local moral worlds or cultures of nurses who care for those who are suffering, we are, as nurses, obligated to understand, as Kleinman (1992) states,

[w]hat precedes, constitutes, expresses, and follows from our actions in interpersonal flows of experience, it is important to understand, what is most at stake for us, what we most fear, what we most aspire to, what we are most threatened by, what we most desire to cross over to safety, what we jointly take to be the purpose, and the ultimate meaning of our living and our dying. (p. 129)

Nurses have the opportunity to bring personal context to the suffering experience. Each nurse, as a person, embodies a private experience of suffering. Suffering evolves from a particular biographical journey through time in relation to professional experiences, threatening some aspect of our personal identities (Ferrell, 2001).

Holding the fragility of life in their hands as part of their everyday work permits nurses to be themselves (Maeve, 1998). This everydayness creates opportunities for nurses to face their own death as well as their patient's death. Nurses engage in the death-and-dying experience through a certain projection of themselves as the meaning of life and death is considered on a daily basis. Nurses involved in the intimate journey to death "cannot hide behind technology or a veil of omniscience as other practitioners. . . . [N]urses are there to hear secrets, especially the ones born of vulnerability" (Fagin & Diers, 1983, p. 117). Giving of themselves and sharing heartfelt emotion are seen as beneficial to their patients, and to give any less might interfere with nurses' ability to know and understand suffering.

The importance of relationships in caring for suffering individuals cannot be underestimated. Relationships in health care are important determinants for health outcomes, for the experiences of family members, and for the quality of work life of health care providers (Rodney, 1997). The quality of nurses' relationships with patients is central to understanding and experiencing suffering. We have only begun to know and understand the phenomenon of suffering and the moral relationship that exists between nurses and patients in relieving the suffering of both. As a professional and an educator I approach suffering by having made some effort to prepare myself for this experience. If nursing is to meet its philosophical goal of caring for the whole person, increased understanding of the nature of suffering within the nurse–patient relationship is crucial.

I have been informed of suffering by the wisdom of cultural and religious traditions and by scholarly opinion that will be integrated throughout this paper. My knowledge also stems from personal experience, much of which I include as clinical experience as a hospice and staff nurse on a number of nursing units. The purpose of this paper is to offer the face of suffering that nurses may experience in caring for dying individuals who are suffering. I hope to portray the nurses' own suffering as a way of engaging with others as intention to understand the suffering experienced in the context of the nurse–patient relationship. I will begin by discussing the research methodology—ethnography—of this particular study.

Ethnography as a Research Approach

Exploring the nurses' world of caring for dying individuals who are suffering requires the ability to plumb the great depths of their experience—a personal world that is difficult to articulate (Lindholm & Eriksson, 1993). While much of this is due to the elusiveness of the language of suffering, to understand the deeply personal and intimate nature of our beliefs, our own experiences, and our relationships is a further complicating factor. It is my belief that the qualitative method of ethnography serves as the preeminent approach in which to study the abstract yet ubiquitous subject of nurses caring for dying individuals who are suffering. Kleinman (1992) suggests that ethnography deepens the study of human suffering by reframing the experience as an interpersonal process in a moral context. The culture of nurses caring for dying individuals—the people, places, and day-to-day experiences of this study—will be articulated, giving life to their realities. The reader will have an opportunity to gain understanding of the human practices of nurses who care for dying individuals. These understandings will include the joys and suffering of the dying person, the interpersonal or intersubjective web of engagements, transformations, communications, and social realities that the nurses, dying individuals, and their families experience on a palliative care unit. Although this study represents only one culture of nurses who care for dying individuals, it is anticipated that others will connect and compare it to their own cultural experiences of caring for dying individuals. It is hoped that this may begin a conversation among all nurses who care for dying individuals so that they too can connect in understanding suffering experiences.

Ethnography as a focus of study has been employed for over a hundred years, finding its roots within the discipline of anthropology, and is arguably the oldest qualitative method (Hughes, 1992). Ethnography as a method of research began as a way to capture the subtleties of human experience and to create understanding of different cultures. Culture, broadly defined, is the learned social behavior or the way of life of a particular group (Germain, 2001). As a nurse who has lived within a palliative care culture for several years, I have witnessed the cultural threads of palliative care nurses. I had a desire both to expand my understanding and to immerse myself as a researcher with both the individuals and the group of nurses who provide care for dying individuals. As Germain (2001) notes, cultural groups have "characteristics such as beliefs, values, ideals, norms (rules of behavior), controls and sanctions for social deviance, language, dress, rituals, interaction patterns, artifacts (technology), socio-political patterns, structure and function and many others" (p. 279). Thus it became my intention to deepen my understanding of the beliefs, values, ideals, and so forth of palliative care nurses through an interpretive ethnographic approach.

Holistic and Contextual Nature of Ethnography

Qualitative ethnography has certain characteristics of interpretive paradigm research, namely, a holistic perspective that seeks to describe as much as possible about a culture or subcultural group (Germain, 2001). An integral characteristic is not only learning from the culture members but also the researcher's immersing herself in the cultural setting. Ethnographers work to become as enmeshed as possible in the lives of members of the cultural group, acting as coparticipants in the research process. Ethnographers subscribe to the belief that human behavior can be understood only in context, in other words, that observed behavior not be separated from the relevant context of meaning and purpose (Germain, 2001). The holistic and contextual nature of nurses' experiences of caring for dying individuals was captured in this study through participant observation, interviews of a dialogic nature, and immersion in the setting where nurses provided direct care to patients and their families. Ultimately, the researcher was concerned not only with nurses' values and beliefs about suffering but also with suffering in the everyday, moment-by-moment experiences of caring for dying individuals. Watching and listening for the implicit and explicit meanings of caring for dying individuals who were suffering was carried out in the clinical unit. This ethnographic study began with watching and listening to the nurse-participants in their naturalistic setting.

Engaging in the Culture

The first step was to gain entry to and become enmeshed in the culture of the palliative care unit. According to Kleinman (1995), the role of the ethnographer is to discover meanings and relationships in "local worlds." To obtain a sense of the breadth and depth of the "local world" one must understand the experiences that flow between and within that world (Kleinman, 1992). Ethnographers begin the process of understanding through observation, seeking to gain an overall sense of the environment and the people who live there. Feeling like an outsider, out of place and awkward, I navigated my way into the work setting in order to establish intimate relationships with members of the culture (Wax, 1977). Once engaged, I attempted to capture meanings and relationships by providing a voice for individual participants through their stories, both spoken and unspoken. Using unstructured interviews (conversations) with nurses as a means to understand the experience, I explored the moral commitments, meanings, beliefs, and values found in their stories. In addition, I engaged in participant observation of the nurses in the context of caring for dying individuals.

The nurses in this study helped me appreciate their basic beliefs, fears, hopes, and expectations about caring for dying individuals through my role of "observer [of] and participant" with the nine nurses who participated in this study (Morse & Field, 1995). At the beginning of each observational experience I explained to the nurses and to the patients and family members for whom the nurses were caring that my role was primarily to be that of an observer; I did not initiate care but did assist, for example, in turning or bathing individuals. Initially, in making these observations I was a bit nervous and very conscious that I might get lost in the detail of the observational experience. I wanted to obtain quality in the data I collected. This process began with establishing reciprocal trust between the participants and me. I always began by establishing rapport through conversation. Often it began with who I was when I was not a researcher or with the status of dying individuals that day. When I felt comfortable, I would absorb as much of the experience as I possibly could. Occasionally, I would leave the room and jot down verbal or nonverbal exchanges or salient points that captured the essence of the experiences. When it was feasible, shortly after an event I would ask key participants about their perceptions of the event and their feelings about it. Remaining focused for a long period of time was mentally exhausting, and I was conscious that I needed to stop when I felt my thoughts begin to wander. Upon leaving the unit my mind was often spinning, and I tried to capture my experiences on the way home by using a tape recorder. The essence of each observational visit was captured in field notes. Field notes written after participant-observation experiences provided rich descriptions of the nurses' behaviors and actions as well as dialogue between nurses and patients in context.

A great deal of time needs to be devoted to gathering the kinds of data that are rich enough to create a "picture of the whole." Hughes (1992) writes that, in ethnography, "the goal of inquiry is rounded, not segmented understanding, it is comprehensive in intent" (p. 443). Through analysis of the data I made an effort not to separate the data gained from the nurses' stories and from their actions/dialogue in practice but to embellish their stories in order to explore in depth how they unfolded in practice. I looked for descriptions, patterns, and relationships through data collected from the key participants.

Experienced palliative care nurses volunteered to be key participants in this study. I will introduce these key participants throughout the manuscript. To maintain confidentiality, the names of all participants and places have been changed. Furthermore, all the nurses volunteering in the study were female, and thus "she" will be used throughout the paper.

Reflexivity

Ethnography has a reflexive character by which researchers engage in and influence the collection, selection, and interpretation of data (Finlay, 2002). Reflexivity places the researcher in the middle of the cultural setting to soak in the local moral world before returning to the place of observation, as it were, with a changed perspective. The study of a culture requires an intimacy with the participants who are a part of the culture. The researcher brings her own culture to the setting and leaves the participants with a changed perspective. This dialectical relationship is summarized by Bruyn (1996), who asserts that "the role of the participant-observer requires sharing the sentiments of people in social situations; as he himself is changed as well as changing in some degree the situation in which he participates" (p. 14). Anderson (1991) discusses the concept that fieldwork is inherently dialectical; the researcher affects and is affected by the phenomena she seeks to understand: "Meaning is not merely investigated, but is constructed by the researcher and informant through active and reciprocal relationships and the dialectical processes of interaction" (p. 116). Reflexivity therefore leads to a greater understanding of the dynamics of particular phenomena and relationships found within cultures.

This dialectical relationship is not just between the researcher and the culture under study; it also occurs within the researcher—a reflexivity of the self. In studying nurses caring for dying individuals who were suffering I expected to connect with the suffering experiences through my own emotions, biases, and beliefs. I brought to the research my experience as a nurse who has cared for dying individuals; myself as a beginning researcher; and my social history, perceptions, and prejudices as part of understanding this culture (Coffey, 1999; Gregory, 1994). Personal insights of suffering, when they arose, were uncomfortable. Understanding how I changed and developed through this fieldwork and the analysis was an important part of this work. Immediate and continuing self-awareness of feelings, thoughts, and interpretations was revealed through the use of a journal. Through continually evaluating my responses I interpreted those responses and questioned how they came to be. Hertz (1997) argues that a researcher must become more aware of how she owns positions and how her interests are imposed at all stages of the research process, from the questions she asks to those she ignores, from problem formulation to analysis representation and writing. Thus while I studied nurses' personal suffering as they cared for dying individuals my responses were affected by my roles both as a researcher and as a nurse. The questions were not only whether my background would influence the research but also whether or not I was aware of this interaction and how transparent I was regarding interpreting my own feelings and responses.

The unfolding of this paper will disclose descriptions and interpretations gleaned from observations and participation in the lives of nurses and their patients on a specific nursing unit. These interpretations were made with the assistance of audiotaped interviews and observations along with my own experience as a researcher. Several pertinent themes will be presented, uncovering aspects of nursing practice that are often tacit and taken for granted. In revealing the experiences of nurses with whom I walked on this journey, it seems most important to capture their beginnings in palliative care. The next section of this paper will reveal the nurses' call to relationship.

Nurses in Palliative Care: A Call to Relationship

Death is not the ultimate tragedy of life. The ultimate tragedy is depersonalization, dying . . . separated from the spiritual nourishment that comes from being able to reach out to a loving hand, separated from a desire to experience the things that make life worth living, separated from hope. (Cousins, 1981, p. 133)

Nurses often speak of the privilege of sharing in the intimate journey of living and dying with their patients. To share in such a special relationship, where high regard for the whole person and his or her being-in-the-world is paramount, can be very rewarding for the nurses who choose to be in those settings. Individuals' dying journeys are, however, not always peaceful. Suffering, pain, and loss are often part of the journey. I often wondered why nurses choose to partake in this journey. Are there special kinds of nurses who are best suited to be on this journey? One might speculate that nurses are *called* to palliative care. Throughout the study I wondered what kinds of persons are drawn to those who are dying, who are suffering, and who are searching for meaning in living and meaning in dying.

Palliative care is a profound experience in which a life-threatening illness brings patients, families, and nurses together in a human relationship that unfolds in unique and mysterious ways. Nurses in this study frequently described caring for dying individuals as a "vocation" or "calling," reflecting a moral and/or spiritual essence to their care (Raffin, 2002). The term *vocation,* which is derived from the Latin word *vocare,* "to call," is broadly understood as defining an individual's felt call to a particular ministry or work (Olson & Clark, 2000). In theological terminology the word *vocation* generally refers to a divine call to undertake a particular activity or embrace a particular stage of life on behalf of God or the community (Olson & Clark, 2000).

Being called to relationship is an appropriate description of evoking a way of being (Chinn, 1994). In this study being called to care is a willingness to be in significant relation, to be responsive to others, to be in spirit together and in human existence together (Raffin, 2002). It is through these relationships that nurses come to know more about the meaning of life, death, and suffering.

Most of the nurses in this study said they were called to palliative care because they wanted to give of themselves to others and to grow as persons. They expected and desired that personal closeness would be the core of their work with dying individuals and their families. The nurse-participants hoped that, in view of their own suffering, religious beliefs, and sense of self-confidence as persons, they would be able to give of themselves. Ultimately, for whatever reason they were called to be palliative care nurses, there was a search for possibilities that fostered human well-being. Barbara said, "Nurses do this kind of nursing because it brings us closer to who we are as people." Barbara shared her beliefs about working in palliative care:

In this work there is a "peace" that occurs, there is a beauty with it, and there's an end to suffering. It's not gross, it's not a bad thing, and it's not always a sad thing. We have a [tradition] on the floor that says you have to wear waterproof mascara, because we cry lots. You get close to people. Sometimes it's a pretty rough death, but there's a release when it's done. It's not bad.

Bringing Authenticity

Nurses, in their call to being with others, search for authenticity. Searching for authenticity means being true to self, accepting responsibility for choices, and being willing to make choices directed by values, personal identities, and life goals (Taylor, 1991). Bringing authenticity to being with others helps people to discover possibilities for becoming their best selves, given their situation. Ruth shared her beliefs about bringing authenticity:

Not all nurses are able to be authentic with dying individuals. Being authentic does not happen overnight. Knowing one's values about dying requires constant reflection that does not happen upon graduation from nursing school. Life experience and a personal understanding about what death really entails is the only way one can really be authentic. Helping someone explore personal intimate meanings of life and death is not a task that can be memorized but rather must be experienced from the depth of one's soul, to reach within and find personal meaning. The connection that is experienced in searching for intimate meaning is what entices nurses to work in palliative care. You have to want that connection to be an authentic palliative care nurse.

In this study bringing authenticity meant that nurses help others to care for their own being. Palliative care nurses help others in the process of dying to discover meaning in their life by encouraging and assisting them in exploring meaning in the past, present, and future. An authentic self, for both nurses and dying individuals, cannot be socially derived but must be inwardly generated. Darlene expressed her feelings of being authentic:

I've cared for so many young women—38, 42—and we've seen them from the diagnostic stage to death, sometimes for a very short period of time. I recognize how precious and vulnerable we are, and that there is a plan out there somewhere for why I'm here. I wouldn't say I'm a religious person in that God has a plan for us. I don't know why, but for some reason there is an explanation as to why this experience is happening to both of us. These experiences force us to look at our beliefs about life and death regularly. Patients look at you, the nurse, to help them sort out these experiences.

The Moral Call of Responsibility and Responsiveness: The Role of Emotions

This call to relationship is a call to responsibility, a responsibility to suffer with the other, to be responsive and sensitive. Responsiveness and sensitivity allow the nurse to be open to the face of the other. The face of the other is a moral connection to relationship (Olthuis, 1997). In seeing the face of the other we understand a special sensitivity to situations. The following reveals Barbara's sensitivity to the face of the other:

Those who suffer often don't say anything. You have to look at their face; they just have to hold on to your hand. You know that gut feeling nurses get? Well, it's that gut feeling. It's a lot of stuff. . . . [I]t's something you feel, something you see. I don't know how you can tell. It's just there. It's the clues that they give you. We don't have to ask if we don't know. We just touch. It's what nursing is all about.

In caring for a dying individual moral sensitivity is paramount, often evoking deep emotions. A nurse's sensitivity, commitment, and intention to understand suffering are central to understanding a patient's experience of dying (Raffin, 2002). Emotions, commitment, intention, and value ascribe importance to human experience. "No one can help anyone without entering with his/her whole self into the painful situation, without risk of becoming hurt, wounded or even destroyed in the process" (Thomasma, 1994, p. 132). The nurse's suffering does not hinder understanding but rather allows her the capacity of seeing a patient's suffering (Raffin, 2002). Emotions call a nurse to a heightened sense of being. Emotions allow the nurse to show her relational being. The nurse who has a sense of genuineness can understand the call in a moment (Cameron, 2004). Emotions can themselves be a source of knowledge. Emotions for a nurse can reflect embodied knowledge of rituals and practices that are often unspoken, tacit, taken for granted.

The following example from Nancy uncovers the moral role that emotions play in this relationship. The face-to-face relationship with this individual opened a moral space, a space for sensitivity to suffering. The care the nurse provided required a high degree of professional skill in her responsiveness. In addition, the nurse's sensitivity to suffering gave her knowledge of what was important at that particular moment.

We had a patient who was bleeding profusely. He had esophageal varices and whatnot, and we were just trying to keep him comfortable. I suctioned him and that made him bleed more, but if I didn't suction him he couldn't breathe. I didn't want to leave him alone. I was holding his hand and basically directing someone to go and get the morphine. I didn't want to leave his room. Even though he wasn't aware that we were there, I just stayed. And I think I actually prayed. I know the nurses were getting frustrated because we couldn't stop the bleeding. We were all just focused on doing whatever we could to make him comfortable. I felt privileged to be there for him even for the short period of time I spent with him

It is evident in this situation that Nancy was present to the face of the other. Emotions did not get in the way of providing good care for this individual. Nancy obtained a feeling of fulfillment from her moral response to the other, a relationship in which she performed professional activities out of responsibility and compassion. In observing other nurses I noted that personal closeness, sharing of emotions, being present with individuals, and knowing who they really were as individuals were most important in their relationships. I sensed that nurses were most fulfilled when professional care was performed out of a moral sense and *through* face-to-face relationships with dying individuals who confirmed the moral worth of their care.

During an observation visit with Barbara we cared for Lillie, an 87-year-old woman with non-Hodgkin's lymphoma. Lillie had been admitted three weeks earlier with pneumonia and hypoxia and was not responding verbally. Oxygen was being administered at 4 liters per minute, yet her respirations were deep and labored and her skin was cool to touch. Barbara came over to Lillie and stroked her head. She immediately assessed Lillie's respiratory rate and checked to make sure she was not experiencing any pain. She repositioned Lillie so that she was in an upright position to enhance her ability to breathe. The physical touch Barbara used seemed to create an atmosphere of familiarity. It made their relationship seem very close. She stood there for a long period, watching Lillie's face. Lillie reached out to grab Barbara's hand.

The physical motion and emotional expression of touch are reciprocal; touch affects both the person initiating it and the person being touched. Touch can reach past technological treatment, allowing the patient to reach out of the solitude of suffering (Gadow, 1991). For Barbara the use of touch was obviously an authentic expression of her moral sense of being with Lillie. In observing Barbara I could see that she authentically knew whether to touch or not touch Lillie; she knew whether to take her hand or place a hand on her shoulder. Barbara came up to Lillie instead of addressing her from the foot of the bed or the doorway. She stood close, making physical contact and talking directly to her patient. She made her presence known to Lillie even when she was performing technical care, and Lillie responded by grabbing her hand.

The nature of the nurse–patient relationship is such that touching is both inescapable and acceptable. Touch is powerful. I often noted patients opening their eyes, breathing more slowly and relaxing, and reciprocating by clutching the nurse's hand. It appears that touch causes the dissolution of boundaries between two persons. When they have difficulty knowing what to say, nurses often use touch, which is the silent expression of being present in the fullest sense of the word. The nurses in the study all agree that touch needs to be genuine to be effective. They believe that patients know when a touch is not authentic and that they can feel a nurse's hesitation.

The nurses described their call as a "giving," a being responsive to others—"to keep us in touch with life as it really is," Barbara claims. Suffering acknowledges our humanness (Caputo, 1993). Nurses in this study acknowledged that the imminence of death breaks through the facade behind which one can tend to hide. Stepping out into the open is refreshing, but it is scary. These nurses say that when they develop authentic caring the rewards are immeasurable (Raffin, 2002). A call to relationship can be experienced by nurses who look into the face of the other. Olthuis (1997) invites us to see the face as "an epiphany of the nakedness of the other, a visitation, a coming, a saying which comes in the passivity of the face, not threatening, but obligating. I encounter a face, my world is ruptured, my contentment interrupted; I am already obligated" (p. 136). In looking into the face of the other, nurses have the potential to see and feel the pain, but they also see the spirit that people discover within themselves. Nurses are expected to care for the whole person—body, mind, and spirit. Being with people on their final journey is a special kind of work that offers the fulfillment of being in relationship with others.

Relational Ethics: Nurses Create a Moral Space for Suffering

Relational ethics is an action ethic, an action that arises from a profound sense of the insecurity to which we are exposed (Caputo, 1989). "Instead of making judgments about the goodness or badness of human actions and character" (Morris, 1978, p. 852), we act in ways that lead to goodness without being certain if we are right. Caputo (1989) writes:

We act not on the basis of unshakeable grounds but in order to do what we can, taking what action seems wise, and not without misgivings. We act, but we understand that we are not situated safely above the flux and that we do not have a view of the whole. . . . We act because something has to be done. (p. 59)

Relationships are the focus of understanding and examining the moral life in nursing (Bergum, 2004). Creating a moral space for suffering speaks to the inherent nature of relationships in nursing. "The healer has to keep striving for the space . . . in which healer and patient can reach out to each other as travelers sharing the same broken human condition" (Nouwen, 1986, p. 93). The moral space is where action takes place. To be responsible in an ethical way, people need to understand other persons as well as themselves. One attends to the moral space created by one's relation to oneself and to the other (Bergum & Dossetor, 2005). Having an awareness of themselves as persons is the containing space—the space where nurses and patients make connections—for others who suffer (Bergum, 2004; Jopling, 2000). It is this relational space that gives moral meaning to our actions (Gaita, 1991).

It is discomforting to be reminded of one's own mortality. Nurses in this study reported that understanding their own suffering enhanced the possibility that they would be competent and trustworthy and that they would give of themselves, listen attentively, encourage hope, and be open and honest (Raffin, 2002). It was their own experience of suffering that enabled them to be compassionate and to share in the plight of another (Gregory, 1994). Personal suffering has a hollowing effect; it allowed them the internal space to be able to contain the suffering of others (Bergum, 2002).

Embodied Experiences of Suffering

The nursing relationship is an intersubjective experience, and intersubjectivity subsumes the notion of embodiment (Maeve, 1998). Embodiment is the giving of one's entire self—the ways in which meanings, expectations, and values are expressed and experienced in the body of the nurse and the patient. While health care providers primarily focus on the patient's body as object (the physical or emotional body needing care), family and friends make the necessary and ethical connection to the patient's lived body and human, everyday lived experiences. "Nurses support the reconnection of the body as an object to the body as lived because they know that the lived body is as ethically important as the object body" (Bergum, 2004, p. 493). Embodied nurses are fully present to others and their experiences and are also aware of their own bodies in relation to the experience (Gadow, 1991). They have a moral obligation to the individual's body as living flesh, and humility and compassion sharpen their senses to act cautiously, reflectively, and with understandings stemming from experience. Since humans are susceptible to pain and suffering, embodiment (in an ethical sense) is a lived bodily relation to the other (Gadow, 1991). The inseparability of the lived body and the object body of individuals who are suffering is known in the moment of suffering when eyes meet and a connection is experienced by both the nurse and the patient. "Commitment to others is felt in the body" (Bergum, 2004, p. 493).

The nurse in an embodied relationship experiences feelings as part of being and becoming in the relationship. In the nurse–patient relationship there is reciprocal sharing and mutual respect in which nurse and patient may be unique but have equivalent worth and dignity (Bergum, 2004). The nurse engages with the patient without reducing *you* (the patient) to the same as *me* (the nurse) or *me* to the same as *you* (Bergum, 2004). In mutual respect of the other the nurse acknowledges the other's suffering experience.

In suffering with, in compassion for, the other the nurse creates a space for suffering. Etymologically, the word *compassion* is derived from *passion* (the suffering of pain, being acted upon, a powerful affection of the mind) and *com-* (in combination or in union together) (Hoad, 2001). *Compassion* means the suffering of pain together. The embodied nurse facing one who is suffering creates an open space in which she listens to the pain, sees the pain, touches and feels the pain. Of course, the intensity of the nurse's experience is different from that of the patient. Intense, immediate emotions may be felt by the nurse; however, they serve to generate a moral process necessary in attempts to comfort and to alleviate the individual's suffering. This moral process or choice is compassion. Jennifer talked of her beliefs about this moral process:

Suffering connects us with our humanity, who we really are as individuals. When a nurse witnesses suffering, she sees a person suffering. This person brings forth the compassion within us. This last summer we cared for a woman who was only 32 years old. She had two children. I'll never forget the 4-year-old outside of her hospital door crying, "Mommy, Mommy, Mommy." You feel so helpless, your heart just stops, you feel so empty. Often there is the immediacy of crying with them—the sadness is overwhelming. It's like a transference, imagining for yourself how devastating that would be. Then your next reaction is to help them. How can I make this experience so that they feel loved, dignified, and worthwhile? How can I lessen their burden of grief? We try and meet them where they are. It's never easy and never routine. Physical pain is much more strategic; a plan of care usually comes to your mind. Not with suffering—it happens in the moment.

Compassion, Imagination, and Courage: A Moral Commitment

Compassion, or suffering with someone, is a quality that is a natural part of being human. Humans have a moral impulse to alleviate suffering (Lindholm & Eriksson, 1993). Compassion for suffering, as a moral response to understanding and alleviating another's suffering, is a moral imperative for nurses (Raffin, 2002). Gregory (1994) suggests that we are obligated to try to understand the meaning of the experience from the patients' perspective. We are obliged to hear their voices.

The moral quality of compassion involves union in another person's suffering—not merely an identification of the suffering but identification with it. The personhood of the sufferer and caregiver coalesces for the purposes of sharing and offering support to the patient who attempts to work through his or her suffering (Gregory & English, 1994). To suffer is to undergo, to endure, to tolerate, and to allow (Hoad, 2001). Jennifer voiced how being in compassionate relationships with patients allows one to be in a unique position to ensure that the sufferer is not alienated, that the experience is acknowledged, and that the path taken to alleviate suffering is open. When we create a space for suffering we suffer together. In relationship with our patients we unite to create an acknowledgment and perhaps an understanding of suffering. Eileen talked about the union of suffering, the changes in relationship that occurred for both her and the patient when suffering was acknowledged:

I remember the feeling of caring for a patient who finally, after several days of [our] being together, revealed to me that he was scared of dying alone. He told me how betrayed he felt by his physical body, how diseased and distasteful he felt he was to others, but that I could look beyond his diseased body and capture his spirit. In this experience he felt whole and that his suffering was acknowledged. He told me that our relationship made him feel valued and worthwhile. When he told me this I remember starting to cry, and he held my hand. I sat there not knowing what to say for what seemed like a very long time. I will never forget this experience and the strength he gave to me as his nurse.

In this relationship a mutual commitment opened the possibilities for responding to suffering in a deeper, authentic, and genuine way, bringing words to emotion. Frank (1992) has discussed this as a coming into "imaginative alignment" with the patient—looking at the world from behind the eyes of the suffering patient as clearly as one can imagine. To do this requires a willingness to share the pain of the other. Nurses can never directly know the suffering of another and must never say, "I know what you are going through." Yet in saying "I can only imagine how hard this is for you" they communicate genuine compassion, assuming that the statement expresses a genuine willingness to invest the emotional energy and to accept the personal risk that such imagination entails (Frank, 1992).

Understanding patients' suffering and where it is located in their bodies and their lives is fundamental to a compassionate response (Gregory & English, 1994). Compassionate care is made possible only by being present and engaging with those who suffer. This care requires a true movement toward the other as a person. Through embodiment and compassion nurses openly engage with dying individuals, where they meet to experience an energetic absorption of these individuals' pain, suffering, and fear and to commiserate with their frustration and anger. Relational engagement occurs in the moment of suffering when this nurse, this patient, and this place allow meaning to emerge through each person in his or her own way (Bergum, 2004). For nurses the cost of this journey is high because it means being exposed to their own suffering, woundedness, and grief. This sense of suffering is recognized by nurses as a call to relationship, a call to be known, to be heard and validated, and an opportunity to recognize their own vulnerabilities and humanness as nurses (Raffin, 2002). This begins with nurses learning what they can regarding their assumptions and beliefs about suffering.

Nurses in palliative care delve deep in search of their own fears and uncertainties (Raffin, 2002). Acknowledging within ourselves our uncertainties takes courage and commitment. Courage, derived from the Latin word *coraticum,* means to act with heart, spirit, intention, purpose, bravery, and valor (Hoad, 1986). Courage makes risk taking possible, carrying one beyond safety and security. Nurses move beyond their moral distress to enact moral courage (Storch, 2004). Moral courage is courage informed by knowledge, past experience, and trust in one's own and another's ability to grow (Raffin, 2002). For example, courage may be required when collaborating with other members of the medical team if they are pursuing care that the nurse may deem not in the best interests of a dying individual. On a busy medical unit palliative care is sometimes regarded as less important than curative or life-prolonging treatments, and courage may be required to convince other members of the team that dying individuals in the hospital deserve respect, dignity, and the right to choose alternative measures of care. It takes courage for nurses to stand up to others on behalf of patients and their families. On an observation visit, for example, I watched Helen approach a physician with courage and compassion.

Helen was caring for Bill, a man with multiple melanomas, which are more common in individuals between the ages of 40 and 60; Bill, however, was 32. Usually in this disease the malignant cells infiltrate the bone marrow, often causing excruciating back and bone pain. Bill had been unresponsive to chemotherapy treatments, the malignant cells were "spreading like wildfire," and the oncologist gave him no hope of remission. The chemotherapy had been stopped, but the family was searching for other treatment options. Bill's back pain was getting worse. Two weeks of trying different pain medication regimes resulted in no improvement. Without warning the health care team, Bill consulted a herbalist and was advised to take certain herbs. The nurses on the evening shift notified the physician, who refused to give an order for Bill to take the herbs. Not wanting to go against the advice of his physician but knowing that he had limited choice, Bill asked Helen to phone the physician again. Knowing that the physician was coming in that morning, Helen chose to speak with him in person. "I know that this physician is not going to change his mind, but I feel obligated, for Bill, to speak to him face to face."

The physician arrived sometime later, and I watched Helen approach him. She stood by as he spoke to another physician. Then Helen said, "Dr. Smith, I was wondering if I could speak to you about your patient Bill. Bill wants to try these herbal remedies." Dr. Smith gave Helen little time to explain Bill's situation. "I will not write an order that I do not agree with. If Bill chooses to take these herbs, I guess that is his decision, but I do not see it as being in his best interest." "Dr. Smith," Helen asked, "what other alternatives can you suggest for Bill? If this gives Bill hope, is that not in his best interest?" Dr. Smith paused, looked at Helen, and walked away to Bill's room. Helen sighed, shook her head, and also walked away. Later she checked the chart. The physician had not ordered the herbs. Helen, in a disappointed voice, spoke out loud: "I guess Bill doesn't have the physician's support, but he has mine."

In giving authentic care Helen courageously spoke out for Bill. Out of a desire to be a caring, moral person Helen supported Bill. She knew this was important to Bill and that it gave him the hope he needed to work through his suffering in this illness experience.

Nurses' Vulnerability

Nurses who care for the suffering and the dying are accustomed to the question "How do you do that?" Ironically, nurses often ask themselves this same question (Maeve, 1998). Vulnerability is often defined as being susceptible; "[one] may be wounded . . . open to attack" (Hoad, 2001). However, vulnerability, like suffering, is one characteristic of being human. By the mere fact that we have body, mind, and spirit we are vulnerable (Sellman, 2005). We have no choice in being vulnerable; rather, our choice lies in whether or not we will be authentic with our vulnerability. Reeder (1995) suggests that authenticity is "listening to hear the discourse of positive and negative desires of our embodied selves, making it possible to hear the desires of another" (p. 199). This embodied discourse, which includes vulnerability, enables people to recognize vulnerability in others and thus share in the human condition. From this perspective people must be aware of their own vulnerability, recognize it in others as they recognize themselves in others, and be willing to enter into mutual vulnerability. Viewing vulnerability as a way of celebrating humanness differs greatly from the popular notion of avoiding and protecting oneself against vulnerability.

Initially, I thought of vulnerability from a more traditional viewpoint. As I observed and listened to the nurses I often wondered if nurses in their vulnerability were helpful to dying individuals who were suffering. Should they convey their suffering to the dying individuals? What would this accomplish? I observed that nurses in their vulnerability, their words and gestures, conveyed the anguish, fear, and bewilderment that they were experiencing.

I watched Nancy care for Joe, an elderly man with end-stage diabetes. Joe had only one lower limb, and it was now infested with gangrene. Nancy was changing his foot dressing, and concern about whether one of his blackened toes would come off in the process consumed her every thought. Joe could not have survived a surgical amputation, so the nurses attentively cared for his body—physically, emotionally, and spiritually. I watched Nancy don a mask and gloves. The smell of dying flesh kept most people away, but Nancy tried her best to convey respect for and acceptance of the smells of Joe's decaying body. She carefully began to remove the dressing, her eyes tentative and fearful as she watched Joe's foot. Her gaze moved from the dressing back to Joe's face, acknowledging his pain and suffering. "Am I hurting you, Joe?" Nancy inquired. Finally, the dressing was peeled away, the toes still intact. The suffering experienced by both Joe and Nancy, although not verbally expressed, was embodied in their shared breath and in Nancy's shaking hands as she continued her nursing care.

Nancy portrays how the vulnerability of another person can touch us not only because we recognize our own vulnerability but also in a moral obligation to practice authentic nursing. Vulnerable patients seek nursing care, and nurses seek those who are vulnerable. Travelbee (1971) describes the commitment that is involved in the relationship:

[One has to] expose oneself to the shocks of commitment and all that entails. It is to care and in the caring to be vulnerable, but it is the vulnerability of the strong who are not afraid to be authentic human beings. It is the ability to face and confront reality, to face reality not as we wish it to be, but as it actually exists. Nurses must possess this trait if they would help others to cope with the reality of suffering. (p. 4)

The vulnerability of nurses' suffering can be enabling. Sharing of vulnerability is authentic, a moral response, an acknowledgment and embracing of another's suffering. That sharing of vulnerability represents a rich synthesis of nurse and dying individual, of embodiment, union, and transcendence, and allows for understanding suffering in people (Raffin, 2002). Observing nurses revealed their vulnerability, uniquely embodied in each experience of suffering.

I was reminded, however, by Darlene that although nurses' vulnerability can be enabling, there are experiences when "patients do not let you into their suffering." Nurses in their own vulnerability are not always able to "break the barrier of suffering." "Even with several encounters with suffering, we are not united in suffering." Many nurses endure the vulnerability they experience because of their commitment to alleviate suffering and to assist people to live as fully as possible.

Nurses on the unit discussed their philosophy as based on the intrinsic worth of each individual for whom they cared. Understanding people's suffering necessitates gaining knowledge of the ideas held by suffering individuals about their identities; their lives past, present, and future; their relationships to others and their environment; their aims; and their anticipated actions (Cassell, 1982). Knowledge of people is partly knowl-edge about how people live as well as what they live for. For these nurses protecting patients' inherent worth is a central moral feature of nursing practice that calls them into relationship with others.

Protecting the worth of individuals who cannot or choose not to speak about their experiences, values, or beliefs presents a challenge to even the most experienced palliative care nurses. Palliative care nurses learn to acknowledge the silence and offer the opportunity to open a conversation. Not all nurses are comfortable with silence; they describe feeling helpless because they sense the loneliness and alienation of their patients. Nurses leave the dying journey feeling that they have walked away from suffering and that the patient has died alone. Helen related this experience:

I remember caring for Beatrice, who would willingly accept my physical com-forts of positioning her body into supported positions and taking ice chips so that her lips were not parched. But she would literally lie there with tears streaming down her cheeks, making no eye contact. I held her hand, and she did not resist, but I could not feel a connection. Nurses openly accept that you cannot connect with every individual, but Beatrice was connecting with no one. After she died we all prayed that our suffering [had] somehow reached hers and that she knew that we were reaching out to her.

In the dying journey there are occasionally patients who choose to die alone, wishing no one to be present in the room with them. Respecting their wish to be alone is distressing to nurses. Being physically present is somehow more comforting to nurses, as they feel they are making a dif-ference. In these relationships the palliative care nurses experience giv-ing to others and receiving from others. The union of giving something of oneself for the purpose of being of service and of doing what is good for another person is fulfilling. Jennifer voiced her feelings of discomfort at having to walk away from a person who asked to be left alone:

When patients want to be left alone to die it's a very different kind of caring and attention you have to give. I mean, it's not your conventional nursing care . . . that you feel proud of. You are not able to visually see that you have done a "good" job. I remember entering a patient's room to do my initial rounds and let him know that I would be his nurse, and he said, "Thank you. Now please leave me alone. I just need to be alone." I had a lot of difficulty physically leaving him alone. I just did not feel that I was exactly meeting the standards of being a good nurse in my opinion. That was his choice and you had to respect it, but you still feel responsible for him, and it's not easy to walk away.

It took strength for Jennifer to walk away from this relationship. Yet her responsibility and responsiveness were kept alive in her desire to honor, acknowledge, and keep open a space for sharing suffering. As I watched Jennifer's distress at longing to go into the room to make sure the patient was all right she allowed me to understand that the space she created for suffering was ever present. Her willingness to accept the patient's suffering from a distance was admirable. Through the experience of responsiveness to the needs of both herself and the other the palliative care nurse discovers and responds to the moral commitment of relationship.

Creating a Space for Suffering That Persists

When individuals' suffering and dying are prolonged nurses experience distress. The nurse-participants spoke of many experiences where suffering persisted. We had repeated discussions about the uneasiness the nurses felt regarding the use or abuse of technology with dying individuals in order to prolong their lives. Brock (1989) explains how life-prolonging treatment has become a reality of much of our clinical practices:

In recent decades medicine has gained dramatic new abilities to prolong life. . . . While . . . life-sustaining treatments often provide very great benefits to individual patients by restoring or prolonging functioning lives, they also have the capacity to prolong patients' lives beyond the point at which they desire continued life support or are reasonably thought to be benefited by it. Thus, where once nature took its course and pneumonia was the "old man's friend," now increasingly someone must decide how long a life will be prolonged and when death will come. (p. 131)

Nurses in this study described experiences in which suffering persisted as a consequence of "heroic measures." It was not unusual for nurses to be left with orders that they believed made little sense. Ruth explained:

I'll never forget this 82-year-old gentleman who had [had] a "radical neck dissection" for cancer of the larynx. He opted for the surgery so that "he could have more time with his family." Postoperatively, he received the standard tracheotomy and feeding tube. After weeks of nausea and vomiting from not tolerating the tube feeding his weight dropped dramatically, and he began to . . . fade away. The look of terror in his eyes when he attempted on several occasions to remove his tracheotomy [tube] was too much for me to watch. I kept asking myself, What was he telling us? Why do we keep reinserting this tube upon the wish of his family? Were we only prolonging the anguish, fear, and suffering of this individual? What kind of death are we creating for this individual? I remember stopping in the middle of inserting the tracheotomy tube, saying to the daughter, who was holding his hands down, "I cannot do this anymore." But someone else did.

The suffering that was apparent in this individual's face, along with his need and vulnerability, shaped Ruth's moral response. To be touched by the individual's suffering helped her to understand that care cannot be strictly equated with treatment given. The suffering that Ruth experienced represents a sense of transformed responsibility through her embodied relationship with her patient. She recognized that the impersonal and dehumanizing act of continually reinserting the tracheotomy tube was only intensifying his suffering and that this treatment was prolonging and intensifying his death. It is in these experiences that nurses claim that medical treatment is serving its own needs and not the needs of the dying individual. It was Ruth's embodied compassion that gave direction to her actions and commitment.

In creating a space for suffering nurses respond and listen to the bodies and personal needs of dying individuals whose greatest fear has become further suffering (Gregory, 1994). Like Ruth, nurses motivated by their embodiment are then moved to take action. When nurses are genuinely present in the moment they are able to read bodily signs, signs they are both consciously and unconsciously aware of, that offer us more than we can see, feel, or think. Nurses open themselves to a process of deep reflection that invites both critical awareness and attunement to one's emotions and bodily experiences. Nurses like Ruth carry with them a sense of professional duty and a feeling in their hearts that move them to thoughtfully consider their experience in the moment, considering moral aspects such as dignity, family needs, and their professional obligations.

Palliative care nurses act in ways that comfort and convey respect so as not to increase the vulnerability that individuals are experiencing. The nurses in this study were concerned with maintaining patients' dignity. This was related in part to prevention of suffering and supporting patients' rights to direct their care, but it also involved the importance of privacy, respectful care of a patient's body, and respect for the personhood of a patient. Ruth's actions portrayed this as she bathed Rebecca.

Rebecca was receiving external radiation treatment for recurrence of cancer of the cervix and vulva. The radiation area on her upper pelvis and lower abdomen was marked, so it could not be immersed in water or washed with soap. While soaking in a tub would likely be the most soothing and would afford the highest degree of cleanliness, it was not possible.

Rebecca was also very weak. The amount of oxygen saturation in the blood is an important physiologic measure in determining the effectiveness of the respiratory system. Earlier, Ruth had measured Rebecca's oxygen saturation level at 89%. With exertion her levels had been known to drop to as low as 70%. The effort of moving to a tub or shower would have been too strenuous for Rebecca. Ruth recognized that the energy Rebecca could expend was minimal; thus her bath had to be a passive one. Ruth decided that a bed bath was the safest for Rebecca.

I watched Ruth as she began to wash Rebecca. She was efficient but not rushed. She encouraged Rebecca to wash her own face, offering the cloth to her several times, as the warm water on her face made Rebecca feel refreshed and gave a healthy glow to her pale, ashen skin. Ruth then washed Rebecca's legs and feet with slow, relaxing strokes toward her heart. Rebecca's eyes closed, and her breathing was deep. Ruth carefully assisted Rebecca onto her side, where she washed her back and buttocks. After drying and applying lotion she again turned Rebecca onto her back. At this time Ruth changed the bathwater and cloth. She then began to focus on Rebecca's lower abdomen and perineum, the most painful and tender area. To this point Rebecca had been calm, relaxed, and serene. To maintain this calmness Ruth also had to remain calm, approaching Rebecca in a caring, gentle manner. I watched her begin squeezing water from the cloth onto Rebecca's abdomen, not rubbing in order to avoid removing the markings. She allowed the air to dry most of the tepid water, finishing with gentle patting with a soft towel. The area remained red and weepy.

The act of bathing is for Ruth "nursing in its finest form." Ruth was present, committed, and absorbed. This was not a routine task to be done but an act that was caring and required skill and judgment. Ruth enacted her skill in a way that drew me to be with her and her patient. The pain I expected Rebecca to experience did not occur. I witnessed and felt a serene flow of caring in this bathing. There were no mechanistic actions. The bathing was a work of art, a caring for Rebecca that enhanced her dignity. I watched Ruth's absorption as she artfully carried out each action of attending to Rebecca's body, knowing the areas that might be

sensitive or painful. Rebecca's body was familiar to Ruth. There was immediacy to this act of nursing.

Engagement and suffering are essential aspects of responsible caregiving (Schultz & Carnevale, 1996). The acts of protecting and preventing further suffering have the potential to transform suffering (Lindholm
& Eriksson, 1993). Alleviation of the suffering means lessening the patient's sense of vulnerability (Rehnsfeldt & Eriksson, 2004). This necessitates an act of commitment on the part of the nurse. Presence transcends
the self and represents an invitation to share the journey and "come
alongside and be allowed to see, to touch, and to hear the brokenness,
vulnerability and suffering of another" (Pettigrew, 1988, p. 12). Through
embodiment—listening and responding to the body—these nurses see
their goal as comforting and/or alleviating suffering. I observed Barbara
in this experience as she listened, responded, and acted in a manner that
considered the dignity and worth of a dying woman and her family.

I was present with Barbara as we repositioned Geraldine to ease
her breathing. At this time a respiratory therapist and a student entered
the room to assess Geraldine's breathing status. The therapist and the
student performed a full assessment, auscultating breath sounds and
checking oxygen saturation levels. The therapist suggested that a high-
flow oxygen mask might improve Geraldine's oxygenation level and her
breathing. I observed Barbara throughout this assessment. She was silent
and listened to the therapist's suggestions until the mention of an oxygen
mask. Barbara acted professionally, thanking the therapist for his assessment but politely reminding him that Geraldine was dying and needed to
be "comforted and not treated aggressively." Barbara humanized the experience, connecting the family's needs, voicing how they might feel seeing Geraldine for the last time with an oxygen mask on. Barbara prom-
ised that she would provide comfort measures to reduce suffering and
alleviate Geraldine's labored respirations. Barbara told me that she felt
the mask would only serve the purpose of medicalizing Geraldine's
death.

Inadequate Time: An Experience of Moral Distress

Inadequate time has become increasingly common and challenging
for these nurses. Time pressures within the context of the nurses' work
on this unit were evident in many ways. Holistic palliative care that includes both dying individuals and their families takes time. There were

several instances when nurses conveyed an awareness of the difference between the care that they value and have been taught to provide and the care that they are able to give. When time is inadequate the result can be moral distress for the nurses and a related negative impact on the dying individuals, who receive care that is not holistic. The experiences of having time to do only basic care and of not being fully present—because their thoughts are occupied with doing and not being—are distressing. Several nurses described staying overtime until someone could be with patients who were dying alone. Many nurses stated that the system was forcing them (because of lack of time and staff) to give care that undermined their own values. Nurses experience feelings that they have not adequately done their job. Muriel related her feeling of pressured care with little time:

The environment doesn't allow us to care the way we need to. Sometimes I've been so caught up in everything around me that I'm really not aware of where I'm coming from. I do things but I'm more like a robot, I'm not a nurse. I had to leave a dying patient who was alone once because another patient down the hall was irate that I wasn't changing his intravenous bag. There was no one nearby to help, and I couldn't stand the irate screaming from down the hall. We couldn't satisfy the needs of the dying individual because there were not enough bodies to go around. That haunts me. It's as bad as having someone in poor pain control that you can't do something for fast enough.

Nurses talked about having time as "really being able to listen[,] . . . [t]o actually stand there and focus on your patient's voice without being interrupted from a million other sources." Darlene talked about finding herself "wishing that dying individuals would just hurry their conversation so that she could move on to the next task at hand." She realized that she was compromising the care of her patients just so she could be viewed as being efficient. Darlene's story portrays her plight with time:

Mary had amyotrophic lateral sclerosis [ALS]. She had lived with her disease for several years and was very clear on how she wanted her care to be given. She would often try to communicate these needs to us, but she could not speak clearly enough for us to understand. Out of frustration she would break into uncontrollable crying, trying to explain how she wanted to be positioned, or to have her curtain opened more, or whatever. It took so long for her to explain what she wanted, and I just couldn't wait. Something so simple as this, and I didn't have the time to figure it out. What kind of care is this?

The rush of time as well as the robbing of time not only become issues of loss for these nurses, they also jeopardize the quality of the dying journey for individuals. The development of a trusting, caring nurse–patient relationship takes time. Many feel that the healing developed through the relationship of getting to know the patients and their families is just not there as it used to be. In fact, some wonder if more harm is done when the dying journey is interrupted when the patient is discharged to another facility. Not only is the process interrupted, but added burdens are placed on families in a way that invites concern and trepidation regarding the remainder of the person's life. The quality of the nurses' work as well as their fulfillment as nurses suffer when they lose the intimacy of the nurse–patient relationship. Ruth shared her perspective:

I find that my role as a palliative care nurse has changed a lot. I feel like most of my time is spent preparing the patient for discharge. There is so little time for getting to know them deeply. It's just that superficial data needed to make sure that their discharge is at least smooth. I think that changes in acute care, with the push to discharge patients, creates a lot of suffering for nurses. They suffer because it's not always the patient's agenda, so we're dealing with something that we are imposing on them and expect them to make decisions at a time when they already have so many decisions to make. We also want to send them to the first available bed in the system. It doesn't matter if it inconveniences the family because it's so far away—it's a bed, a bed out of acute care.

Nurses on this unit recognize the important role that time plays for families in finding strength and/or meaning in their loved one's dying journey. Nurses suffer when family members feel fear, separation, and anxiety. As a dying individual's time on the unit is often shorter, these nurses sense that their role in helping families find strength and meaning is even more important than in other settings. They want to feel confident that families are prepared to go home with their loved one or to find comfort when he or she is moved to another facility. Corley, Minick, Elswick, and Jacobs (2005), in proposing a theory of moral distress, argue that the explicit goals of nursing are "demonstrably ethical" (p. 382). When these goals to protect patients from harm, to provide competent and timely care, and to maintain a healing environment are blocked, these nurses experience moral distress.

Spirituality in Suffering: The Nurse's Moral Commitment

What Is Spirituality?

Spirituality is an inherent, integrating, and often extremely valued dimension of the dying journey of individuals and their families (Johnston Taylor, 2001). Heightened spiritual awareness and concerns are part of the dying journey (Francis, 1986; Fryback, 1993; Hall, 1997; Reed, 1987) and often a time of life review and search for meaning and purpose. Spirituality generates love (Bryson, 2004). Etymologically, the word *spirituality* originates from the Latin word *spiritus*, meaning "breath," "wind," "air," or "spirit," suggesting that spirit energy is essential for life (Banhart, 1988; Hoad, 2001). From an existential perspective, spirituality is what moves us outside ourselves to find the meaning of life (Bryson, 2004). However, spirituality continues to exist in us when life seems to lose meaning. Reed (1992) proposed that spirituality is involved in meaning making through intrapersonal, interpersonal, and transpersonal connections. In essence, spirituality generally connotes "harmonious relationships with or connections with self, neighbor, nature, God, or a higher being that draw one beyond oneself. Spirituality provides a sense of purpose, enables transcendence, and empowers individuals to be whole and live fully" (Fehring, Miller, & Shaw, 1997, p. 663).

Existential Suffering

Suffering has been viewed as a mirror that reflects spirituality when individuals face the basic conditions of life and their normal understanding of life is challenged (Lindholm & Eriksson, 1993; Raholm, Lindholm, & Eriksson, 2002). Existential suffering, also referred to as spiritual suffering, has been revealed when individuals feel that parts of their lives have lost their meaning, when they have come to doubt the usefulness of their religious beliefs, and/or when who they were in the past is now lost. Psychological suffering is a part of existential suffering that occurs when individuals cannot understand why they are suffering—because of lack of cognitive ability, when no explanation exists for suffering, when people do not believe their suffering, and/or when what the future holds for them is unknown (Rousseau, 2001).

Persisting unbearable suffering, the suffering that by its crippling character stops individuals from growing, can reflect uncertainty and confusion in the understanding of life (Eriksson, 1992). Dying individuals sometimes have disturbing questions to which there seems to be no answer. Unanswerable questions sometimes draw nurses into spaces where they have never been before, and they can experience distress when these questions are addressed to them. The inward journey deep into the souls of dying individuals and their families is one way in which the essence of spirituality in suffering is provided space to be explored. A different type of listening, curiosity, and uncovering by health care professionals is needed to help diminish their pain and assist them in finding their own healing path. The following example shows several nurses' anguish in addressing and responding to difficult spiritual questions.

David, a 40-year-old husband and father of two children, had been diagnosed with lung cancer one year earlier. Since the time of his diagnosis he had experienced anger, fear, and emotional outbursts of anxiety and blaming others for his disease. The many months of emotional denial and anger had served him well through his treatments of radiation and chemotherapy; David was familiar and comfortable with anger, while other feelings such as hope or sadness were unknown and terrifying. As it became apparent that his disease had not responded to medical therapies, his anger led to emotional and physical outbursts that became frightening to his family and nurses.

Although the nurses respected David's right to denial, his outbursts became more frequent and severe and an issue of safety for both his family and his caregivers. Nurses had difficulty imagining their way through David's suffering. Several nurses insisted that he acknowledge and confront his illness and fears. They found themselves feeling distant, not wanting to enter into a suffering relationship or delve into questions of an existential nature. These nurses were not able to honor David's suffering, sensing that they were creating more pain for him and his family. The uncertainty of David's suffering and their inability to confront it immobilized the nurses. Their fears of making it worse resulted in David's suffering being untouched until the time of his death.

Spiritual care for these nurses was not addressed in the face of suffering. Fear immobilized them, making them unable to delve into reflection about their own spiritual care practices. These nurses needed to make known their own beliefs and assumptions that might have hidden biases that inhibited them from initiating conversations of spiritual suffering with David. Unawareness of their own beliefs might have hindered the possibilities for acknowledgment of different expressions of suffering.

In confronting unanswerable spiritual questions nurses need to consider their role as listeners and witnesses to others' suffering. Listening to suffering human beings' unanswerable questions is not easy. In seeking an understanding of moral practices in suffering our challenge is to recognize and respond to the call of individuals in need. In attuning ourselves to the call of the vulnerable other an ethical moment arises (Cameron, 2004). In these circumstances the nurse's intention should be to be present, to listen, and to stay with the unanswerable questions. This moral sensitivity opens a space where spiritual concerns in suffering may be heard, encountered, acknowledged, and witnessed.

The nurses stated that when they are present they gain insight from addressing a person's experience of suffering. This insight has been referred to by Frank (1992) as the "pedagogy of suffering," meaning that one who suffers has "something to teach and thus has something to give" (p. 150). Nurses on this unit revealed that their frequent encounters with mortality encouraged them to look for signs that their patients were suffering and expressing their spiritual selves. Nancy spoke about how she knew when her patient needed to express his spiritual distress:

You can usually tell when your patients have spiritual concerns or questions. Oftentimes they will talk about their life experiences at various stages in their lives, such as past relationships, past suffering, past deaths of individuals that they have been close to, things like that. You get the sense that their reminiscing in the past is now bringing them to the present, where they are now questioning their personal experience of dying. These are the kinds of clues that I usually take to mean that they are questioning their beliefs and sometimes expressing their faith to you. I always try to just drop whatever I'm doing and listen. Missing these kinds of openings would only convey a lack of respect, [a sense] that they and their spiritual needs are not important.

In all of the examples provided thus far the nurse's presence has made the difference in helping these individuals express their spiritual needs. Acknowledging and embracing the expression of spirituality in therapeutic conversations with patients and their families serves to alleviate their suffering as they struggle to address a fundamental spiritual need, the need to search for meaning.

Searching for Meaning in Suffering

Suffering creates one of the greatest challenges to uncovering meaning (Borneman & Brown-Saltzman, 2001). Heidegger (1962) and Frankl (1987) both stressed that meaning is essential for life and that humans are intentional, looking for or creating meaning, as meaninglessness is impossible to endure. Mount (2003) adds that meaning is not an end in itself but a means to an end: "That end is an experience of community, attachment, union with self, with others, with the Other, however perceived" (p. 94).

One does not find meaning in a vacuum; it has everything to do with relationships and spirituality and is intertwined with the beliefs that one holds about one's suffering (Johnston Taylor, 2001). Nurses who are part of the journey of dying individuals and their families can help them to review their life, integrate their experiences, and perhaps make sense of what is happening in their suffering. In the face of suffering spirituality can "go sour" (Bryson, 2004). It is a time when people become angry at God and express feelings that spirituality is false belief. The challenge for caregivers is to redirect spiritual energies toward the discovery of meaning. Nurses themselves find meaning in the search for meaning (Raffin, 2002).

People who are suffering may be able to find meaning in that suffering before healing takes place (Bryson, 2004). While the process of finding meaning depends greatly on an inward journey, it also relies on the "telling of" the suffering that is being endured and the effects of this suffering (Frank, 1992). The telling may reveal itself in language or be conveyed by the eyes, through the hands, or just in the way the body is held (Frank, 1992). The telling is the connectedness in the shared journey of finding meaning in suffering. Jennifer told of finding meaning in suffering in her embodied connection:

I remember this patient—my very first time with him—I walked in and there were these piercing blue eyes that looked at you, and there I was with my clipboard, and I felt really uncomfortable with his eyes. He had a trach[eotomy] with humidity, and his breathing was labored. He was so air-hungry and had been this way for a week now. Everything had been tried, and nothing was easing his breathing. I put down my clipboard, and he grabbed my hand, and I sensed that he was frightened. It seemed like he didn't want me to leave the room. Knowing that he had no family, I asked if there was anyone I could call, like a priest. His eyes closed, and I sensed that he was comfortable with this. I didn't leave the room; instead, we prayed together that peace would come and that his suffering would end. The priest came, and he didn't let go of my hand. Not just any hand would do. I stayed until he died.

In her embodied connection Jennifer shared in an unspoken search for meaning during this man's last hours of life. Her spirituality was the key to moving beyond this loss and finding ways of maintaining this connection in the face of suffering. In her presence Jennifer served to affirm herself as a participant in this search for meaning. Bryson (2004) reminds us that one of the most important gifts that a nurse brings to her patient is to be authentic, to be "real." The nurse brings compassion, joy, hope, and commitment to quality of life but does so from a patient's reality. In entering these relationships a nurse chooses to pursue the best, given her potential and the context of the situation.

It is important to note, however, that not all individuals will find meaning in suffering (Johnston Taylor, 2001). Meanings are contingent because of our human experiences. The very enterprise of making meaning is never assured. Individuals who have struggled throughout their life to find meaning may not in the last days of life find meaning (Johnston Taylor, 2001). The nurses discussed how individuals whose physical symptoms are unmanaged, without remission, may not be able to address meaning and other spiritual issues, as they are more likely to focus only on physical needs. There are others who struggle to understand despite their pain and suffering.

Many persons, however, grow from their search for meaning. Palliative care nurses, in their embodied relationship with patients, can help dying individuals to find their "whys": "The caregivers' willingness to promote the patients' quest for transcendence promotes holistic healing, the integration of body, mind and spirit" (Bryson, 2004, p. 323). All of the nurses in the study discussed the suffering they experienced in helping dying individuals and their families search for meaning to the questions "Why me?" and "Why him or her?" As previously discussed, these questions are not for nurses or others to answer. Rather, the response is to stay with the patients in their time of questioning and doubt. Many times, providing an answer only stifles patients' exploration of suffering and its meaning (Jevne, 1991). The urgency and despair under which such questions are often asked intensify the challenge of the search for meaning.

Barbara said, "It is so unfair, so painful for patients to suffer and search for meaning as they bring forth painful memories and regrets. How much more difficult can it get?" It is in experiences such as the above that nurses are committed to those who are vulnerable in their search for meaning. The following example, related by Barbara, reveals the nurses' call to relationship in searching for meaning in suffering:

I'll never forget the experience of a young man who was dying of cancer. The experience of loss was insurmountable to all involved. Our patient was young and in his short life [had] suffered much physical pain and indignity because of his illness. His physical pain was unrelenting and not controlled before he died. The emotional loss of losing his wife and daughter and feeling their suffering was tragic. It had not been a long time since he had been diagnosed, the progress of the disease was rapid, and because of his uncontrolled physical pain quality time was not available to focus on the meaning of his illness or suffering. His death was not peaceful, and the outward emotion of letting go for the daughter was very hard. The intense emotions had a congregation of nurses in the room at the time of death to support each other. A few hours after the death the family left for home. Almost immediately upon leaving the hospital the wife and daughter were killed in a car accident—a senseless accident that we will never forget. The[ir] death was so overwhelmingly shocking that many of the nurses present needed to visit the emergency room to be with [the] extended family in their grief. The enormity of the suffering of so many individuals will never be forgotten. Many of the nurses gathered together later to pray that the family was now together and that suffering was over.

In the face of suffering and death these nurses have—through the use of prayer, compassionate listening, and presence—opened a door for the search for meaning to occur. Even though not all of the nurses expressed faith in God or a higher power, their spirituality helped them to reflect on their own relatedness, their love for each other, and the privilege of caring for individuals facing death. In varying ways faith was a key support for each of them to the degree that they had developed this resource (Olson & Clark, 2000). Facing one's own mortality brings us closer to humanity and our faith.

The nurses' embodied relationship, spirituality, and perhaps faith help those who are searching for meaning to review their life, integrate their experiences, and perhaps make sense of what is happening in suffering. Nurses in their own search for meaning enhance the care of the dying individuals and their families and enable the potential for healing in suffering to occur.

The Connection of Colleagues

Nurses need mentoring and emotional support because of their vulnerability and their potential to relieve their own suffering as embodied witnesses (Gregory & English, 1994). Throughout this paper the nurses have revealed the importance of the need to create a moral space for suffering. Joint transcendence, the mutuality of a healing relationship between nurse and patient, and the release of compassion can promote self-healing and harmony in both (Watson, 1988). But what happens to the nurse when the suffering of her patient continues, is prolonged, and is not dignified? Who supports and cares for the nurse when the patient dies or when many patients die within a short time of one another? Who helps the nurse when she has not been able to help the patient die a good death, when pain and symptoms are not controlled? Who does the nurse reach out to in her own vulnerability?

In times of need the nurses on this unit turned to each other. I asked these nurses to describe their colleagues. I was interested in exploring the qualities of nurses who are able to support each other time and time again in the face of death and suffering. Muriel shared her beliefs about her colleagues and the mutual reciprocity that they shared:

Palliative care nurses are the most wonderful, caring people that I know. They are authentic in their support. The falseness of our behavior vanishes when we are a part of death and suffering. Emotions are authentic, undisguised. I feel comfortable in sharing my own emotions, to reveal them to these wonderful human beings. They make me feel special.

Caring for dying individuals can be stressful work that requires a supportive environment if nurses are to endure this specialty for a prolonged period of time (Vachon, 2001). Colleagues and caring leaders who trust, accept, protect, and value a philosophy of palliative care are most important in providing this space. Colleagues need to share their humanness with one another, to be familiar with each other's philosophy of life and death and accepting of each other's strengths and weaknesses. Together they must work as a team, drawing strength from each other's resources (Vachon, 1995). They share responsibilities, ventilate, validate feelings and thoughts; they cry, laugh, discuss, inspire, and confirm each other. Barbara said:

The nurses are wonderful, so supportive. We get together a lot; even last night we were all together and we shared whatever we needed to. It helps us get rid of anxiety, stress, when other people can talk about what they have gone through with the same person, or what they've gone through in another situation. It really helps. So you have a few laughs, or we have a few tears sometimes, and we go on. We do have lots of tears every so often; there's no place to hide. But there's always somebody that puts their arms around you and says you're doing a good job, or you've done okay, or can they help you. They're wonderful, they're wonderful.

During rough times the nurses sensed that they were becoming more secure as a group. They felt that there was always someone in whom they could confide and from whom they could gain strength, inspiration, and confirmation. An abundance of humor, joking, and laughter helped to relieve tension in tragic experiences. Humor among patients, families, and staff most commonly serves to build therapeutic relationships, relieve tension, and protect dignity and a sense of worth. Humor is particularly significant in managing stressful situations and maintaining a sense of perspective (Kinsman & Gregory, 2004). The nurse in a difficult situation can count on her colleagues to "step in if she needs to step out." Jennifer commented:

My colleagues will come in and pitch in if you have a hard time. They'll come in with you or they'll deal with procedures, events, or whatever you need. It's that support again. Nobody ever, ever condemns you for your beliefs or how you do things on the floor. They always pat you on the back for doing a good job.

The nurses in this study learned most about themselves from others: colleagues and patients. Through their interactions with others they have recognized their own limitations and learned that no one, including themselves, is perfect and that interdependence leads to every chance of succeeding. Most nurses, they said, are dedicated and committed to giving and following a palliative care philosophy. Of course, there are others who, because of a lack of experience or perhaps limited self-awareness, are fearful of a suffering individual. They distance themselves from those individuals, making it difficult for the others. But the nurses on the unit understand. They do their best to guide and teach less-experienced nurses. Beverly explained:

Nurses on the unit know what it is like to be fearful of pain, suffering, and your responsibilities as a nurse. We have had nurses who are scared to give too much analgesic; they don't want to be responsible for making someone too drowsy. It's scary to think that you have that much power. But you learn that it only lasts for a short period, and, in the end, the patient is much more comfortable. We support one another in these circumstances for the good of our patient's well-being.

Most of these nurses see their role as being in a human–human relationship. Their professional knowledge and skills are a part of who they are as individuals. Being visible as a person, giving of oneself, and exposing oneself to one's own vulnerability are part of who they are as individuals. Being competent, enduring, engaging the suffering, and portraying a professional image provide both personal and professional satisfaction. In creating a space for suffering with others nurses strive to be present in order to listen to and acknowledge spiritual questions. They are open to the possibilities of finding meaning in suffering. Nancy expressed this eloquently:

Suffering is not bad; it is an expression of our humanity that calls to another. If the other responds in love and authenticity, we can find wholeness and peace in our suffering. Left untouched, suffering can destroy our body, mind, and spirit.

Nurses talked about the connection and healing that are created together. They are born out of a relationship to suffer together, to commit, endure, tolerate, and allow together.

Creating a Space for Continuing Conversations of Nurses' Suffering: The End and Onward

The Nature of Nurses' Suffering

In a sense this journey to understand nurses' experience of caring for dying individuals who are suffering is akin to rock climbing—both difficult and exhilarating. Both activities force you into uncharted territory. Both share common qualities of uncertainty, anxiety, exposure, and loneliness and yet allow you to take responsibility and cultivate each step even though you are roped to a wonderful team.

As nurses in palliative care live a philosophy that centers on actions that promote whole-person care, they do not simply care for dying individuals' physical bodies but "tend their spirit, gently, respectfully, and knowingly" (Moules, 2000a, p. 4). In practice nurses live out their beliefs, values, theories, knowledge, and experience in their actions. Acts of compassion, presence, embodiment, and respect are integrally a part of who they are as persons and as palliative care nurses. Borgmann (1992) suggested that, as in German tradition, the word *practical* is synonymous with *moral,* and thus practice and the decisions that govern practice and conduct within it are moral decisions. "Practice involves us morally, practically, and spiritually" (Moules, 2000a, p. 5).

The nature of palliative care nursing is such that, every day, practitioners face some of the most fundamental and poignant issues confronting humanity (Perry, 1998). Nurses are invited to share in the intimate journey of living and dying where suffering is present. This sharing often entails a commitment to developing a meaningful relationship as a way to know and understand the patient's experience. The relationship, although rewarding, often places the nurse in a vulnerable position. That is, nurses themselves are not unaffected.

Whenever possible, nurses accept this vulnerability as a part of their obligation to dying individuals and their families. They do not walk away from the suffering of the dying but are called to it. Obligations call to us; we do not summon them. "Obligations do not ask for my consent. . . . [S]omething demands my response. If an obligation is mine it is not because it belongs to me but because I belong to it" (Caputo, 1993, pp. 7, 8). Nurses are morally obligated to enter into the suffering of others, the joys, illnesses, and deaths, and nurses learn to accept that suffering is a part of living and dying. "There is something about suffering that stops us in our tracks" (Caputo, 1993, p. 29). In this study I witnessed that, whenever possible, nurses use every layer of themselves when invited into the personal realm of dying individuals. Near the end of dying individuals' lives I watched nurses become intensely engaged. Patients invite nurses to participate with them at a deeper level in trust that nurses will help to make life or death more comfortable and dignified. This invitation is a moral call to relationship.

Nurses bear many different responsibilities and exhibit great strength, which is necessary for coping with the innumerable pressures placed on them, and in many situations nurses encounter "obligation." The sphere of obligation is constituted by "a power that overpowers them, that constrains them to take notice, and sends shudders through their flesh" (Caputo, 1993, p. 8). Nurses do not escape the eyes of those who suffer. Whenever possible they embrace the experience and temporarily become the conscious of the unconscious, a means of knowledge and confidence for those who are overwhelmed, and a voice for those too weak or withdrawn to speak.

In this study I have come to understand and respect that palliative care nursing as a discipline uniquely blends varying forms of knowledge—empirical, relational, and personal—in practice. First and foremost, the nurses in this study have affirmed the respect for others' knowledge that comes from living with the experience of suffering and dying. They have helped me to understand the importance of reciprocity of relationships in practice. Suffering is reciprocal and is experienced through embodied relationships, nurtured and supported in the space that is created between the nurse and the patient. In this space the nurses see, feel, and touch the dying individual's suffering.

Suffering also has the potential to disconnect and alienate dying individuals from the deepest and most fundamental aspects of themselves. Dying individuals who are experiencing pain and difficult symptoms experience what Kearney (1996) calls "soul pain." Nurses assume a responsibility to assist and alleviate the physical, emotional, and spiritual symptoms of their patients and to try to acknowledge these experiences, but they are not always successful, as suffering may not always be relieved. The locus of suffering rests with dying individuals (Gregory, 1994). Ultimately, only patients can ease their own burden of suffering; this process is ultimately a personal matter (Cassell, 1982). The nurses' compassion may allow dying individuals to work through the suffering, but the experience itself may not be alleviated or eliminated.

Changed Understanding: Can We Truly Understand Suffering?

Prior to this study I believed, and the literature suggested, that nurses did not really understand suffering when caring for dying individuals. My thinking has been refined and changed by this study in many ways. I have begun to question the notion of understanding suffering, whether one can truly understand another's suffering. Understanding presupposes the notion of certainty. In the dying journey the path is bumpy, it is uncertain. This study has fostered my belief that each individual's suffering on this journey is unique and happens in the moment. The intention to understand an individual's suffering is what matters to nurses. The *Oxford Companion to Philosophy* (Honderich, 1995) describes intention as being directed toward action that is conceptualized in relation to others. During conversations with the nurses and on the observation visits I witnessed an intense desire to be in relationship with the intention of understanding the dying individuals' expressions of suffering. Perhaps the intention to understand suffering is more realistic than the notion of understanding suffering, as the certainty of understanding suffering does not exist. This act of intention is compassion. This intention to understand, I believe, has resulted in a different conception of understanding suffering. Understanding in this sense is not spoken words about what suffering means but rather an intention to embody and commit to another's suffering. Through this commitment one is oriented to interpreting the moment of the suffering individual's experience, which is often unspoken. Such a relation uses forms of knowledge that are not abstract but rather immediate, local, intuitive, emotive, informed, and embodied (Bergum, 1992).

This study revealed the importance of relational (inherent) knowledge in understanding the experience of suffering. The text (writings) uncovered suffering in an embodied relationship: the mutual sharing of vulnerability, trust, and connectedness that brings nurses and dying individuals closer to suffering and to humanity. Inherent knowledge of suffering is constructed through understanding the person not as an objective body (a thing, a heart, a breast) but as "a living person where the body and self are one" (Bergum, 1994, p. 73). Nurses must link their abstract knowledge of suffering (pain, loss) to their inherent constructed knowledge of this person as "a living person." Of importance for these nurses was the ability to focus on suffering that was expressed in the moment and that occurred in relationship rather than suffering analyzed from a chart or even heard from another colleague. This knowledge is "irreplaceable and unique to relationships, patients, and nurses" (Bergum, 1994, p. 74) and is the knowledge of intending to understand suffering. Understanding suffering in the moment takes it to a deeper level where the intertwining of physical and metaphysical closeness fosters the unity of body and soul (Kitson, 1987). It is through attentive listening, touch, eye contact, and a sharing of vulnerability that palliative care nurses come to know the experience of suffering.

The importance of this relational (inherent) knowledge was also revealed when the nurses discussed their dissatisfaction with the health care environment, which threatened the possibilities of developing and sustaining embodied relationships. Without these relationships knowledge of suffering is disengaged, felt to be more objective and superficial. Nurses without these relationships suffered in silence. In a system where time to develop relationships and quality of care is lacking, the sharing of one's vulnerability (suffering) is not possible. Nurses in this study said that with time pressures and a heavy workload true commitment was not always easy. There are times when significant situational constraints interrupt this goal. Situational constraints are "aspects of structural and interpersonal work environments that impede our standards of practice and thus jeopardize the quality of patient care" (Rodney & Starzomski, 1993, p. 24). Helen said that the luxury of "seeing your patients through the journey of dying in a responsible way no longer exists." The intention to understand suffering as well as these nurses' fulfillment as nurses suffer as a result.

In summary, commitment is a moral expression of responsibility—responsibility that occurs from a call to relationship with others. I believe that an embodied relationship is necessary if inherent knowledge is to be constructed. Inherent knowledge is imperative for ethical action (compassion) to occur. An understanding of suffering without inherent knowledge is shallow and inauthentic and distorts nurses' reasons for being called to relationship in palliative care nursing. Creating an open space for suffering to occur can be achieved only at the cost of suffering oneself, as is eloquently expressed by Caputo (1993):

Pain and suffering belong to our pact with life. They are unavoidable if ominous companions and they cannot be written out of the script of life. Disasters are constituted by suffering, but not all suffering is a disaster. My suffering, the suffering of the I is something for me to work through, to get beyond. (p. 29)

This research supports nurses who care for the suffering. Other nurses are urged to consider the importance of hearing and acknowledging suffering in the moral space. Nurses and patients need to know that their suffering has been recognized. It is only in this recognition and listening for suffering that possibilities for healing may occur. In the very practice of nursing we live intention or obligation. Obligation, as portrayed by Caputo (1993), is

[s]omething that overtakes us, that comes over and seizes us by the collar. . . . [It is] something that we do not do (only) by claim but that lays claim to us, that we

do not (only) constitute . . . but that is constituting us[,] . . . commanding and demanding our respect, our response. (p. 83)

Obligation is not safe and predictable, and ethics cannot provide this safety, for an obligation is both full history and the particular moment (Moules, 2000b). Ethics calls nurses to make the best decisions possible. The best decisions in caring for dying individuals who are suffering are made by acknowledging and listening to the sounds of suffering in the moral space created between the nurse and patient. Caputo (1987) wrote that it is suffering that takes us to the mystery and prevents us from confusing what we find with idealized poetic notions or reveries:

The face of suffering is a mask through which something deeper resonates, leaving its echo behind. . . . [T]he task . . . is not to decipher the speaker beneath the mask but to alert us to the distance which separates them and to preserve it and keep it open. (p. 280)

Suffering is a vital part of the human lives of dying individuals and is embedded in nursing practice. Suffering calls us as nurses to relations with dying individuals, to look in with intention and respect.

References

Anderson, J. M. (1991). Reflexivity in fieldwork: Toward a feminist epistemology. *Image, 23*(2), 115–118.

Barnhart, R. (Ed.). (1988). *The Barnhart dictionary of etymology.* New York: Wilson.

Bergum, V. (1992). Beyond rights: The ethical challenge. *Phenomenology and Pedagogy, 10,* 75–84.

Bergum, V. (1994). Knowledge for ethical care. *Nursing Ethics, 1,* 71–79.

Bergum, V. (2002). Ethical challenges of the 21st century: Attending to relations. *Canadian Journal of Nursing Research, 34*(2), 9–15.

Bergum, V. (2004). Relational ethics in nursing. In J. Storch, P. Rodney, & R. Starzomski (Eds.), *Toward a moral horizon: Nursing ethics for leadership and practice* (pp. 1–14). Toronto: Pearson Education Canada.

Bergum, V., & Dossetor, J. (2005). *Relational ethics: The true meaning of respect.* Hagerstown, MD: University Publishing Group.

Borgmann, A. (1992). *Crossing the postmodern divide.* Chicago: University of Chicago Press.

Borneman, T., & Brown-Saltzman, K. (2001). Meaning in illness. In B. Rolling Ferrell & N. Coyle (Eds.), *Textbook of palliative nursing* (pp. 415–424). New York: Oxford University Press.

Brock, D. (1989). Death and dying. In P. Veatch (Ed.), *Medical ethics* (pp. 329–356). Boston: Jones & Bartlett.

Bruyn, S. (1996). *The human perspective in sociology.* Englewood Cliffs, CA: Prentice-Hall.

Bryson, K. (2004). Spirituality, meaning and transcendence. *Palliative and Supportive Care, 2,* 321–328.

Cameron, B. (2004). Ethical moments in practice: The nursing "how are you?" revisited. *Nursing Ethics, 11*(1), 53–62.

Caputo, J. D. (1987). *Radical hermeneutics: Repetition, deconstruction, and the hermeneutic project.* Bloomington: Indiana University Press.

Caputo, J. D. (1989). Disseminating originary ethics and the ethics of dissemination. In A. Dallery & C. Scott (Eds.), *The question of the other: Essays in contemporary continental philosophy* (pp. 55–62). Albany: State University of New York Press.

Caputo, J. D. (1993). *Against ethics.* Bloomington: Indiana University Press.

Cassell, E. (1982). The nature of suffering and the goals of medicine. *New England Journal of Medicine, 306,* 639–645.

Chinn, P. (1994). *Being called to care.* Albany: State University of New York Press.

Coffey, A. (1999). *The ethnographic self.* London: Sage.

Corley, M., Minick, P., Elswick, R., & Jacobs, M. (2005). Nurse moral distress and ethical work environment. *Nursing Ethics, 12,* 381–390.

Cousins, N. (1981). *Anatomy of an illness as perceived by the patient.* New York: Bantam.

Eriksson, K. (1992). The alleviation of suffering: The idea of caring. *Scandinavian Journal of Caring Sciences, 6,* 119–123.

Fagin, C., & Diers, D. (1983). Nursing as metaphor: Occasional notes. *New England Journal of Medicine, 309,* 116–120.

Fehring, R., Miller, J., & Shaw, C. (1997). Spiritual wellbeing, religiosity, hope, depression, and other mood states in elderly people coping with cancer. *Oncology Nursing Forum, 24,* 663–671.

Ferrell, B. (2001). Preface. In B. Rolling Ferrell & N. Coyle (Eds.), *Textbook of palliative nursing.* New York: Oxford University Press.

Finlay, L. (2002). Outing the researcher: The provenance, process and practice of reflexivity. *Qualitative Health Research, 12,* 531–545.

Francis, M. (1986). Concerns of terminally ill adult Hindu cancer patients. *Cancer Nursing, 9,* 164–171.

Frank, A. (1992). The pedagogy of suffering. *Theory & Psychology, 2,* 467–485.

Frankl, V. (1987). *Man's search for meaning.* London: Hodder & Stoughton.

Fryback, P. (1993). Health for people with a terminal diagnosis. *Nursing Science Quarterly, 6,* 147–159.

Gadow, G. (1991). Suffering and interpersonal meaning. *Journal of Clinical Ethics, 2,* 103–107.

Gaita, R. (1991). *Good and evil: An absolute conception.* London: Macmillan.

Germain, C. (2001). Ethnography: The method. In P. Munhall (Ed.), *Nursing research: A qualitative perspective* (pp. 277–306). Sudbury, MA: Jones & Bartlett.

Gregory, D. (1994). *Narratives of suffering in the cancer experience.* Unpublished doctoral dissertation, University of Arizona, Tucson.

Gregory, D., & English, J. (1994). The myth and control: Suffering in palliative care. *Journal of Palliative Care, 10*(2), 18–22.

Hall, B. (1997). Spirituality in terminal illness: An alternative view of theory. *Journal of Holistic Nursing, 15,* 82–96.

Heidegger, M. (1962). *Being and time* (J. Macquarrie & E. Robinson, Trans.). New York: Harper & Row. (Original work published 1927)

Hertz, R. (1997). Introduction: Reflexivity and voice. In R. Hertz (Ed.), *Reflexivity and voice* (pp. vii–xviii). Thousand Oaks, CA: Sage.

Hoad, T. (Ed.). (2001). *Oxford concise dictionary of English etymology.* Oxford: Oxford University Press.

Honderich, T. (Ed.). (1995). *Oxford companion to philosophy.* New York: Oxford University Press.

Hughes, C. (1992). Ethnography: What's in a word—process? product? promise? *Qualitative Health Research, 2,* 439–450.

Jevne, R. (1991). *It all begins with hope: Patients, caregivers and the bereaved speak out.* San Diego: LuraMedia.

Johnston Taylor, E. (2001). Spiritual assessment. In B. Rolling Ferrell & N. Coyle (Eds.), *Textbook of palliative nursing* (pp. 397–406). New York: Oxford University Press.

Jopling, D. (2000). *Self knowledge and the self.* New York: Routledge.

Kearney, M. (1996). *Mortally wounded: Stories of soul pain, death, and healing.* New York: Scribner.

Kinsman, D. R., & Gregory, D. (2004). Humor and laughter in palliative care: An ethnographic investigation. *Palliative and Supportive Care, 2,* 139–148.

Kitson, A. (1987). Raising standards of clinical practice: The fundamental issue of reflective nursing practice. *Journal of Advanced Nursing, 12,* 321–329.

Kleinman, A. (1992). Local worlds of suffering: An interpersonal focus for ethnographies of illness experience. *Qualitative Health Research, 2,* 127–134.

Kleinman, A. (1995). *Writing at the margin. Discourse between anthropology and medicine.* Berkley: University of California Press.

Lindholm, L., & Eriksson, K. (1993). To understand and alleviate suffering in a caring culture. *Journal of Advanced Nursing, 18,* 1354–1361.

Maeve, M. (1998). Weaving a fabric of moral meaning: How nurses live with suffering and death. *Journal of Advanced Nursing, 27,* 1136–1142.

Morris, W. (1978). *The American heritage dictionary of the English language.* Boston: Houghton Mifflin.

Morse, J., & Field, P. (1995). *Qualitative research methods for health care professionals.* Thousand Oaks, CA: Sage.

Moules, N. (2000a). Funerals, families and family nursing: Lessons of love and practice. *Journal of Family Nursing, 6,* 3–8.

Moules, N. (2000b). *Nursing on paper: The art and mystery of therapeutic letters in clinical work with families experiencing illness.* Unpublished doctoral dissertation, University of Calgary, Calgary, Alberta.

Mount, B. (2003). The existential moment. *Palliative and Supportive Care, 1,* 93–96.

Nouwen, H. (1986). *Reaching out.* New York: Doubleday.

Olson, J., & Clark, M. (2000). Characteristics of health promoting faith community nurses. In M. Clark & J. Olson (Eds.), *Nursing within a faith community: Promoting health in times of transition* (pp. 226–236). Thousand Oaks, CA: Sage.

Olthuis, J. (1997). Face to face: Ethical asymmetry or the symmetry of mutuality? In J. Olthuis (Ed.), *Philosophy at the threshold of spirituality* (pp. 131–158). New York: Fordham University Press.

Perry, B. (1998). *Moments in time: Images of exemplary nursing care.* Ottawa, ON: Canadian Nurses Association.

Pettigrew, J. (1988). *A phenomenological study of the nurse's presence with persons experiencing suffering.* Unpublished doctoral dissertation, Texas Women's University, Denton, TX.

Raffin, D. S. (2002). *Accompanying the dying: Nurses create a moral space for suffering.* Unpublished doctoral dissertation, University of Alberta, Edmonton.

Raholm, M., Lindholm, L., & Eriksson, K. (2002). Grasping the essence of the spiritual dimension reflected through the horizon of suffering: An interpretive research synthesis. *Australian Journal of Holistic Nursing, 9,* 4–13.

Reed, P. (1987). Spirituality and wellbeing in terminally ill hospitalized adults. *Research in Nursing and in Health, 10,* 335–344.

Reed, P. (1992). An emerging paradigm for the investigation of spirituality in nursing. *Research in Nursing and in Health, 15,* 349–357.

Reeder, F. (1995). Passages through the heart: A hermeneutic of choice. In A. Omery, C. Kasper, & G. Page (Eds.), *In search of nursing science* (pp. 194–204). London: Sage.

Rehnsfeldt, A., & Eriksson, K. (2004). The progression of suffering implies alleviated suffering. *Scandinavian Journal of Caring Sciences, 18,* 264–272.

Rodney, P., & Starzomski, R. (1993). Constraints on the moral agency of nurses. *Canadian Nurse, 10,* 23–26.

Rodney, P. (1997). *Towards connectedness and trust: Nurses' enactment of their moral agency within an organizational context.* Unpublished doctoral dissertation, University of British Columbia, Vancouver.

Rousseau, P. (2001). Existential suffering and palliative sedation: A brief commentary with proposal for clinical guidelines. *American Journal of Hospice and Palliative Care, 18,* 151–153.

Schultz, D., & Carnevale, F. (1996). Engagement and suffering in responsible care giving: On overcoming malificence in health care. *Theoretical Medicine, 17,* 189–207.

Sellman, D. (2005). Towards an understanding of nursing as a response to human vulnerability. *Nursing Philosophy, 6,* 2–10.

Storch, J. (2004). Nursing ethics: A developing moral terrain. In J. Storch, P. Rodney, & R. Starzomski (Eds.), *Toward a moral horizon: Nursing ethics for leadership and practice* (pp. 1–14). Toronto: Pearson Education Canada.

Taylor, C. (1991). *The ethics of authenticity.* Cambridge, MA: Harvard University Press.

Thomasma, D. (1994). Beyond the ethics of rightness: The role of compassion in moral responsibility. In S. Philips & P. Benner (Eds.), *The crisis of care* (pp. 123–143). Washington, DC: Georgetown University Press.

Travelbee, J. (1971). *Interpersonal aspects of nursing* (2nd ed.). Philadelphia: F.A. Davis.

Vachon, M. (1995). Staff stress in hospice/palliative care: A review. *Palliative Medicine, 9,* 91–122.

Vachon, M. (2001). The nurse's role: The world of palliative care nursing. In B. Rolling Ferrell & N. Coyle (Eds.), *Textbook of palliative nursing* (pp. 647–662). New York: Oxford University Press.

Watson, J. (1988). *Nursing: Human science and human care.* New York: National League for Nursing.

Wax, M. (1977). On fieldworkers and those exposed to fieldwork: Federal regulations and moral issues. *Human Organization, 36,* 321–328.

Contributors

Shelley Raffin Bouchal, RN, PhD, CHPCN©, is a nurse with certification and research interests in palliative care and ethics. Currently she is an assistant professor in the Faculty of Nursing at the University of Calgary. Prior to becoming a professor she practiced as a clinical nurse specialist in a hospice. Her current teaching is focused in the areas of qualitative research, adult health and illness, palliative care, and ethics with undergraduate and graduate students. Her current research and scholarly writing focuses on palliative care professionals, spirituality, and ethics. Currently she is coauthoring a book on Canadian nursing ethics intended for undergraduate students. She finds interdisciplinary research with other palliative care professionals to be most engaging and applicable to practice.

Bonnie Ewing, PhD, RN, is an assistant professor at Adelphi University, Garden City, New York, where she obtained a master's degree in community health nursing and a PhD. She has been a maternal child health nursing administrator and has taught obstetrics, pediatrics, and community nursing. She co-founded a chapter of the Make-A-Wish Foundation in Suffolk County, New York, where she assisted with the fulfillment of wishes for children with life-threatening illnesses. Presently, Dr. Ewing is teaching nursing administration, health promotion, and disease prevention.

Nancy E. Johnston, RN, PhD, is an associate professor in the School of Nursing at York University, Toronto, Canada. Her current teaching is focused in the undergraduate and graduate areas of qualitative research, mental health, leadership, and global health. Her research interests include suffering, social exclusion, resilience, and the recovery of meaning in the face of adversity and loss. In addition to her teaching and research responsibilities she works with community health centers to expand outreach activities and develop programming of relevance to immigrants and other marginalized and racialized groups.

Ingrid Harris, PhD, received her doctorate in philosophy from McMaster University in Hamilton, Ontario, Canada, where she taught courses in existentialism, contemporary continental philosophy, and business ethics. She studied hermeneutics, phenomenology, and existentialism with G.B. Madison. She received her BA (Hon.) from Queen's University in Kingston, Ontario, and completed her master's program at Simon Fraser University in Burnaby, British Columbia. Dr Harris's published work includes *Is There a Canadian Philosophy? Reflections on the Canadian Identity* (Ottawa: University of Ottawa Press, 2000), coauthored with G.B. Madison and Paul Fairfield. Her current interests include philosophy of religion and theology.

Kathryn H. Kavanagh, BSN, MS, MA, PhD, is a medical anthropologist who has taught for many years in both nursing and anthropology. Her primary interests are health and healing across cultures. After conducting a series of summer field schools on the Pine Ridge Reservation in South Dakota, Kathy taught for Northern Arizona University on the Navajo and Hopi Reservations. She currently teaches courses in medical anthropology, indigenous healing traditions, American Indian cultures, and the anthropology of foodways in the Baltimore area. Widely published in cultural aspects of health and healthcare, she continues to write on various diversity-related topics.

Craig M. Klugman, PhD, received his BA with Honors from Stanford University, his MAs in medical anthropology and bioethics from Case Western Reserve University, and his doctorate in medical humanities from the University of Texas Medical Branch. Originally trained as a science journalist, he now teaches at the University of Nevada, Reno, where he chairs the Program in Health Care Ethics. He teaches courses in medical ethics, bioethics, public health ethics, and medical humanities. His current research examines teaching and ethics, bioethics rhetoric, ethics and politics, rural bioethics, and ethics and economics.

Index

279

Interpretive Studies in Healthcare and the Human Sciences

Series Editors

Nancy L. Diekelmann, PhD, RN, FAAN, Helen Denne Schulte Professor
   Emerita, School of Nursing, University of Wisconsin–Madison
Pamela M. Ironside, PhD, RN, FAAN, Associate Professor, Indiana University
   School of Nurshing

Volume 1

First, Do No Harm: Power, Oppression, and Violence in Healthcare
Edited by Nancy L. Diekelmann

Volume 2

Teaching the Practitioners of Care: New Pedagogies for the Health Professions
Edited by Nancy L. Diekelmann

Volume 3

Many Voices: Toward Caring Culture in Healthcare and Healing
Edited by Kathryn Hopkins Kavanagh and Virginia Knowlden

Volume 4

*Beyond Method: Philosophical Conversations in Healthcare Research and
   Scholarship*
Edited by Pamela M. Ironside

Volume 5

Listening to the Whispers: Re-thinking Ethics in Healthcare
Edited by Christine Sorrell Dinkins and Jeanne Merkle Sorrell

Volume 6

Meaning in Suffering: Caring Practices in the Health Professions
Edited by Nancy E. Johnston and Alwilda Scholler-Jaquish